U.S. Nutrition Policies in the Seventies

A Series of Books in Food and Nutrition

EDITOR: B. S. Schweigert

U.S. Nutrition Policies in the Seventies

edited by

Jean Mayer

Harvard University

W. H. Freeman and Company
San Francisco

"Toward a National Nutrition Policy" by Jean Mayer,
was first published in *Science*, Vol. 176 (April 21, 1972),
pp. 237–241. (Copyright 1972 by the American Association
for the Advancement of Science.)

Library of Congress Cataloging in Publication Data

Mayer, Jean.
    U.S. nutrition policies in the seventies.

    (A Series of books in food and nutrition)
    Includes bibliographical references.
    1. Nutrition policy—United States. I. Title.
TX360.U6M39   362   72–6548
ISBN 0–7167–0599–0
ISBN 0–7167–0596–6 (pbk.)

Printed in the United States of America

International Standard Book Number: 0–7167–0599–0 (cloth)
                                  0–7167–0596–6 (paper)

2 3 4 5 6 7 8 9

Dedicated to the members and staff of the first White House Conference on Food, Nutrition and Health (1969) in remembrance of a common endeavor in behalf of our fellow citizens.

Contents

Preface

Although the report of the December, 1969 White House Conference on Food, Nutrition and Health and the follow-up report (1971) have been published fairly widely, they are hardly appealing fare for readers who are not thoroughly acquainted with our country's nutrition problems. The style of these reports is forbidding: because each panel attached great price to specific wording (often arrived at as a result of prolonged discussion and tenuous compromises), the reports conserve the White House Conference flavor—a mixture of exhortation and officialese. Furthermore, the desirability of making the reports available to the conference members, the Congress, the executive branch, and the public as soon after the meetings as possible prevented the preparation of introductory material that could have established the background of many recommendations.

It became clear that an entirely different type of presentation was needed by students of U.S. nutrition policies who are seeking to become acquainted with the thinking of those distinguished Americans who are directly concerned with the future of our food supply and our state of nutrition. Accordingly, I invited a number of members of the White House Conference on Food, Nutrition and Health, most of them chairmen of panels at the conference, to undertake to examine, in the chapters of a simply written book, some of the crucial policies that should be developed and applied within the decade of the seventies. Although the authors speak with the experience of the conference and its one-year-after follow-up—and although all of them would acknowledge the intellectual contribution of fellow panel members and conference members—they speak as individuals, expressing their own interests, prejudices, and ambitions for the nation and for their own professions. No attempt was made to bend their views to fit into a closely coordinated *opus*. That there would be some duplication of subject matter and some differences of opinions is unavoidable. But the object of this book is not to present a fine blueprint—which in any case would not be followed closely—but to invite reflection on many of the important problems we face in the field of nutrition. The reader will, I am sure, think of many areas which could or should have been included; this is also unavoidable: the number of topics had to be limited. One important field that was not touched either at the conference or in this book, is the activity of the United States in the field of nutrition abroad. In spite of a seemingly growing mood of isolationism in the United States, all Americans of good will hope that such an activity will continue and, indeed, grow. (The complexity of this issue deserves to be treated in a separate book.)

Even though a number of contributors to the present book, including the editor, have spent much of their lives doing research, no chapter is devoted to nutrition research policy. One hopes that nutrition research—particularly concerning degenerative diseases, toxicology, and educational methods—will continue to be vigorously pursued (and supported). New facts may well emerge that will change the directions and priorities of nutrition policies, but this book must be predicated on the idea that the policies one can envisage now, in early 1972, have to be based on present knowledge and that it is unlikely that a sudden breakthrough will suddenly transform our whole outlook on U.S. nutrition policies.

Finally, although a brief chapter does grapple indirectly with the influence of the agricultural priorities of the U.S. Department of Agriculture on the status of farmers, migrant laborers, and the nutrition activities pursued by the department, no attempt has been made to evaluate in detail the relation of the economics of farm production and the subsidies program on basic food prices; nor have we attempted to explore in depth the contribution of labor, processing, distribution, advertising and profit policies to the structure of retail prices (though this obviously influences the nutrition pattern of Americans). We have concentrated instead on four important areas: policies concerning the protection of the vulnerable groups; policies concerning foods and the consumer; nutrition education policies; and certain governmental policies affecting the quality and safety of our food supply.

After a general introduction, giving an overview of the evolution of food and nutrition problems, we shall, in Part I, Improving the Nutrition of Those Most Vulnerable to Hunger and Malnutrition, examine possible methods of surveillance of the state of nutrition of the nation; we shall examine special policies concerning infants, pregnant and nursing women; we shall see how the prevention and alleviation of those diseases which have a strong nutritional component and affect tens of millions of Americans can be promoted. We shall pay particular attention to those nutrition policies that are directed at those population groups that for historic reasons are wards of our government.

In Part II, Monitoring the Wholesomeness and Nutritional Value of Our Foods, we shall look at new policies concerning manufacturing of "old" and "new" foods, and the safety of these foods; and we shall deal with the way the consumer perceives what he or she buys as a result of grading and labeling policies, advertising, and general consumer policies.

In Part III, we shall look at educational policies: those directed at the education of the public, with particular reference to the very poor, as well as those directed at the training of professionals and para-professionals.

Finally, in Part IV, we look at public policies effected by government at all levels: income maintenance, nutritional programs for the very poor—both of these essential if there is going to be any policy at all regarding our poorest citizens; state and local programs; and finally, at some crucial aspects at the federal level, with particular reference to the main agencies, the USDA and the Food and Drug Administration.

In the past three years, food and nutrition policies have become a subject of great interest to many Americans, of almost obsessive concern to some. It is our collective hope that this book will make a contribution to the quality of the debates concerning national nutrition programs.

Jean Mayer

November 1972

U.S. Nutrition Policies
in the Seventies

Introduction

Toward a National Nutrition Policy

Jean Mayer

The White House Conference on Food, Nutrition and Health, a watershed in American social history, was held in December, 1969, in Washington, D.C.[1-4]* Enough time has elapsed now to pause and consider what the situation was in 1969 and what it is now (in mid-1972), what progress has been made and what remains to be done.

The relation between nutrition and a number of social problems has long been recognized; however, in the past American scientists who were concerned with the clinical aspects of nutrition generally focused their attention on the underdeveloped countries of Africa, Latin America, and the Far East. In these countries, the problems are acute, and relatively easy to quantify, and the work is supported by a number of international and American agencies. Also, the "apolitical," establishment-approved character of international work made it more congenial for academicians than was domestic research that raised disturbing social and political issues within our own society.

It was only in the nineteen-sixties that malnutrition became a national issue. The disgraceful state of hunger and poverty in the United States was brought to the attention of the American people not by nutritionists but by the Southern Christian Leadership

*Superscript numbers refer to sources listed at the end of the Introduction and at the ends of chapters.

Conference led by Martin Luther King. By dedicating themselves to bettering the life of poor blacks, Reverend Doctor King and his followers created a new climate of concern about many of our urban problems, our educational problems, and, above all, about poverty in America.

That the national conscience was awakened slowly is attributable in part to the failure of professionals in the health field to recognize the extent of this nation's nutrition problems. Indeed, it was not the experts but rather a small, heterogeneous group of concerned citizens who took the first steps toward eliminating hunger among the black agricultural workers in the deep South.

In the sixties, the growing demand for man-made fibers had left the owners of the great cotton plantations with few options—either they replaced their cotton with corn crops, which require little manpower, or they committed their fields to the soil bank in exchange for a subsidy. In the wake of this turnover, no provision was made for poor blacks and their families who were wholly dependent on the plantations for their meager livelihood. Hunger and malnutrition, and at times, actual starvation, were to be their fate.[5-12] As poor blacks became unneeded in agriculture, and at the same time, eligible to vote, reactionary officials in the South seemed determined to drive them North. Certainly, little was done to help the blacks survive.

Awakening Little by little, however, a growing number of concerned Americans became aware of these conditions. A board of inquiry was established to identify "hunger counties," those areas where malnutrition had become a way of life. A number of concerned organizations came together, under the leadership of the Field Foundation, and created a "National Council on Hunger and Malnutrition in the United States," of

which I was elected the first chairman. Several members of Congress, including Joseph Clark, George McGovern, and the late Robert Kennedy, took up the cause. A number of dedicated individuals, like Leslie Dunbar, Walter Reuther, Robert Choate, John Kramer, and Dorothy Height, spoke of the problem all over the country. Finally, the newspapers and radio and television networks took cognizance of the problem; a number of pioneering articles written by journalists such as Nick (Nathan) Kotz[13] were followed by a powerful CBS television documentary entitled "Hunger in America" that was based on the findings of the board of inquiry[6] and of the "National Council." This hour-long program marked a turning point in the fight against hunger for it shocked the nation into the realization that ill-fed Americans could no longer be ignored.

It then became evident publicly that poverty, which is so real to so many people in our country, had too often been masked by our tendency to look only at those statistics that point to steadily rising average income and an ever-increasing gross national product. Despite protests to the contrary, there has been scarcely any redistribution of income in the United States over the past 30 years. Now, as 30 years ago, 20 percent of our population possesses only 5 percent of the total wealth, and half of these possess no more than 1 to 2 percent. The Department of Agriculture estimated in 1969 that a minimum of $106 a month was required to provide a sound diet for a family of four. Yet, at that time, 20 million to 30 million Americans did not have $106 a month for food. They lived in a variety of geographic areas and came from a number of different ethnic and cultural backgrounds. The unemployed agricultural workers of the deep South, many Mexican-Americans both in the rural areas of the Southwest and in the barrios of the larger Texas cities, American Indians on a number of reservations, and many in Appalachia fell within this category. In addition, there were (and are) the migrant and other seasonal farm workers, some 400,000 Americans, primarily blacks in the East, Mexican-Americans and blacks in the West. As a group, these laborers are deprived of the benefits of most social and economic legislation instituted to protect the rights of other types of workers. They are ineligible for the food-stamp program because they fail to meet residency requirements. Private hospitals will admit them only if they can pay their bills in cash; the net result is an infant mortality rate of 63 per thousand and an incidence of stillbirth of 70 per thousand— statistics that are comparable to those for the inhabitants of underdeveloped countries.[14,15] The average annual income of migrant workers in Colorado is approximately $1,885 per family.[16]

In the large cities of America, the two groups most vulnerable to malnutrition were (and are) the aged and a growing number of women with small children, abandoned by their husbands, and unable to obtain alimony and child support. Malnutrition is equally prevalent among groups living in America's more remote states and territories. The Alaskan natives, including Eskimos, Indians, and Aleuts, live on land that not only has marginal economic potential, but that is continually being threatened by commercial interests and various forms of pollution. Kwashiorkor (a protein-deficiency syndrome, particularly affecting small children) is rampant in American Samoa; marasmus (a syndrome of slow starvation, again particularly affecting small children) seems widespread in Micronesia, where hurricanes periodically cause extensive devastation to housing and to the crops of an entire season. In the Virgin Islands, generally thought of as a tourist's paradise, the welfare payments

for a family of four were, on the average, $19 a month in 1969.

Attempts at Solution On the whole, the food-assistance programs instituted by the federal government to meet the needs of all of these groups had been poorly designed and administered. When the first White House Conference on Food, Nutrition and Health convened in December, 1969, there were essentially three major food programs in operation: the food-commodity program, the food-stamp program, and the school-lunch program.

The food-commodity program disposed of surplus food while maintaining farm income and stabilizing agricultural prices; it was not a nutrition program as such. Among the 23 items offered under direct distribution, only a small number were, in fact, available. In Boston, for example, where no more than six or eight components were available, bulgur wheat, corn flour, and lard were the main components of a potentially disastrous diet. The manner in which food was delivered to the poor was another serious drawback of the commodity program: the rural poor had to collect promptly a complete month's supply of food, 30 pounds, in the basement of the county courthouse, which was often several miles away; urban recipients (usually elderly women or women with small children) had to carry the allotment from the local welfare office to what might be a seventh-floor tenement apartment. Finally, by providing the poor with foods that bore little resemblance to those purchased by the consumer at the supermarket, the commodity program stigmatized the poor and widened the gap between the haves and the have-nots in our society.

In contrast, the food-stamp program offered greater convenience and more variety in the selection of foods. However, its effectiveness was seriously hampered by unrealistic and unreasonable methods of operation. Those who could not pay $45 in cash on the first day of the month were dropped from the program. In addition, eligibility for welfare was a prerequisite for participation in the food-stamp program, thereby automatically barring the elderly and a great many people who would not apply for welfare. Furthermore, eligibility for welfare, particularly in the South and Southwest, depended entirely on the whim or good will of the local sheriff or county judge; in most cases, these magistrates derived their jurisdiction from a patchwork of welfare legislation reminiscent of the Elizabethan poor laws of 1601.

The third program, the provision of nutritious school lunches, contributed primarily to the well-being of middle-income people and scarcely helped the poor. Plate lunches were provided for some 24 million middle-income children in elementary and secondary schools; yet, the program fed only two million of the six million children who were desperately poor.

Thus, on the eve of the White House conference, only five million or six million people, out of a potential 25 million, actually benefited from the commodity program, the food-stamp program, or the free school-lunch program.

Changing Character of Food Poverty was obviously the most urgent problem for the conference to consider, but it appeared to me as chairman and chief organizer that the changing character of our food supply was another factor that should be considered. This nation's food products have been virtually transformed under the impact of forces that the public has yet to recognize fully. Food manufacturers, distributors, and retailers are well aware that theirs is not basically a "growth" industry. The failure of the Americans to exercise, coupled with their rising concern over the dangers of obesity, have resulted in an extremely slow increase in the overall consumption of food. Thus, in an effort to increase sales, the food companies are marketing service and convenience in the form of frozen foods and packaged meals. The work that was once performed by the unpaid housewife is now being done by organized labor—food has thus become subject to the same seemingly inexorable inflation that is characteristic of the prices of all industrial goods. This is true despite the fact that food is basically a commodity obtained with less land, fewer farmers, and more efficient methods than ever before in history. Faced with increasing prices, the consumer has been driven to find cheaper substitutes for the primary foods: meat, for instance, may be increasingly displaced by textured vegetable protein. These substitutes can be judged acceptable only if they are enriched with an equivalent quantity of a long list of vitamins and minerals—a complex operation that is just beginning to be studied. Our inadequate knowledge of human nutrition also makes it necessary to ensure that only a fraction of the unprocessed foods be replaced by new "engineered" foods.

Indeed, the organic food fad so prevalent among the young has focused attention on yet another product of our advanced technology—the highly processed nature of our food supply. In 1941, only 10 percent of our foods were highly processed; today, that amount has risen to 50 percent. Yet, until the White House Conference, it could be said that the major improvements in the nutritional content of foods had taken place primarily in the nineteen-forties: unfortunately, in the period after World War II, the commitment of both government and industry to establish and revise standards of nutritional quality had not been sustained. For example, the addition of iron, thiamine, riboflavin, and niacin to bread and flour was instituted in 1941. However, many bread substitutes, flour mixes, and most milled rice were (and are) still not enriched. In fact, a great many of the cereal-based products, which the public thought were enriched, were not.

The nutritive value of snack foods, an increasingly important component of our daily intake of food, was extremely low, and there was essentially no leadership in encouraging or requiring its improvement. Each year, the advertising industry concentrated a major portion of its efforts on the promotion of our least nutritious foods: candy, soft drinks, beer, and a host of crisp-fried snack items that are consumed in great quantities, particularly by our young people. Even though there were no standards of identity (that is, standardized, officially prescribed recipes) for such products, and the food industry was thus free to add to their nutritive value, to fortify and enrich these foods, few such efforts were made.

Malnourishment, whether caused by poverty or improper diet, contributes to an alarming situation in the United States today. Since 1950, that portion of the nation's income devoted to health services had risen from 12 billion to 70 billion dollars. Yet, during the same period, there had been absolutely no increase in the life expectancy of males at age ten, and a very insignificant increase for women. Indeed life expectancies for adult males in almost 30 nations were greater than they were in the United States.

White House Conference The aim of the 1969 White House Conference was thus to evaluate the state of nutrition of the American people and to formulate the basis of a national nutrition policy. The recommendations put forth by the conference had to cover four principal areas of concern: (1) food assistance for the poor, (2) nutrition and health programs, (3) the regulation of food production and supply, (4) and nutrition education.

At the conference, more than 30 panels of experts from the academic, medical, industrial, and agricultural worlds, as well as qualified representatives of consumer and poverty organizations prepared preliminary recommendations. Because the conference represented such a diversity of viewpoints, it was rather like a gigantic exercise in sensitivity training. Among the 4,000 delegates were hundreds of poor persons; students; representatives from all large social organizations; the chief executives of all large food companies; consumer advocates; government officials, including the President; academic and government nutritionists; and a host of other concerned citizens. The meetings forced everyone to listen to points of view they had never listened to before. It is noteworthy that a broad measure of consensus was ultimately reached.

A follow-up conference, held in February, 1971,[3,4] which had been planned along with the original conference, served to measure programs and emphasize deficiencies.

The conference was extensively covered by the press and by other media. Fifteen thousand reports were distributed free of charge by the conference. In retrospect, it is apparent that the conference has been a very effective planning and motivating device. (It has also been economical; over 120,000 of the 500,000 dollars jointly allotted to the White House Conference by the Ford, Rockefeller, and Kellogg Foundations were returned to the foundations.)

What has transpired since the White House Conference?

Hunger Programs First, the food-stamp program has been radically revised. In general, the amount of food stamps available to poor families—$106 per month, for a family of four—was sufficient to provide an adequate diet in 1969. The price of stamps has been reduced, and free stamps are offered to those in the lowest income brackets. The number of people receiving food stamps has risen from two million to well over ten million. And, now that cuts in the program have been warded off, that figure should rise further, to about 14 million in the near future. The 1969 payment of $106 has been raised to $112. The latter sum, however, is no longer sufficient; a family of four needs at least $120. In fact, it would be desirable to shift the food-stamp standard from the U.S. Department of Agriculture's "economy" diet to the low-cost diet of $134.

Second, the commodity program is gradually being ended; in many areas, it has already been replaced by the revised food-stamp program. However, in December, 1971, direct food distribution still covered three million to four million people, primarily in counties that had previously had no food assistance program of any type. In 1969, nearly 500 counties were without family food programs; today every county in the United States has some form of assistance.

Third, the school-lunch program has been expanded to cover over eight million poor children as compared with only two million prior to the conference. In addition, a total of 14 million to 15 million people out of a potential 25 million now are receiving one or the other form of family food assistance.[3,4]

Despite these gains, further action must be taken, not only to improve the quality of existing programs but also to implement many of the other recommendations proposed by the conference participants. The school-lunch program, in particular, is faced with several serious problems.

The depressed state of the American economy has increased the number of children who desperately need to be included in the program. In 1969, 6.6 million children were classified among the very poor; a year later the number had risen to nine or 9.5 million, at least one million of whom still do not receive a free lunch. Supplementary appropriations are essential if we are to reach these additional students.

At the same time, many communities seem reluctant to implement school-lunch (and breakfast) programs. A major problem is insufficient good will on the part of school committees or boards in cities such as Boston.

Other difficulties are (1) the absence, at the local level, of flexibility and of resources such as professional assistance and food services equipment (a failing that could be corrected by the adoption of an adequate revenue-sharing plan) and (2) the lack of sharply defined directives from Washington. (The regulations set by the Department of Agriculture generally contain such a multitude of loopholes that local school districts that are unwilling to institute free lunches are simply not required to do so.)

In terms of general nutrition programs, the federal government has moved much more slowly. The Department of Health, Education, and Welfare has been particularly tardy in expanding health services, including nutrition services. The President's Family Assistance Plan, if implemented correctly, could be an effective way to provide food assistance through income maintenance. However, a great many other programs, particularly those relating to the health of children, should have been developed without waiting for an overall rise in the income of the poor, a rise that will be appreciable in only five or six states once the plan is enacted. Comprehensive health-care programs that incorporate effective nutritional services should be provided immediately for all children.

The elderly present a problem of special urgency. On the whole, they are poor. They are also handicapped by a number of chronic diseases and often have lost their teeth; they lack mobility and tend to be isolated; many are malnourished. They fear being sent to nursing homes much as young men fear being drafted. They need nutritional services that also enable them to have daily contacts with the outside world.[14,15] "Meals on

Wheels" programs (delivering at least one good meal every day) and daily community meals were programs recommended by the Section on Aging of the White House Conference on Food, Nutrition and Health, and repeated by the Nutrition Section of the White House Conference on Aging.[8] A bill to implement these proprosals has been passed by Congress and provides 100 million dollars in fiscal 1973 and 150 million dollars in fiscal 1974.

Consumer Programs With regard to informed labeling, quality grading, and food safety, progress is evident in some areas and totally absent in others. The question of improved food labeling and date coding has engendered considerable interest over the past year. Consumers regard labels as their primary source of information about the contents, safety, and nutritional value of the food they buy. Given our existing nutrition-education program, it is not difficult for the average citizen to select simple meats, vegetables, and fruits, and produce a balanced diet. But what if the choice involves such new foods as frozen pizza or a spinach soufflé? How should these products be classified? And how should they be labeled? In recent months, various attempts have been made to devise an accurate and useful method of presenting food information to consumers through product labeling. An experimental scheme has now been adopted by the chain of Giant Food Stores in Washington, D.C., Baltimore, Maryland, and the northern Virginia area. The content and percentage of recommended dietary allowances, in terms of calories and vitamins and minerals—ten different nutrients—are printed on the label of house brands distributed by the chain. The old system, where the only indications on the label were those favorable to the product, has been replaced by a complete listing of the calories per portion, the amounts of protein and fat, and quantity of several vitamins and minerals.

All of these nutrients appear in the same order on the label of every item, along with the specific concentration for that particular product; for instance, the listing on a can of pork and beans may indicate the content of vitamins A and C to be zero. In addition, the labels will give the percentage content of the valuable (named) ingredient: percentage of beef in "beef stew," percentage of turkey in "turkey pie," percentages of pork and of beans in "pork and beans." It is to be hoped that this system or a comparable form of informed labeling will soon be adopted by food manufacturers and retailers across the country. Legislation to this effect has been introduced in the United States Senate.

Food Safety With regard to food safety, an effective approach to the complex question of toxicity has yet to be found. The Food and Drug Administration (FDA) is unable to carry out all the research required in this area, and until recently no independent research groups had been established to study such problems as the safety of new chemical additives and to make recommendations to federal regulatory agencies. A large U.S. Army installation in Arkansas has now been deactivated and will be put at the disposal of the FDA. This will enlarge the "in-house" capabilities of the FDA and will somewhat relieve the pressure on it. With respect to nutrition advice, the Food and Nutrition Board of the National Academy of Sciences-National Research Council performed a valuable service in regard to a number of nutritional problems during and since World War II; however, it seems unable to provide on a day-by-day basis the advice required by the FDA now with the speed expected (and required) by consumers, manufacturers, and federal agencies.

The current controversy surrounding the mercury content of fish underscores the need for authoritative, yet understandable, information about food safety. Mercury is an element of the earth's crust and is present, in varying trace amounts, in every food. However, if this natural toxicant is consumed in excessive amounts, it can cause death. Somewhere there is a safe limit of intake of mercury. How long it will take to determine that limit remains to be seen, but, in the interim, some guidance must be provided. (As an experimental scientist, I would be reluctant to offer advice on the basis of incomplete evidence. Yet, it is clear that when a case of food toxicity becomes public knowledge, a host of commentators begins to voice opinions that influence the eating habits of the American consumer. Given this situation, it is better to act on the conjecture of scientists than on the conjecture of nonscientists.)

The safety of the more than 1,500 chemical additives now present in American foods should also be studied more closely. Most of these substances fulfill definite needs: they inhibit the growth of molds or microorganisms; they permit the development of convenience foods; they preserve vitamins or polyunsaturated fatty acids, etc. Others, however, like many dyes, have been introduced for no compelling reason. In evaluating each compound, its safety must be balanced against its potential nutritional, economic, or esthetic usefulness. The risk-to-benefit ratio has to be examined case by case.

Long-Range Problems Efforts to establish new guidelines for food enrichment and fortification have progressed at a disappointingly slow pace. The organized scientific bodies seem unwilling to make recommendations on the basis of information currently available and then to make clear that their judgments may be modified in three to five years if subsequent research dictates such action. In addition, virtually no steps have been taken by the food industry to reduce either the sugar content or the saturated-fat and cholesterol content of foods. The technology of the food-processing industry has made it possible to alter the fat and sugar content of a great variety of foods, but without public pressure few changes can be expected. There is evidence, however, that this pressure is now being felt in some areas; the meat industry, for example, is being urged by nutritionists to shift its emphasis to leaner meat or even to substitute polyunsaturated fats for part of the meat fats in formulated meat products.

Ultimately, each person must have a basic understanding of the principles of nutrition if we are to ensure a healthful diet for all Americans. Recently, there has been widespread discussion of the importance of instituting nutrition education in the schools and universities, and in communities. However, few attempts have been made to make use of the insights of the social sciences in order to change people's behavior. A public-information campaign concerning nutrition should be instituted immediately on the basis of existing knowledge and resources; later, the effectiveness of this program can be improved through further research into the socio-economic and cultural factors that influence the individual's choice of food.

A national nutrition policy cannot succeed unless substantial federal funds are appropriated for applied nutrition research, nutrition education, and food control. Each year, the people of the United States spend approximately 125 billion dollars on food, yet the FDA must carry out its varied program of food inspection on an annual budget of 34 million dollars. Furthermore, the FDA has only a few hundred inspectors to oversee 60,000 to 80,000 food plants in this country. In regard to informing the public about nutrition, only a few million dollars have been allocated by the federal government to counterbalance the expenditures of well over a billion dollars that are annually devoted by food companies to promote what are often the least nutritious foods. Unless a minimum of 0.2 percent of the nation's food bill is expended on each one of the three programs—food control, nutrition research, and public education—the United States cannot even begin to achieve an adequate and comprehensive nutrition policy.[3,4]

Greater public awareness of our social problems will be a decisive factor in eradicating hunger due to poverty. For the first time in the history of mankind, we have the technical potential to fulfill all the food needs of this nation, now and for many years to come. However, this tremendous agricultural productivity does not, by itself, ensure an adequate diet for all Americans; it must be coupled with laws based on compassion for the poor, an understanding of the extent of their needs, and finally, the determination to end their hunger.

In contrast, the broader problems of food policy are far more difficult to solve. They will be present continuously not only in this country but, to a far greater extent, in those areas of the world where population pressures are intensifying so rapidly. These issues necessitate a thorough reexamination of policies and habits concerning food. This rethinking should begin in the scientific and medical community, which, oddly enough, has appeared reluctant to accept the call for change. To an extent, their reticence reflects a lack of training in basic and applied nutrition science. Nutrition is a relatively new science; until very recently, it was not taught at all in medical schools, and even now, it is not taught in the vast majority of them. However, a national nutrition policy cannot become a reality unless advanced academic training in nutrition is required for medical personnel, other health scientists, and educators.

Health problems are like many other social problems whose vastness and complexity defy any but slow and experimental solutions. Our nutrition problems, though vast, are by no means hopeless. The White House Conference demonstrated that a blueprint could be established. Progress since then shows that action is possible, but it will take concentrated action by experts as well as by large, vigorous groups of citizens if the momentum is to be conserved.

REFERENCES

1. *Final Report, White House Conference on Food, Nutrition and Health,* 1970. Government Printing Office, Washington, D.C.

2. **Mayer, J.,** 1970. Letter of Transmittal sent with the Final Report of the White House Conference on Food, Nutrition and Health. *Postgraduate Medicine* 47(2): 248–251.

3. *Follow-up Report, White House Conference on Food, Nutrition and Health,* 1971. Government Printing Office, Washington, D.C.

4. **Mayer, J.,** 1971. One Year Later. *Journal of the American Dietetic Association* 58:300–302.

5. **Mayer, J.,** 1965. The Nutritional Status of American Negroes. *Nutrition Reviews* 23:161–164.

6. *Hunger, USA,* 1968. New Community Press, Washington, D.C. pp. 1–100.

7. *Dietary Levels of Households in the U.S.,* 1968. Agricultural Research Service 62–17, Government Printing Office, Washington, D.C.

8. **Owen, G. M., and Kram, K. M.,** 1969. Nutritional Status of Preschool Children in Mississippi. *Journal of the American Dietetic Association* 54:490–494.

9. **Verghese, K. P., Scott, R. B., Teixeira, G., and Ferguson, A. D.,** 1969. Studies in Growth and Development XII. Physical Growth of North American Negro Children. *Pediatrics* 4:243–247.

10. **Zee, P.,** 1970. A Nutritional Survey of Preschool Children from Impoverished Black Families, Memphis. *Journal of the American Medical Association* 213:739–742.

11. **Jones, R. E., and Schendel, H. E.,** 1966. Nutritional Status of Selected Negro Infants in Greenville County, South Carolina. *American Journal of Clinical Nutrition* 18:407–412.

12. **Schaefer, A. E.,** 1969. The National Nutrition Survey. *Journal of the American Dietetic Association* 54:371–375.

13. **Kotz, N.,** 1971. *Let Them Eat Promises.* Doubleday, New York.

14. **Mayer, J.,** 1970. Nutrition in the Aging. *Geriatric Digest* 7:7–13.

15. Recommendations of the Nutrition Section, White House Conference on Aging, 1971. Washington, D.C.

16. **Chase, P. H., and Martin, H. P.,** 1970. Undernutrition and Child Development. *New England Journal of Medicine* 282:933–939.

PART 1

Improving the Nutrition
of Those Most Vulnerable
to Hunger and
Malnutrition

Chapter 1

Infants, Children, and Adolescents

Samuel J. Fomon and Mary C. Egan

Those responsible for development of future policies relating to the nutritional status of children must be guided by five general principles:

1. The nutritional needs of children must be considered within the framework of their needs for total health and general well-being. (Little success can be anticipated if nutritional needs are met in isolation from other basic needs, such as those for shelter, clothing, education, and emotional security.)

2. The needs and expectations of the child must be considered in the context of the needs and expectations of the family. (The particular physiologic needs of pregnant women, infants, children, and adolescents must be recognized; however, programs aimed at improving the lot of preschool children or of pregnant women that ignore the needs of other family members are likely to fail completely or to achieve only limited success. Policies should be developed in such a way as to contribute to the integrity and solidarity of the family unit.)

3. The dignity of the individual must be safeguarded. (Although food-assistance programs are necessary as interim or emergency measures, we must work to bring about more satisfactory solutions

to the problems of those who lack the money to buy food.)

4. Recognition of the importance of essential nutrients for promotion of health and normal growth and development should not overshadow the significance of food and feeding as a means of establishing warm relationships within the family and outside it. (The family meal provides a channel for communication between parents and children, thereby strengthening family ties and reinforcing the role of parents as providers not only of food but of love and security. To accomplish this goal, nutrition policy must be created with considerable sensitivity to cultural patterns.)

5. Nutrition services for children should include attention to the assessment of their nutritional status; provision of a safe food supply adequate in quality and quantity; nutrition counseling for specific nutritional problems; and sound nutrition education for children, parents, and all other caretakers of children such as teachers, day-care staff, health personnel.

Scope of the Problem

In the United States in 1970 there were nearly 71 million persons less than 18 years of age. Of these, nearly 3.5 million were infants less than one year of age; more than 18 million were from one through five years of age, about 25 million from six through 11 and about 24 million from 12 through 17. The complexity of the problem is evident when one considers that nutritional needs may be substantially different between younger and older children, between boys and girls and between more rapidly and less rapidly growing children of the same age and sex.

Nutritional problems of children are related not only to age and sex, but to income

level of the family, cultural patterns, and parental education. For example, anemia caused by lack of iron is much more prevalent among children between six months and two years of age than among school-age children, and more prevalent among children from low-income families than among those from families with higher incomes. In 1969, ten million children under 18 years of age lived in families with incomes below the poverty level. About 5.5 million individuals less than 21 years of age lived in families helped by Aid to Families with Dependent Children. However, in ten states, the average monthly payment per recipient was less than $30—an amount grossly inadequate to provide for all essentials and, in fact, not even sufficient to purchase the relatively small quantity of food needed by a typical 12- to 15-year-old girl according to the U.S. Department of Agriculture's low-cost food plan.

Attitudes Toward Food

Abundant evidence from animal studies suggests that food habits established in infancy and early childhood are likely to persist throughout life. Feeding practices during early life thus deserve careful examination.

In much of the United States today, infants and small children may be subjected to subtle pressures that lead to overeating. When a breast-fed baby ceases to suck and swallow, his mother will assume that he is satisfied. By contrast, the bottle-fed baby is frequently encouraged to drain the last drop from the bottle; thus an artificial endpoint has been introduced with respect to the amount of food consumed. Similarly, many parents praise the toddler who "cleans his plate" and "drinks his milk" and, in fact, may impose minor punishment (no dessert) if he does not consume what is set before him. A definite possibility exists that such long-continued reinforcement with respect to eating all of the food that is set before a person may contribute to overeating in adult life. Instead of limiting food intake to the amount needed to allay hunger, an individual may eat all that has been served to him, being otherwise faced with feelings of guilt because food is being "wasted."

Experimental evidence of several types suggests that many small meals may be preferable to a few large meals. Inclusion of snacks in the diet is therefore probably desirable so long as the choice of snack foods contributes to a balanced and nutritionally adequate diet and is not conducive to development of dental caries.

Breast Feeding

In comparison with other technologically advanced nations, a relatively small percentage of infants in the United States are breast-fed. The pattern has changed but little during the past ten years: about 25 percent of infants are breast-fed at the time of discharge from the hospital after birth, 15 percent at age two months and less than 10 percent at age four months. Reasons for the low frequency of breast feeding are unquestionably complex and deserve study; they almost certainly include the need of many women to work outside the home and the convenience of formula feeding. As already mentioned, breast feeding may be an important means of preventing overfeeding. Many pediatricians and nutritionists suspect that there are other nutritional advantages and important psychological advantages of breast feeding. With the development of more sophisticated research techniques, future studies may help to determine the true value of breast feeding.

Feeding Outside the Home

Each year, increasing numbers of children are being fed outside the home—in day-care centers, Head Start centers, summer camps, settlement houses, and schools. The need for such services is apparent when one considers that approximately 30 percent of children under 18 years of age live in families in which both parents work. About 300,000 children live in residential institutions, including facilities for neglected children, juvenile delinquents, and the retarded or mentally ill.

In 1969 slightly more than 500,000 children were receiving care through licensed or state-approved group day-care services. However, it is apparent that such services are reaching only a small fraction of those who might benefit and that increased resources are needed. In expansion of day-care facilities, it is particularly important to consider the urgent need to provide adequate care for infants and children less than three years of age. These groups have heretofore received only limited attention in the planning of day-care service.

Day-care centers and family day-care facilities often make it possible for parents to work and support their families. In addition to helping meet the special needs of working parents, such programs can be useful in helping to meet the nutritional requirements of the children, most of whom receive meals and/or snacks during the time they are in the center.

In regard to feeding the children, those responsible for a program should take into consideration the nutritional requirements of the child, his need for socialization, and also the cultural patterns and food practices, of the child and his family. The development of healthful food habits should be encouraged; the children should be fed in a safe, clean, pleasant environment; a continuing nutrition-education program should be provided for the children, the parents, and the staff.

As is true of all aspects of group-care programs, food service should be directed at complementing rather than replacing the family's efforts. Every effort should be made to assure that children receive nutritionally adequate diets. In the process, however, nothing should be done to usurp the rights of parents or to erode the integrity of the home.

Promotion of Physical Fitness

For prevention of obesity in children and adults, and perhaps for improvement of other aspects of health, desirable patterns of physical activity need to be established during childhood. To prepare people for a physically active adult life, we need to emphasize from early school age those physical and recreational activities that can be pursued throughout life. Few adults are able to engage regularly in team sports such as football, basketball or soccer; however, many are able to participate regularly in handball, swimming, volleyball, and tennis.

Programs of physical education should emphasize development of the skills necessary for physical activities that can readily be pursued by adults. Appropriate facilities for such activities should be included in planning school buildings and school yards. School facilities should be made available for both children and adults during non-school hours, preferably under supervision.

Prevention of Specific Disorders

At least four nutrition-related disorders are sufficiently widespread and sufficiently well understood that efforts at prevention should be given high priority. They are iron-deficiency anemia, dental caries, atherosclerosis, and obesity.

Iron-Deficiency Anemia Iron-deficiency anemia is almost certainly the most prevalent nutritional disorder among infants and children in the United States. Several factors help to explain the relatively frequent occurrence of this preventable disorder: first, an erroneous belief exists among many physicians and nutritionists that iron is not absorbed before two or three months of age and that it is therefore useless to give iron during the first months of life. In fact, iron is absorbed efficiently by young infants and subsequently is utilized in formation of hemoglobin. Second, many professional workers as well as parents are unaware that most unfortified foods provide rather limited amounts of iron. For practical purposes, iron-fortified foods for infants are restricted to certain commercially prepared formulas and to iron-fortified cereals. Finally, it seems likely that infants born to women with moderate-to-severe iron deficiency are poorly endowed with iron at the time of birth.

Because it is not possible to identify all infants who will become anemic if their diets are not supplemented with iron, it is recommended that every infant, from the early weeks of life until at least 18 months of age, receive a dietary supplement of iron either in the form of medicinal iron or in an iron-fortified food, such as the iron-fortified formulas and cereals.

The major effort in the prevention of iron-deficiency anemia in infants and young children should be an intensive educational campaign that is directed toward parents and professional workers. The campaign should stress (a) the need of the infant and child of preschool age for iron and (b) the role of iron-fortified formulas and iron-fortified cereals in the prevention of iron-deficiency anemia.

In regard to infants of needy families (who are especially likely to develop iron-deficiency anemia), the provision or distribution of iron-fortified formulas, iron-fortified cereals, or medicinal iron should be considered.

In addition, it seems important for nutritionists to pay particular attention to the amount of iron in the diet of girls and women between 11 and 45 years of age. Because the amount of iron ingested by the pregnant woman may influence the iron stores of the fetus, attention to intake of iron and maintenance of normal hematologic indices is especially important throughout the childbearing age.

Dental Caries   The prevalence of dental caries can be reduced through ingestion of appropriate amounts of fluoride and through a decrease in the consumption of sucrose. Efforts must be made to bring about fluoridation of public water supplies where this is not yet being done and to encourage the intake of fluoride in the form of tablets or drop preparations by persons whose drinking water is not fluoridated. Educational efforts should be directed toward decreasing the intake of sucrose, especially in the form of sticky candy eaten between meals. For between-meal snacks, fruits, vegetables, and whole or skim milk are preferable to foods rich in sucrose.

Atherosclerosis   Considerable evidence now exists to indicate that dietary intake of cholesterol and of long-chain, saturated fatty acids contributes to development of atherosclerosis. Dietary habits with respect to intake of foods rich in these substances are extremely difficult to change in the adult population. We must begin with the child of school age and perhaps even with the pre-

school child to develop attitudes toward specific foods that will help to avoid undue risk of atherosclerosis in adult life.

Obesity   It is not enough merely to change food attitudes as they relate to food choices. We must also develop sound attitudes toward the total amount of food consumed. The child classified by many parents as a "good eater" is the one who cleans his plate quickly and with obvious pleasure and then requests a second (or third) serving. We ourselves need to recognize (and we need to teach parents) that a good eater is one who knows when his needs for food have been fulfilled. Only confusion can result if excessive food intake is encouraged during infancy and the preschool period and then (when obesity develops) is condemned in children of school age. Prevention of obesity must begin in infancy.

Nutrition of the Prepregnant Girl

It is during prenatal life and infancy that malnutrition is likely to exert its greatest effect on physical and mental growth. The mother's diet and nutritional status at the time of conception is the culmination of her lifetime nutritional experience and an important determinant of successful childbearing.

The importance of preparing the young girl for future pregnancy can hardly be overemphasized. Too often attention has been focused on improvement of the nutritional status of the pregnant woman to the exclusion of the prepregnant girl. In 1967 about 8,600 babies were born to girls less than 15 years of age and more than 357,000 were born to girls 15 through 18 years of age. Perinatal mortality is high and congenital abnormalities are relatively frequent among infants born to these young women. In addition, pregnancy creates additional nutrient demands and thus may compromise the growth potential and health of the adolescent girl herself.

As noted in the report *Maternal Nutrition and the Course of Pregnancy*[1] lifelong good health and sound nutrition are the best biologic preparation for successful childbearing. This is one more reason why every effort should be made to help parents and other caretakers of children feed their children and safeguard their health from preconception through childhood and adolescence. This means (*a*) assuring access to comprehensive health and medical care (including nutrition services); (*b*) informing parents and other caretakers as well as children themselves about the nutritional needs of children and how to meet them; (*c*) providing practical help for parents in home management, budgeting, consumer education, and child care; (*d*) if necessary, providing enough financial assistance to buy food.

REFERENCE

1. Committee on Maternal Nutrition, Food and Nutrition Board, National Research Council, 1970. *Maternal Nutrition and the Course of Pregnancy.* National Academy of Sciences, Washington, D.C.

Chapter 2

Pregnant and Lactating Women

Howard N. Jacobson and Susan H. Mills

Pregnancy is too often regarded as a natural state that will somehow always take care of itself, and motherhood is too often classed with apple pie as a valuable national institution that has always survived and will continue to do so with no outside interference. The relationship of poor health to malnutrition and of malnutrition to poor outcomes of pregnancy is not widely understood. Thus, the need for national policies has been easily overlooked, and the lack of attention to the health needs of pregnant and lactating women goes unremedied.

For the past 15 years, any efforts towards research in the field of nutrition for pregnant and lactating women, and hence any push toward national nutrition policies for pregnant women, have been almost entirely abandoned because of the disillusionment that arose following the unrealistic expectations of the late forties and early fifties. Rather than face that disillusionment again, most professionals in the fields of health and nutrition, have let their fight lapse into easygoing disinterest. Only in recent years has the desire for research on nutrition in pregnancy been reborn, and along with this research has come the realization that it is vitally important to establish and implement a national nutrition policy.

One of the lessons of the recent past is that problems related to pregnant and lactating women cannot be considered as isolated phenomena. One cannot speak of nutritional policies for mothers without acknowledging that young girls become mothers, and that inadequate nutrition for children means malnourished mothers. Thus, nutritional policies for children must be correlated with those for mothers. One also must see the influence of the mother on her family's education; her concepts of nutrition and health are inevitably imposed on the other members of the household. Furthermore, one must realize that in most families, the mother will feed her children before herself, so that if there is inadequate food to begin with, her food needs will be far less than satisfied; should she be pregnant, her unborn child will suffer the consequences. To sum up, although we must seek the establishment of a national policy with guidelines specifically designed for pregnant women, it is imperative that we understand the close interrelationship of the mother, the family, and the total society; they cannot be dealt with as separate entities.

Developing a Policy for Maternal Nutrition

Before considering the short and recent history of policies for maternal nutrition, it must be said that at present there is no accepted overall approach to national health problems. In 1970, a Senate subcommittee officially disclosed this, stating:

> There is no national health policy to provide form and direction to Federal health programs and expenditures. Furthermore . . . there is no central body or group within the executive branch that is responsible for developing health policy and evaluating Federal performance in light of that policy . . .[1]

Given this lack of governmental structure, the difficulties and frustrations encountered by the various groups that have met to discuss national nutrition problems are more easily appreciated. It is clear that the complexity of the task of creating national nutrition policies is compounded by the need to simultaneously establish a national health structure within which new nutrition policies can be implemented.

The present trends toward developing nutritional policy for pregnant women began in 1962, when a report to the President entitled "A Proposed Program for National Action to Combat Mental Retardation" was published.[2] The shocking and largely unseen problems of pregnant women were brought to national attention as a result of this report, whose purpose was to "explore the possibilities and pathways to prevent and cure mental retardation." One of the principal findings was that the "prevalence of mental retardation (in children) tends to be heavily associated with lack of prenatal care, prematurity, and high infant death rates."

A short time later, the positive value of health care for mothers was emphasized again in the First Report of the 1958 British Perinatal Mortality Survey, under the auspices of the National Birthday Trust Fund, published in 1963. This survey gave special attention to the importance of prenatal care and of the maturity of the pregnancy to the survival of the fetus and infant.[3]

These two reports provided the impetus for a series of studies that revealed an alarmingly high infant mortality rate in the United States; for more than ten years, this rate had consistently persisted at levels above those reported in many Western European countries. Thus followed an intensive search for explanations, which, in turn, stimulated a renewed interest in the possible role of maternal nutrition.

In 1965, the Children's Bureau of the

Department of Health, Education, and Welfare requested that a committee be formed to synthesize available scientific information relating to nutrition and maternal and child health services. In response, the Food and Nutrition Board of the National Academy of Sciences-National Research Council (NRC), organized the Committee on Maternal Nutrition in 1966, and made it responsible for: (1) reviewing current knowledge, (2) providing opportunities for interdisciplinary conferences, (3) identifying areas for further study, and (4) making recommendations and pointing out implications for medicine and public health.

This NRC Committee on Maternal Nutrition completed its work in 1969, and its findings were published in the summer of 1970 in three separate forms: a final report, *Maternal Nutrition and the Course of Pregnancy;*[4] a *Summary Report;*[5] and an *Annotated Bibliography on Maternal Nutrition.*[6]

One of the early and most important difficulties encountered by the NRC committee in preparing the materials for presentation— and one which still remains—was the lack of an official and agreed-upon conceptual framework that expressed in positive terms what the nature and purpose of maternity care in the United States should be. Therefore, in order to establish an authoritative and acceptable basis for their recommendations, the NRC committee adopted the World Health Organization's definition of maternity care. That definition is:

The object of maternity care is to ensure that every expectant and nursing mother maintains good health, learns the art of child care, has a normal delivery, and bears healthy children. Maternity care in the narrower sense consists in the care of the pregnant woman, her safe delivery, her postnatal care and examination, the care of her newly born infant, and the maintenance of lactation. In the wider sense, it begins much earlier in measures aimed to

promote the health and well-being of the young people who are potential parents, and to help them to develop the right approach to family life and to the place of the family in the community. It should also include guidance in parentcraft and in problems associated with infertility and family planning.[7]

Within that framework, the committee set about to develop its recommendations. The committee considered methods and manners in the application of existing knowledge, education of the public and of the health professionals who provide the services, kinds of additional knowledge and information required, and the manpower needed to carry out the recommendations.

The committee realized that all of its recommended changes and improvements would have to be made within the context of rapidly changing national health services. To move from a situation where there are essentially no nutrition services to one in which recommended nutrition services will have become normal and routine is an enormous task.

This challenge of implementation raised questions about *who is responsible* for seeing that change happens as rapidly as possible and in an orderly, integrated, comprehensive, and suitable way. The Committee on Maternal Nutrition took it for granted that most of its specific recommendations would, in the normal course of events, become the responsibilities of the Maternal and Child Health Services (Children's Bureau) of HEW or of the National Institute of Child Health and Human Development (NICHHD), as was found to be appropriate to their respective goals. The members, aware of the complexities of the role of the mother, and hence of maternal nutrition, knew that their proposals entailed responsibilities far wider than those normally associated with those two agencies. They thus stated,

To reach such an objective [to ensure safe, healthy pregnancies and healthy babies] on a national scale has implications for policies that affect the availability of food, especially for families with inadequate food budgets; for public health and nutrition services and educational programs at the federal, state, and local levels of government; for nutrition education through schools and public communication channels; and for nutrition education of those in the professions concerned with maternity care.[5]

The NRC Committee strongly felt that the nutritional needs of mothers and their families must receive constant attention from all who have overall responsibilities for the health and nutrition status of the nation. Therefore, although its assigned task had been completed, and this *ad hoc* committee would naturally be discharged, the members searched for a way to keep the problems of maternal nutrition before the public.

The White House Conference—Enunciation of a Policy

Evidence of growing nationwide concern for the problems of nutrition and health was demonstrated by the sudden calling of the White House Conference on Food, Nutrition and Health in 1969. Here, it seemed, was the logical place to continue to focus public attention on the problems of maternal nutrition.

Specifically, this conference was called so that panels of experts and other concerned citizens could explore "implications for policies that affect the availability of food, especially for families with inadequate food budgets."[8] In his statement of June 11, 1969, President Nixon clarified the purpose of the conference—

In calling the White House Conference on Food, Nutrition, and Health, we are both re-affirming our commitment to a full and healthful diet for all Americans and exploring what we yet need to know and do to achieve that goal. For despite our achievements, much remains to be done. All of us have been shocked as we have become more aware that millions of Americans are malnourished because they are too poor to purchase enough of the right kinds of foods. We also know that many Americans who have enough money to afford a healthful diet do not have one. Many of our youngsters have erratic diets which may be deficient in certain nutrients. Many more of us eat not wisely but too well.

The White House Conference on Food, Nutrition, and Health is intended to focus national attention and national resources on our country's remaining—and changing—nutrition problems. It will assemble the Nation's best minds and expertise, from our business, labor, and academic communities. I shall ask them to consider the following questions:

1. How do we insure continuing surveillance of the state of nutrition of our citizens?

2. What should be done to improve the nutrition of our more vulnerable groups—the very poor, pregnant, and nursing mothers, children and adolescents, the aging, and those such as Indians for whom we have a direct and special responsibility.[8]

Among the 26 panels at the conference was the Panel on Pregnant and Nursing Women and Infants. Like the NRC Committee on Maternal Nutrition, this panel realized that there was no national health policy, no structure within which to work or to provide recommendations. Therefore, before the panel could begin to take up any specific problem (such as possible ways to assure that pregnant women would have the food recommended for them), it was first necessary to establish national goals, objectives, and priorities to provide "form and direction" for the panel's specific recommendations. The preliminary statement of national goals and objectives adopted at the White House Conference in December, 1969, is presented below. It is the only such state-ment that speaks positively to the needs of women and that has been ratified by a Na-tional Conference convened for that purpose.

The Panel's Preliminary Statement

The Panel considers that pregnancy and child-birth are unique events that link the present generation with future ones. The factors that affect reproduction affect not only mothers but families and children as well. They are critical to a sound society. There must be a national affirmation that every woman has the right to high quality and high standard health care. This includes a food intake that will prepare her for and carry her through a healthy preg-nancy and childbirth and permit her infant to flourish. It affirms that the right to adequate nutrition is an inseparable part of the basic right to health care and that women require and are entitled to sufficient amounts of nutri-tious food.

The nutritional needs of mothers and in-fants, the charge of this Panel, should be met only by future programs that meet the nutri-tional needs of all family members through-out their life cycle. Thus, we strongly urge an approach that develops integrated programs for family units, and we reject the continua-tion of fragmentary programs for specific population groups.

Problems of hunger and malnutrition must be treated within the family context and not as problems exclusive to specific age or eco-nomic groups or family members. Any pro-grams to alleviate hunger and poverty must be designed for that end and not for poor people who would be so identified by their use of a given program. Nutritional needs cannot be met in isolation from other basic needs, e.g. for shelter, clothing, health care, education, love, and environmental support to modify conditions of social deprivation.

Vital statistics of the United States indicate a major shortage of national resources for medical and nutritional support committed to the pregnant woman and the infant. Data on the numbers of pregnant women who lack adequate maternity care, the prevalence of

preventable complications of pregnancy, the incidence and trends in premature births, and the incidence of deaths in infancy indicate serious prejudice by our national posture to the health of women and the growth and de-velopment of infants and children.

Further, factors known to be necessary for favorable outcomes of pregnancy and the in-tegrity of families such as health services and adequate diets have been found all too often to be neither available nor accessible to those mothers and families most in need. Thus, President Nixon recently stated: "Too many mothers and young babies do not receive life-saving care." When attention has been turned toward ways to solve our national health prob-lems it has been found that, as the National Advisory Commission on Health Manpower reported in 1967[9]: "the organization of health services has not kept pace with advances in medical science or with changes in society it-self. Medical care in the United States is more a collection of bits and pieces (with overlap-ping, duplication, great gaps, high costs, and wasted efforts), than an integrated system in which needs and efforts are closely related." This is equally true of Federal programs for food and nutrition. The Panel affirms that health services and nutrition are inseparable.[8]

This policy statement should be studied carefully, for it served as the basis for all of the final recommendations made by the panel. Among the central issues in this state-ment is that:

. . . every woman has the right to high quality and high standard health care. [The Panel] affirmed that the right to adequate nutrition is an inseparable part of the basic right to health care and that women require and are entitled to sufficient amounts of nutritious foods.[8]

Attitudes similar to those of the panel were beginning to develop throughout the United States as the seriousness of nutrition problems became more apparent and better reported. For example, in the Report of the

Joint Commission on Mental Health of Children, entitled *Crisis in Child Mental Health*, published in Spring, 1970, mothers' and infants' rights are reaffirmed:

> Every infant must be granted the *right to be born healthy*; yet approximately 1,000,000 children will be born this year to women who get no medical care during their pregnancy or no adequate obstetrical care for delivery; thus many will be born with brain damage from disorders of pregnancy. For some, protein and vitamin supplementation might have prevented such tragedy.[10]

The American Medical Association supports the health needs of mothers and children and so stated in two contexts. First, in the "President's Report to the House of Delegates" of the AMA, delivered on June 21, 1970, President Dorman states, "I should like to set a specific minimum health standard for the American Medical Association to attain and maintain. That is—a healthy child and a healthy mother.[11]

Secondly, in the *Journal of the American Medical Association* (July 13, 1970), the AMA's Council on Foods and Nutrition reported:

> Malnutrition, because it can have so many manifestations, is insidious. Depending on how it is defined, it can be found under many situations. Classical malnutrition exemplified by vitamin deficiency diseases is but a small segment of the spectrum. The less dramatic manifestations of malnutrition—poor performance in pregnancy—are widespread and of great importance.

Another point made in the statement of the Panel on Pregnant and Nursing Mothers and Infants is that the health and nutrition needs of pregnant women must be placed within the context of the other basic needs of the family.

> . . . The nutritional needs of mothers and infants . . . should be met only by future programs that meet the nutritional needs of all family members throughout their life cycle . . . Problems of hunger and malnutrition must be treated within the family context and not as problems exclusive to specific age or economic groups or family members.[8]

The panel noted that experience has shown that in a family with limited income, food spending is the first spending to be reduced, and because of the tendency of mothers to eat last, solutions to the problem of maternal malnutrition must take into account the basic needs of the entire family.

The third major point in the panel's statement is that "health services and nutrition are inseparable." This point has broad implications, for it necessarily brings welfare, national health policy, subsidies, education, and a multitude of other issues into question in any discussion of nutrition policies. The interrelationship of these subjects is stressed throughout most of the recommendations proposed by the panel. For example, Recommendation II, Food Buying and Health, states:

> Nutrition education must be beamed at Americans in general rather than at the poor alone . . . The Panel is convinced that programs must recognize the right of families to preserve the food patterns integral to the cultural, ethnic, and religious groups from which they draw their identity.

The individual rights and human dignity of family members must be respected, and the panel recognized this. Thus,

> The Panel cannot emphasize too strongly that the primary criteria for evaluating any programs designed to meet the nutritional needs of family units must be made in human terms; the preservation of human dignity, the maintenance of adequacy,* the realization of the goal of a sound and healthy citizenry.

*See Chapter 25 for an explanation of "adequacy."

In keeping with their policy statement, the panel devoted an entire recommendation to the pregnant adolescent, for her situation is so often overlooked and yet so crucial. The constellation of problems encountered by pregnant school-age girls extends far beyond the area of responsibility of any single service agency, and in the legislative middle-ground between child and adult, these problems seem to get buried. More than other pregnant and lactating women, pregnant teen-agers find themselves facing not only nutritional needs but social difficulties. Because they are so young, these needs are often greatly increased. The NRC Committee on Maternal Nutrition, in recognition of the difficulties faced by the pregnant adolescent, stated:

> The psychological impact of pregnancy on the adolescent girl may well be more detrimental to her lifetime well-being and that of her child than are the effects of biological immaturity. Society, because of its punitive attitudes towards early pregnancy, especially if it occurs out of wedlock, is prone to withold the understanding and support that are so important under these circumstances. Restrictive practices may force the young pregnant girl to discontinue her education, may make it difficult for her to obtain medical care, and in many states may even prevent her from getting married. These social and psychological difficulties are superimposed on the emotional adaptions and problems characteristic of adolescence.[5]

The Panel's Recommendations   Thus, when the White House Conference made its recommendations, it stated:

> The Panel believes that the increasing numbers of pregnancies among adolescent girls and the decreasing age at which girls become pregnant, jeopardize national health goals and compromise the status of the present generation as well as those to follow. The nutritional status of many adolescents in the United States today is such as to contribute unfavorably to the outcome of pregnancy as reflected by maternal mortality, maternal morbidity, perinatal and infant mortality and morbidity.[8]

The panel report also recommends changes in local policies of schools regarding disqualification of pregnant teen-agers, availability of family planning information, and "in the curricula of our schools . . . instructions in health, nutrition, social and physiological aspects of human reproduction and the importance and means of achieving responsible parenthood."

The questions of financial allocations, food stamps, welfare, and income supplementation, are also linked to the issues involved in the formation of nutrition policy. Such issues are confronted, in part, in Recommendation III, Relief from Malnutrition.

Nutritional insufficiency and income insufficiency are inseparable problems. Within the present food distribution system in the United States, adequate nutrition is impossible without adequate income, although income alone cannot guarantee superior nutrition. Experience and evidence indicate that when income is limited, the family unit may feel that certain priorities stand higher than the food budget. So any food program, to succeed, must consider the other demands on the family budget. Any long-range programs developed to eliminate hunger and malnutrition must include provisions to insure family income adequate to all basic needs. Also, it is socially and economically undesirable to create a permanent food delivery system, operating outside the market, for the poor alone.

The panel concludes that any nutrition programs sponsored by Federal or other governmental units must insure a flow of dollars for the family rather than a flow of food. Only in this way can the twin goals of human dignity and adequate nutrition be met. Recommendation:

A National program for adequate income maintenance must be developed at once to replace both the present welfare and food distribution programs. The dollar value of an adequate income for a family of four shall be no less than the lowest subsistence budget estimated by the Bureau of Labor Statistics which was $5915 in 1967. The dollar value must be continually adjusted to fluctuations in the consumer price index as identified by the Bureau of Labor Statistics.

The lowest subsistence budget of the Bureau of Labor Statistics (BLS) was chosen because it is constructed on a set of desiderata that the panel believed conformed to the aspirations of all citizens of the United States, among which are the "maintenance of health and social well-being, the nurture of children, and participation in community activities."[13]

The place of the individual citizen in our society is the point of issue in determining what the level of financial help and support for people should be. The Joint Commission on Mental Health of Children says that people should have "the right to acquire the intellectual and emotional skills necessary to achieve individual aspirations and to cope effectively in our society."[10] If this is true, and if the BLS desiderata are generally acknowledged, then the definition of the rights and roles of citizens will determine how national resources must be allocated to achieve these goals. Further, the allocation of the nation's resources would seem to be the crux of any solution affecting national maternal nutrition policies. Indeed, all nutrition policies depend on how the nation allocates its resources and decides its policies regarding the rights of its citizens to health (including, directly, health care, and indirectly, food, clothing, and shelter). In his Economic Report to the Congress (February 2, 1970) President Nixon expressed the financial policy decisions that face the nation:

We have placed the Nation's larger decisions in the context of a picture of the total resources available and the competing claims upon them. A summary of this analysis is contained in Chapter 3 of the Annual Report of the Council of Economic Advisors; I hope it will be studied carefully and its precedent carried forward in future years.

That analysis is neutral about which options and claims should be chosen. The purpose of the analysis is to help everyone observe the discipline of keeping claims and plans within the limits of our capacity, and to make sure that excessive claims do not prevent us from achieving our most important goals.

Even in our own highly productive and growing economy, resources are limited. There will be competition between private and government uses for our national income, competition among programs within government budgets, and competition among borrowers for the limited national savings.

Our problem, in short, will be to choose wisely what to do with our output and incomes. Large as they are, the claims upon them, what people expect of them, are even larger. If we add the expenditures that consumers will want to make with larger incomes; the investment that businesses must make to assure rising productivity; the housing construction needed to meet the current shortage and the demands of a growing population with rising incomes; the likely expenditures of State and local governments; the costs of present Federal programs plus the proposals already recommended by this Administration—we find that the total would nearly exhaust the national output until 1975. And that total would not include tens of billions of dollars of new programs that are commonly urged upon the Government.

We shall have to think carefully about how to choose the claims upon the national output that will be met, since we cannot meet them all. This choice is not made exclusively or even mainly by the Federal Government. It is mostly made by the individuals who produce the output, earn the income, and decide how it should be spent. Nevertheless, a Federal Government with a budget of $200 billion has a great influence on how the national output is used. This influence is not confined to the output the Federal Government uses itself. The taxes the Federal Government collects, the grants it makes to State and local governments, its borrowing or repayment of debt, influence the purchases of private citizens and of State and local governments.[15]

After the Conference—Implementing the Recommendations

The closing of the White House Conference on Food, Nutrition and Health left the nation with a set of recommendations regarding the formation of health policies. But recommendations had been made before. The questions that had plagued the members of the Committee on Maternal Nutrition began to raise their heads again.

1. What is the function of private organizations, like the National Research Council, in the development of national policies?

2. To what national organization might such a private council report? What organization or agency has the national mandate and authority to ask for and receive recommendations on policies for the nation?

3. Until a national organization or agency with such clearly designated responsibility and authority has been established, how can and should private organizations proceed?

4. To whom is a report of recommendations addressed? Who has ultimate responsibility for its implementation?

5. Who does make policy?

As the nation ponders its new understanding of the importance of health and nutrition, and of, in fact, the right of its citizens to them, it will become more aware of the important relationship of nutrition to the pregnant woman, of the link of her health and happiness with the delivery of an infant who will develop into a normal and healthy child. The nation will then realize that motherhood is not as easy as apple pie, but that it requires the attention and study denied to it for many years. As an enlightened citizenry becomes more aware of these things, it will also recognize the tremendous need for the development of concrete national policies regarding the pregnant woman and the nutrition of her family. A viable health policy must be formulated, and it must take into account all other aspects of life; questions about the rights of people to housing, food, education, dignity, sense of worth, purpose, future expectations, must be answered. The development of answers to these rock-bottom questions, and then the translation of these answers into objectives and policies for the health and nutritional well-being of pregnant women and their families are the challenge for the seventies.

REFERENCES

1. *Federal Role in Health,* 1970. Report of the Committee on Government Operations, United States Senate, made by the Sub-Committee on Executive Reorganization and Government Research, April 30.

2. President's Panel on Mental Retardation, 1962. *National Action to Combat Mental Retardation.* U.S. Government Printing Office, Washington, D.C.

3. Butler, N. R., and Bonham, D. G., 1963. *Perinatal Mortality: The First Report of the British Perinatal Mortality Survey.* E & S Livingstone Ltd., Edinburgh and London.

4. *Maternal Nutrition and the Course of Pregnancy,* 1970. National Academy of Sciences, Washington, D.C.

5. *Maternal Nutrition and the Course of Pregnancy: Summary Report,* 1970. National Academy of Sciences, Washington, D.C.

6. *Annotated Bibliography on Maternal Nutrition,* 1970. Prepared by the Committee on Maternal Nutrition, Food and Nutrition Board, National Research Council, National Academy of Sciences, Superintendent of Documents, U.S. Government Printing Office, Washington, D.C.

7. *The Organization and Administration of Maternal and Child Health Services,* 1969. Fifth Report of the World Health Organization Expert Committee on Maternal and Child Care. WHO Technical Report Series No. 428, Geneva.

8. *White House Conference on Food, Nutrition and Health: Final Report,* 1970. U.S. Government Printing Office, Washington, D.C.

9. *Report of the National Advisory Commission on Health Manpower,* Vol. 1, 1967. U.S. Government Printing Office, Washington, D.C.

10. *Crisis in Child Mental Health,* 1969–1970. Report of the Joint Commission on Mental Health of Children, Harper & Row, New York.

11. **Dorman, G. D.,** 1970. "President's Report to the House of Delegates." *Journal of the American Medical Association,* 213:268.

12. "Malnutrition and Hunger in the United States," 1970. Report of the Council on Foods and Nutrition to the AMA Board of Trustees. *Journal of the American Medical Association,* 213:272.

13. *Three Standards of Living for an Urban Family of Four Persons,* 1969. Bulletin No. 1570–5, U.S. Department of Labor, Bureau of Labor Statistics, U.S. Government Printing Office, Washington, D.C.

14. *Economic Report of the President,* Transmitted to the Congress, February, 1970. U.S. Government Printing Office, Washington, D.C.

Chapter 3

The Obese:
Background and Programs

Albert J. Stunkard

During the past 25 years, interest in weight reduction in our country has grown from a mild concern to an overriding preoccupation. At present, interest in obesity almost assumes the dimensions of a national neurosis. It would be a pleasure to report that this concern has resulted in new and more effective measures of obesity control or even in more effective use of old measures. But we have no evidence of any decrease in the incidence of severity of obesity. The major result of our national preoccupation has been to worry large numbers of mildly obese persons, whose condition presents no real health hazard. It has done nothing about the prevalence of severe obesity among the poor.

What do we know about this condition and what should be done about it?

Who is Obese?

In a society that repeatedly reminds us of the "problem" of obesity, it is hard to realize how recently this condition has been viewed as a problem at all. Rarely, if ever, has a large segment of any people had more than enough to eat for any prolonged period. Throughout history, as in many under-developed areas today, underweight has been the norm, and obesity has been restricted to privileged classes. In many cultures, obesity was and is a status symbol. The legendary yearly weighings of the Aga Khan suggest that the size of a leader can become a source of pride for an entire community. Under the circumstances, we might expect obesity to be more prevalent among privileged groups, and recent studies from a number of cultures suggest that this is indeed the case.

But in the United States, just the opposite situation prevails. In our society, most people can get more than enough to eat, and obesity has long since ceased to be a symbol of high status. In fact, it is regarded with increasing disfavor and disdain. Instead, leanness has displaced obesity as a mark of distinction, so that we see a paradoxical inversion of the relationship between social status and body weight found in much of the world. In the United States, obesity is associated primarily with a lack of wealth and status: a study in one large Eastern city revealed that one-third of lower-class women were obese as compared with one-twentieth of upper-class women. This association between obesity and lower-class status has been found as early as the first year of school and may well begin in infancy.[1] Furthermore, there are very strong associations between all kinds of social influences and obesity. Social mobility, most ethnic and religious variables, and number of generations in this country all are closely linked to presence or absence of obesity. The consistency with which social factors are associated with obesity shows how important they are to our understanding of the condition.

Two findings indicate that, far from being merely casually associated with obesity, social factors are actually responsible for the differing prevalence of obesity in different social groups. First, obesity is many times more common among lower-class six-year-olds than it is among upper-class six-year-olds, a difference that must reflect the differing child-rearing practices of the two groups. Second, obesity is far more common among adults raised in the lower class than in those of upper-class origin.

Before we go further, let us define the disorder. Obesity is a condition characterized by excessive accumulation of fat in the body. In some circles, much is made of the standard height-weight tables; and people are frequently termed obese when their body weight exceeds by 20 percent the standard weight listed in these tables. But since muscle, for example, can contribute to significant degrees of "overweight," this measure often provides only a rough index of obesity in individuals who are only mildly overweight. We look forward to the time when research will offer new and more accurate means of assessing the total amount of body fat. In the meantime, we have no difficulty in recognizing the condition in the severely overweight, for whom it presents serious health hazards.

Health Hazards of Obesity

The life expectancy of the obese is lower than that of the nonobese; this decrease in life expectancy is directly proportional to the degree of obesity. As might be expected from these facts, the mortality rate of obese persons with any medical illness is higher than that among nonobese persons. And the obese are far more likely to suffer from a variety of medical conditions. Diabetes is three times as common among obese persons as in the general population; high blood pressure and gallbladder disease are twice as common; arthritis, lung disability, angina, and sudden death are all far more common. The obese are more likely to have postsurgical complications and mortality. Finally, coronary heart disease—the major killer of Americans today—is more common among obese persons and is more severe the greater the obesity.

These associations with other disorders place obesity near the top of the list of U.S. public health problems. Yet obesity is quite different from other major health problems, for we are not sure that obesity, in itself, has serious ill effects. Rather, it is the way one becomes obese in America—by diminished physical activity and by the consumption of a high-calorie, high-fat diet—that has been implicated in coronary heart disease and other degenerative illnesses.

One of the reasons obesity attracts so much attention is that, in contrast to so many other illnesses, all or almost all, of its ill effects can be reversed. Many obese persons lose their diabetes and their high blood pressure completely when they lose their excess fat. And life-insurance studies tell us that obese persons who successfully lose weight, and keep it off, increase their life expectancy to what it would have been had they never been obese. In its significant and prompt response to a simple treatment—weight reduction—obesity contrasts dramatically with most serious medical problems.

Successful therapy of obesity would have almost unlimited health benefits. But before considering the matter of treatment let us look at a special problem, "juvenile-onset obesity."

Juvenile-Onset Obesity

The consequences of obesity that begins in childhood are sufficiently distinctive that this problem deserves special mention. A growing body of evidence suggests that the fat tissue of persons who become obese in childhood differs in a fundamental way from that of persons who become obese during adult life. Fat tissue is composed of connective tissue in which are imbedded specialized cells for fat storage. We now have good reason to believe that the number of these cells in fat tissue is determined very early in life,

and that overeating during this critical early period gives rise to fat tissue that contains very large numbers of fat cells. Thus, the fat tissue of those with juvenile-onset obesity is quite different from that of persons whose obesity began in adult life. For with increasing age, fat tissue progressively loses its ability to grow by increasing cell number. After childhood, any increase in body fat is achieved by an increase in the size of the individual cells. Furthermore, loss of body fat during weight reduction results entirely from a decrease in the size of the fat cells rather than from a decrease in their number.

These findings have important implications for the person with juvenile-onset obesity. When he attempts weight reduction he must deal with a double burden—more fat cells and bigger ones. Those with adult-onset obesity can return to normal simply by emptying their relatively smaller number of fat cells of excess fat. The juvenile-onset obese, on the other hand, may need to deplete their excessive number of fat cells to abnormally low levels of fat in order to reach a normal body weight. Perhaps their special kind of fat tissue explains why those with juvenile-onset obesity find it harder to lose weight, and keep it off, than do other obese persons. Only about 15 percent of obese children become normal-weight adults; and among obese persons who have not lost weight by age 20, the odds against successful weight reduction rise to 28 to one.

Our reasons for singling out the juvenile-onset obese for special attention derive not only from their differing body composition and treatment history, but also from their emotional problems. Such problems are far more prevalent among those with juvenile-onset obesity than among those with the adult-onset variety; and these problems tend to be far more closely linked to obesity than is true around middle age. A very large percentage of the juvenile-onset obese have disturbances in body image; they view their bodies as repulsive and loathsome and feel that others can look upon them only with contempt. Furthermore, the unusual and even bizarre eating patterns that afflict some obese persons are almost all found in those whose disorder began in childhood.

Treatment

Results The results of treatment for obesity are poor. Most obese persons will not enter treatment; of these who do enter treatment, most will not lose a significant amount of weight; of those who do lose weight, most will regain it.

These poor results are not due to failure to implement any simple therapy of known effectiveness, but to the fact that no simple or uniformly effective treatment exists. Obesity is a chronic condition, resistant to treatment, prone to relapse, for which we have no cure.

Despite these ominous facts, some obese people have been able to lose their excess weight and to maintain a normal weight for long periods of time. Such successful treatment of obesity requires far-reaching changes in life style, including alterations of dietary patterns and patterns of physical activity. Changes in life style of this degree are achieved only by highly motivated persons.

Much anguish is caused obese persons by their failure to recognize these facts and by their repeated failures in weight reduction. Furthermore, attempts at weight reduction are often accompanied by anxiety and depression, at times severe enough to warrant discontinuation. Many obese persons today might well be better off if they learned to live with their condition and stopped subjecting themselves over and over to painful and frustrating attempts to lose weight.

What are the treatments of obesity? All legitimate methods of weight reduction are based on some rather simple facts. The immediate cause of obesity is the consumption of more calories in food than are expended in bodily metabolism and activity. Caloric surplus is stored as fat in specialized fat cells. Weight reduction is achieved by reversing this process and expending more energy than is consumed in caloric form. This is achieved by decreasing food intake, increasing physical activity, or both.

Diet The simplest way to reduce food intake is to follow a low-calorie diet. Best long-term results are achieved with a balanced diet that contains foods usually available. It is important that the foods be ones that can easily be continued during the period of weight maintenance following weight reduction. In many ways this is precisely the most difficult kind of diet to follow during the period of weight reduction. Many obese persons find it easier to stick to novel or even bizarre diets, of which there have been a profusion in recent years—high-fat diets, low-fat diets, high-protein diets, low-protein diets, banana diets, milk diets, "Mayo diets," "Rockefeller diets," rice diets, "macrobiotic" diets, and even a diet in which (in defiance of the laws of thermodynamics) "Calories Don't Count."

Whatever effectiveness these diets may have is due in part to their monotony—almost anyone will get tired of almost any food if that is all he gets to eat. If he is able to stick to one of the bizarre diets, he will very likely tire of it, eat less, and lose weight. In consequence, however, once the person stops the diet and returns to his usual fare, he will usually regain the lost weight promptly and often be left with a small surplus to mock his efforts.

One variant of dieting is total starvation, which, for some reason, many obese persons find relatively easy to tolerate. After two or three days without food, hunger ceases, and the dieter is able to get along quite well, as long as he remains in an undemanding environment. Because of the possibly serious medical consequences of total starvation, this environment should be a hospital. Total starvation results in rapid weight loss, and for some massively obese persons or those who must lose weight promptly for medical reasons, it may have some small rationale. It is worthy of note, however, that weight loss by total starvation is almost invariably regained.

Medicine A variety of medicines has been used in the treatment of obesity. One class of drugs, the amphetamines (especially Dexedrine* and Preludin*) suppresses appetite. The result is decreased food intake and weight loss. When used in conjunction with reducing diets in a carefully planned, medically-supervised treatment program, they may have limited usefulness. This usefulness is seriously limited, however, by the fact that the initial dose loses its effectiveness after a few weeks. The drug's effectiveness can be restored by increasing the dose—a course that has been so frequently pursued by unscrupulous "diet doctors," and unsupervised dieters, as to cast serious doubt on the place of these medications in the treatment of obesity. The amphetamines can have seriously deleterious effects upon the central nervous system. In this day of widespread drug abuse, the mild and transient value of amphetamines in obesity is probably outweighed by the danger posed by their abuse.

No other medicine used to treat obesity has even the small virtue ascribed to the amphetamines; and in no medical condition are patients subjected to more shady practice or downright fraud than in the treatment of obesity. The small number of "diet doctors" (and diet-pill manufacturers) manage to reach a very large number of persons. The pills without a pharmacologic effect are useless, those with an effect are dangerous. In recent years the popular press, the Food and Drug Administration, and a Senate subcommittee have exposed some of these operations. The most common abuse is excessive prescribing of amphetamines. Another is giving thyroid preparations to patients who have no proven thyroid disorder, thereby suppressing the activity of the subject's own thyroid gland. These charlatans also prescribe cardiac glycosides when there is no heart disease, and diuretics in the absence of disturbed water–electrolyte balance. The desperation of many obese persons has led them wittingly or unwittingly to take serious risks. Some have died as a result.

Given the slight benefits achieved, and the larger dangers, it is probably reasonable to contraindicate any medication in the treatment of obesity.

A problem closely associated with that of diet pills is that of "reducing machines," which often purport to reduce body fat in certain areas. There is no argument that physical exercise has value in the treatment of obesity; to the extent that reducing machines increase physical activity, they may have a place in the treatment of obesity. Unfortunately, many such machines do not require increased physical activity. And those that do provide a type of activity so dull that most persons would prefer a walk around the block. Of machines that promise "spot reduction" of fat in certain areas of the body and weight reduction without effort, on the other hand, the most charitable assessment is that they are ineffective. Their manufacturers are subject to penalty for fraud; though legal action is the exception rather than the rule, prosecution is rarely more justified than in the case of those who prey on the anxiety and despair of the obese.

Of the two most generally applicable means of producing weight reduction, restriction of caloric intake is far more widely used than is increase of caloric expenditure. Indeed, some authorities have even argued

*Registered trademarks.

against physical activity in weight-reduction programs on the ground that the caloric expenditure induced by even large amounts of physical activity is relatively low, while such increased physical activity will lead to a compensatory, or more than compensatory, increase in caloric intake. In support of these contentions, they point out that working off a pound of fat requires walking for 36 hours, or splitting wood for seven hours, or playing volley ball for 11 hours.

But it now appears that this counsel is in error. Increased physical activity can and probably should be a vital part of any weight-reduction program. For the energy expended in physical activity is the same whether the activity is performed in a day or a year . Walking for 36 consecutive hours is out of the question for even the most dedicated weight reducer. But walking an extra half hour a day for ten weeks is not only quite feasible, but could add immensely to his general health and pleasure. And the obese person receives a special bonus in this area. For since the caloric expenditure in most forms of physical activity depends largely upon body weight, the obese will expend more energy and thus burn more body fat on the same amount of activity than will those of normal weight.

The second reason that physical activity is useful in weight reduction is precisely that increased physical activity does *not* always result in a compensatory increase in food intake, as conventional wisdom would have it. It is true that such compensatory increases *do* occur in both animals and man, but only when their physical activity exceeds certain minimum levels. Sedentary animals and man not only do not show such compensation, but increased activity may actually decrease their food intake. This combination of increased caloric expenditure and decreased food intake makes an increase in physical activity a highly desirable part of any weight-reduction

program and a factor to consider in any national program for prevention of obesity.

Self-Help   One obstacle to the control of obesity is the scarcity of medical manpower. This scarcity means that even the more effective therapies now available can help only a small proportion of the obese population. The experience of Alcoholics Anonymous suggests that patient self-help groups may provide at least a partial solution to this problem.

In the field of obesity, self-help groups are enjoying a widespread and growing popularity. Furthermore, recent studies suggest that they may be as effective in weight reduction and the maintenance of weight loss as are the usual forms of medical management. The leading organization, TOPS (Take Off Pounds Sensibly), has a national membership of over 300,000 in over 10,000 chapters and is clearly making a significant contribution to the control of obesity. Its contribution could undoubtedly be increased by more effective liaison with the medical profession. In the future, the organization could offer an appropriate means of introducing new weight-reduction technologies as they become available.

Psychological Factors   Just as psychological factors play a role in the overeating that leads to obesity, they are also important in any weight-reduction regimen. The persons around the dieter—his family, friends, and physician—can play a very important part in easing his burden and can contribute to a favorable outcome. The physician who treats his patient with respect and helps reduce his tensions is more apt to help him reduce successfully or preserve confidence and self-esteem should treatment fail.

Recognition of the importance of psychological factors in weight-reduction has led to the hope that psychiatric treatment might prove of value. Time and experience have dimmed this hope. Perhaps psychiatrists saw only the more disturbed obese persons, or perhaps traditional psychiatric treatment is ineffective in the disorder, but there is no evidence that psychiatric treatment is useful for controlling obesity in most persons.

A new form of management, on the other hand, has recently challenged the pessimism about the usefulness of psychological measures in the treatment of obesity. Although it is experimental, behavior therapy has produced results sufficiently encouraging to warrant more intensive investigation of this treatment modality. Almost all of the 300 to 400 patients treated to date have been part of nine or ten research programs that have carefully compared the results of various types of treatment with those of behavior modification. Weight losses in patients treated by behavior modification have significantly exceeded those treated by other methods. Although the number of patients is small, rarely in the history of medicine have trials of treatment been carried out more rigorously or resulted in as clearcut a demonstration of effectiveness.

Recommendations

What action should be taken? The most important recommendation is for more research on obesity.

Research In recent years, we have learned a great deal about obesity. But as is so frequently the case in the early stages of scientific investigation, the new knowledge has as yet little practical effect on our ability to control the disorder. Instead, it has revealed how oversimplified our earlier views were. We now recognize the complexity of the problem. We know that to be successful with our current treatments, obese persons must make far-reaching changes in their life-styles. Very few obese persons can make such changes.

Although it has so far contributed little to our treatment capabilities, obesity research has had other important effects. For one, it has laid bare the ineffectiveness and wastefulness of many of the traditional approaches to weight reduction. We are still only indifferently successful in our efforts to control the disorder, but at least we can spare obese persons—and ourselves—much time, effort, and suffering.

Furthermore, we are beginning to see the outlines of an effective strategy for progress. This strategy requires two kinds of research: first, we must have targeted, applied research designed to improve our current treatment methods. This goal should be achieved as quickly as possible, although we must accept the fact that our results will be limited in scope and applicability. But even modest improvement in the treatment of obesity could have a major impact on our nation's health. Second, we must have basic, untargeted research. Here we cannot hope for speed, but the effort is sure, one day, to yield a safe, economical, and effective method of controlling obesity.

Promising investigations are now being conducted under the auspices of at least four different disciplines:

Biochemical research in fat and carbohydrate metabolism is making rapid progress and should be supported, since it is one of the paths most likely to lead us to our ultimate goal of the control of obesity. Study of adipose tissue and its relationship to biochemical control mechanisms seems a particularly rewarding approach.

Neurophysiological studies to elucidate the brain mechanisms that regulate food intake and energy balance have recently made remarkable strides. There is every reason to believe that more such research will vastly expand our understanding of these processes. One aspect of this work deserves special attention: better understanding of the role of physical activity in regulating energy balance could lead directly to practical measures for control of obesity.

Psychological studies have made a promising start in applying behavior therapy to obesity control. Further efforts in this direction should be pursued.

Sociological studies of the effectiveness of such self-help groups as Alcoholics Anonymous and TOPS in treating chronic disorders suggest that their approaches merit careful consideration. The immediate need is for systematic trials and evaluations of their techniques.

Infancy and childhood should be a major focus of preventive and therapeutic efforts. Obese children usually become obese adults, and obesity that begins in childhood is associated with added sequelae and complications. Dietary and exercise patterns established in youth persist into adult life. The pattern of physical inactivity and consumption of a high-fat, high-calorie diet that so frequently accompanies juvenile obesity predisposes not only to adult obesity but, even more importantly, to coronary heart disease.

Federal school-lunch and breakfast programs are in a particularly good position to demonstrate and teach proper nutritional practices.

Education and Regulation   A two-pronged program of education and regulation should be undertaken. Interested public and private agencies should intensify educational efforts directed towards both the general public and the medical profession. The goal should be to publicize the most recent and most reliable information about obesity and to combat today's widespread misinformation and faddism.

Where misinformation extends to questionable practices and even outright fraud, the Food and Drug Administration and other federal agencies must intervene more forcefully than has been their custom. We need to expand programs designed to control inappropriate diets, drugs, and "reducing machines," and to combat the practices of unscrupulous entrepreneurs.

Adequate Income   We also must recognize that it is very difficult (if not impossible) to prepare diets that are nutritious, and that will prevent obesity and other illness, from foods now available to the poor. Therefore, an income adequate to purchase nutritious foods should be guaranteed all Americans.

REFERENCES

1. **Moore, M. E., Stunkard, A., and Srole, L.,** 1962. Obesity, Social Class, and Mental Illness. *Journal of the American Medical Association* 81:962–966.

Further Reading

2. **Mayer, J.,** 1968. *Overweight: Causes, Cost, and Control.* Prentice-Hall, Inc., Englewood Cliffs, N.J.

Chapter 4

Atherosclerotic Disease, Diabetes, and Hypertension: Background Considerations

Robert B. McGandy and Jean Mayer

No more fitting introduction to this topic can be found than the following statement of the panel on Adults in an Affluent Society: The Degenerative Diseases of Middle Age in the Final Report of the White House Conference on Food, Nutrition and Health.

> Among the affluent it is clear that we have developed a society that is characterized by:
>
> 1. overconsumption of calories with food choices that are not necessarily the wisest on the basis of available nutritional information,
> 2. underexercising and failure to develop life-long habits to combat the ills of sedentary life.
>
> These are important factors promoting excess weight, atherosclerosis, and other degenerative diseases. In spite of much information about these diseases, the medical and allied professions have been unable to make substantial progress in their control.

The several points made in this statement can be rephrased. Our system of treatment-oriented medical care has not been able to influence the course of these diseases on a scale large enough to be reflected in national health statistics. On the other hand, reshaping our life-style, although an obvious and sensible approach to prevention, is not yet a significant commitment or goal of our system of medical care. Worse, there are not yet significant community resources to aid persons who, either on their own or on a physician's advice, desire to improve their mode of living; in some cases, there are impediments.

The three diseases we will discuss here are chronic illnesses that are a major affliction of our society. They all are or act through diseases of the circulatory system; their etiology is still uncertain; they are all amenable to a course of treatment in which diet looms large; and studies show them to be clearly interrelated, although the exact nature of their entanglement is, again, not yet known. All three, in the early stages, can respond favorably to changes in diet and life-style. All three, when sufficiently advanced to require a doctor's care, will be treated with medication and diet, weight reduction and exercise. All three are associated with another malady of technologically advanced societies: obesity. And each of the three, when more than one is present in the patient, will benefit from treatment and control of either of the others.

Atherosclerosis

Atherosclerosis, a disease in which cholesterol and other fats accumulate in walls of arteries, is directly responsible for the great majority of severe disability and death in the United States and other affluent societies. The disease is essentially universally present in our population from adolescence onward, though the rate of its progression and the frequency of its clinical complications* are in-

*When the atherosclerosis becomes severe in the arteries supplying oxygen and nutrients to heart muscle, angina pectoris may appear or a blood clot may form and lead to a coronary thrombosis ("heart attack"). When the arteries supplying the brain are severely involved, a "stroke" may result. These are the major sites at which fatal complications occur.

fluenced by a very large number of both known and unknown factors. Many of these factors are determined by our dietary habits and our way of life.

A few statistics will convey some idea of the magnitude and malignancy of the problem. Of every 100 American males, 20 will develop clinical athersclerotic heart disease (mostly heart attacks) by age 60. And of those stricken, one-third will die within minutes to a week of the initial attack—a grim statistic little influenced by our present sophisticated medical management. Of the two-thirds who survive, many will be disabled to the point of impairment of their contribution to their families or to society; those survivors have five times the risk of dying within the next five years as do men of the same age but without previous evidence of atherosclerotic heart disease. Currently in the United States, there are annually some 160,000 deaths under age 65—mostly males— from atherosclerotic heart disease. In the population as a whole (and at all ages) there are now over 600,000 deaths from this cause and another 200,000 from atherosclerosis of the arteries supplying the brain.

The Prospects for Prevention   What are the characteristics of those individuals who, on the average, have more advanced atherosclerosis and are more prone to develop the clinical complications? These characteristics, commonly called "risk factors," fall into two major categories, which in practical terms separate primarily hereditary from mainly environmentally determined characteristics.

The hereditary factors are:

Sex. The frequency of atherosclerotic disease is much less among premenopausal women, but by age 60 to 65 the two sexes are about equally affected.

Family History. A maternal or paternal history of premature atherosclerosis does increase the risk among the offspring; however, in part, such predisposition is accounted for by the environmentally regulated factors listed below.

Body Build and Behavioral Patterns. These factors, too, are contributors to severe atherosclerosis among some individuals. But to some extent at least (weight control, avoidance of stressful situations, for example) they are also amenable to some environmental amelioration.

The environmental factors are:

Obesity. Overweight, the result of too many calories and too little energy expenditure, characterizes a high proportion of our own population. While obesity per se is associated with an increased risk of death from atherosclerotic disease, its deleterious effect is expanded because obese individuals also have higher levels of blood fat and blood pressure—both factors that in themselves are closely associated with atherosclerosis. Furthermore, correction of obesity leads to lowering of blood pressure and blood fats.

Blood Cholesterol and Other Fats. The higher the levels, the greater the risk. The amounts of these substances circulating in the blood stream are regulated primarily by the quantity and quality of dietary fats. The uniformly high levels of blood fats among American men and women from adolescence onward can be reduced by restricting the use of saturated fat and cholesterol. In addition, other dietary components (trace metals, carbohydrates) may also influence the development of atherosclerosis.

Blood Pressure. At least in part regulated by diet (particularly the intake of sodium from table salt). An elevated level of blood pressure is an important risk factor. Of great importance to prevention is that elevated blood pressure can be readily treated—both by diets of lowered salt content and by drugs.

Sedentary Living. This is an important factor in overweight as well as predisposing to impaired blood supply to the heart, which decreases the efficiency and reserve capacity of that vital organ. A low level of physical activity is a characteristic of our American life style which, with proper motivation, can be reversed.

Diabetes and Gout. Both are diseases in which diet is an important facet of medical management; both are also associated with an increased risk of atherosclerotic disease.

Cigarette Smoking. Heavy cigarette smoking has been linked with enhanced atherosclerosis. It is certainly a habit amenable to change—given proper motivation.

These are the main characteristics that have been consistently demonstrated to be associated with atherosclerotic heart and brain disease. All of the factors in the second category are amenable to change. And while it may seem perfectly reasonable that favorable changes in these aspects of our contemporary way of life would retard or prevent the development of atherosclerosis, there is yet no convincing proof that this is so.

Hypertension

Hypertension, or high blood pressure, is the most common cardiovascular disease. It is a factor in increasing the risk of death from coronary heart disease or stroke, and it afflicts some 20 million Americans. In the comprehensive study made in Tecumseh, Michigan, in a "typical" American population, 27 percent of the men and 37 percent of the women were categorized as having hypertensive disease.[1] Many people are not aware that the disease is so common, or, unless it has been diagnosed by their physician, that they themselves may easily be its victims.

Although the cause, or causes, of hypertension cannot in most cases be identified, it is clear that obesity is closely associated, and that, in many patients, the obesity actually may be the cause of certain forms of hypertensive disease. Data on the prevalence of obesity in the United States make somber reading. In children and adolescents measurements obtained by using densitometry or calipers to measure actual body fat indicate a prevalence over 20 percent, at least in the East. In regard to adults, the Metropolitan Life Insurance Company considers 29 percent of U.S. men 40 to 49 years old to be 10 to 19 percent over ideal weight, and 32 percent to be 20 percent overweight or more. For women, the corresponding figures are 19 and 40 percent. For both sexes, the percentages are even higher in the age group 50 to 59.[2] Clearly, then, obesity and hypertension affect tens of millions of Americans.

In the United States a quite significant correlation exists between overweight and hypertension in the 30-to-59 age group, but it then decreases with age. International data indicate that the correlation is higher in countries where obesity is common and that the increase in blood pressure with age is greater in denser populations. The correlation between blood pressure and weight is higher in women than in men. It is higher in patients with a family history of both problems, in the very obese, and in younger age groups. Weight and blood pressure correlate more closely than skinfold thickness and blood pressure, so that both body type and weight may be factors.

These correlations differ somewhat in different population groups, but for the United States in general we can reasonably assert that between one-fifth and one-third of all hypertensive adults are also markedly overweight or actually obese.

Weight reduction often will favorably affect hypertension, but that response is not universal. However, there are enough examples of successful reduction of blood pressure with weight loss to indicate the wisdom of weight-reduction therapy.

The mechanism of the association between obesity and hypertension is not known. Obesity alone can increase oxygen consumption at rest, increase work when moving, and thus increase cardiac output and peripheral resistance. This forces the left ventricle to do more work. Hypertension has different effects on the cardiovascular system, but the increase in pressure and peripheral resistance also causes an increased left ventricular work load. This synergistic increase of the work of the heart is obviously dangerous and explains why the combined risk of the two conditions, when they are simultaneously present, may be greater than the sum of the risks due to each condition.

Preventive Measures Obesity has been suggested as a *causal* factor in hypertension in some patients. These patients may be unable to respond to the increased cardiac output demanded by obesity without increasing their blood pressure. The importance of weight reduction in this type of patient is obviously even greater than in other hypertensive subjects.

Restriction of salt intake is also of benefit to many patients with hypertension, and evidence is accumulating that high intakes of salt from infancy on may be important in initiating and aggravating hypertension, particularly in those who already exhibit the disorder or who have a genetic predisposition to the disease.

Groups of people who have low intakes of salt appear to have a low incidence of hypertension. West Indian Negroes, who eat a great deal of salt pork and salt fish, have a much higher prevalence of hypertension than the whites and Indians in the same area. L. K. Dahl, dividing adult subjects into three groups according to their salt intake, found that 10 percent of those consuming large amounts were hypertensive, compared with 7 percent of the "average" group and 1 percent of the group accustomed to small amounts of salt in their diets.[3]

A high dietary concentration of salt can induce permanent hypertension in rats, although some difference appears among strains. Very young rats appear to be more immediately sensitive to the effect of high salt diets than older animals, a finding of some concern when one considers that many foods manufactured for human infants are salted, not in accordance with the sodium content of their ideal food, breast milk, which contains 7 milliequivalents per liter, but to please the mother's taste. The calculated requirement of salt for infants from birth to one year of age is 1 milliequivalent per kilogram. Yet one study has shown the average salt intake of healthy American term babies fed cows' milk and processed foods to be 6.3 milliequivalents per kilogram.[4]

It is worth noting that populations living on diets habitually low in salt show no ill effects; Eskimos, Chinese, American Indians, Lapps, and Masai are among the groups studied.

It would seem that the course of wisdom would be to lower the salt content of processed foods in general, and to educate the American public to explore the many other methods of flavoring foods. (Parenthetically, there arises here the question of iodized salt and goiter. What source of iodine other than iodized salt is available easily and cheaply to patients on a restricted sodium diet?)

Diabetes

Diabetes ranks fifth as a cause of death in the United States. The American Diabetes Association has estimated that the minimal number of diagnosed and undiagnosed cases of diabetes runs to about 10 million. It is a disease of advancing age: 70 percent of known diabetics reported by the Bureau of Census Survey of 1964–1965 were 45 or older;[5] less than 1 percent were diagnosed before age 25. Since the discovery of insulin, diabetes has been relegated from the category of short-term, fatal diseases to that of long-term, chronic illnesses which predispose to death from other causes—high on the list being the atherosclerotic diseases, particularly of the heart and small blood vessels;

diseases of the eye, kidney, and nervous system; and often hypertension, which exposes patients to the added risk of heart attack or stroke.

Diabetes mellitus, the acute form of the disease, is marked by excretion of sugar in the urine, usually the result of faulty pancreatic activity, which in turn causes an inability to metabolize carbohydrates. Diabetes has historically been treated by prescribing diets low in carbohydrates and calories—indeed, low in some cases to the point of starvation. With the advent of insulin therapy combined with dietary management, it has been possible to liberalize the starvation diet and still maintain patients for many years in comparative good health. An increasingly large number of patients of the Joslin Clinic are being awarded the clinic's 25-year medal for survival.

Treatment and Control   Now, data from studies on diabetes and related diseases and on the metabolism of different carbohydrates are raising fundamental questions about the basic assumptions of earlier accepted diet therapy. Disaccharides (the simple sugars such as sucrose) and polysaccharides (the starches) are digested in different areas of the intestine and metabolized at different rates. Their end effect on the blood contents is also different. Sucrose increases the triglyceride level; starch tends to lower both triglycerides and cholesterol. Since diabetics are prone to death from heart disease, the desirability of a low-carbohydrate diet, which of necessity is also a high-fat diet, is called into question. There is general agreement that sucrose and the other simple sugars should be avoided in the diabetic's diet—indeed, there is some evidence to suggest that sucrose plays an etiologic role in those individuals who are genetically susceptible to the disease.[6] Many diabetics, however, have been reported to be on good control on diets containing large proportions of starch. Opinions among clinicians vary as to the optimal amount of carbohydrate intake, but most tend to limit it to about 40 percent of calories. Any lower value means a diet very high in fat, with all the dangers attendant on a group already prone to atherosclerotic disease.

It would, then, appear to be prudent to modify the fat component of the diet to achieve the lowest possible levels of serum cholesterol and triglycerides. The fats may be manipulated by limiting consumption of egg yolks, whole milk, and most cheeses, and replacing butter and beef, pork, and mutton with polyunsaturated oils and margarines and fish and poultry. Triglycerides may be lowered by excluding simple sugars from the diet, controlling intake of starches, and also through weight reduction, when it is necessary.

For diabetes, as for atherosclerosis and hypertension, obesity is a predisposing factor. A large proportion of United States patients with adult-onset diabetes are obese, and achievement of the weight desirable for normal adults of the same age and body build can often control the disease, if not too severe, without drug therapy .

There is no longer any rationale for under-feeding the diabetic patient, but it is important to maintain a desirable weight. For this reason, regular exercise is important. Exercise can be instrumental in reducing blood cholesterol, as well as in simply controlling weight, and has been shown to act like an additional dose of insulin in patients who have already been given a base-line dose. It is important, however, that the dietary regimen be carefully timed and regulated in conjunction with the schedule of physical activity.

Understanding and Prevention

It is obvious that there continues to be an urgent need for further research into the basic problems surrounding the inception,

progression, and terminal events of athero-sclerotic disease. Further clarification of the roles of the several risk factors, both alone and in combination, is desperately needed. Atherosclerosis has its onset in childhood and adolescence; diabetes and hypertension also may be influenced by diet patterns from infancy. Much more attention must be paid to the habits of eating and activity that are established in infancy, childhood, and adolescence.

In addition to the need for research, there are now strong reasons to undertake large-scale well-controlled field studies to apply the great body of knowledge we already have. The potential reduction in premature death and disability from favorable alteration of various aspects of our way of life is considerable. Modification of diet (in regard to fats and calories), modification of physical activity, medical management of elevated blood pressure, attention to cigarette smoking—all of these measures can be undertaken on a scale and in a way that will allow for careful evaluation of outcome. The White House Conference put the highest priority on a national commitment in this direction.

It will take many more years before such field trials produce results upon which firm recommendations can be made to the American public in general and upon which a new philosophy of health *promotion* will be based. But there is now a very large number of people who are clearly at great risk of death from atherosclerotic disease, the inevitable course of which will be little altered by current medical care. Present knowledge amply justifies efforts to modify those facets in their way of life that the best scientific evidence implicates in the disease.

The current problem in practicing prevention is how to help these individuals, how to offer them effective aid in altering dietary and exercise habits. Physicians simply do not have the time or expertise for such services. There seems to be a clear need for community- and hospital-based counselling services staffed by qualified health professionals. Instruction in effective adherence to palatable, acceptable diets—whether it be for the control of calories, saturated fats, simple sugars, or salt, is time-consuming; it demands a sound knowledge of food purchasing and preparation.

A major block to the modification of diet is the present chaotic state of labeling and identification. Quantities of fats, sugars, calories, salt are not uniformly specified. Foods useful for special diets are not labeled and identified clearly. The present situation not only presents insoluble dilemmas to the patient and to the nutritionist responsible for guidance but also has retarded the development and marketing of the many modified foods that would be helpful to this facet of preventive medicine. Meaningful labeling and identification of foods are clearly needed.

Furthermore, community facilities for physical reconditioning must be made available on a national scale, as should be centers for the modification of smoking habits.

Both the implementation of present knowledge and the acceptance of a philosophy of health maintenance and health promotion present an enormous challenge to this decade. These are the goals called for in the report of the White House Conference.

REFERENCES

1. **Johnson, B. C., Epstein, F. H., and Kjelsberg, M. O.,** 1965. Distributions and Familial Studies of Blood Pressure and Serum Cholesterol Levels in a Total Community. Tecumseh, Michigan. *Journal of Chronic Diseases* 18:147–160.

2. New Weight Standards for Men and Women, 1959. Metropolitan Life Insurance Company, *Statistical Bulletin*, November-December.

3. **Dahl, L. K., and Love, R. A.,** 1957. Etiological Role of Sodium Chloride Intake in Essential Hypertension in Humans. *Journal of the American Medical Association* 164:397–400.

4. **Puyau, F. A., and Hampton, L. P.,** 1966. Salt Intake of Infants. *American Journal of Disease in Childhood* 111:370–373.

5. **Hodges, R. E., and Krehl, W. A.,** 1965. The Role of Carbohydrates in Lipid Metabolism. *American Journal of Clinical Nutrition* 17:334–346.

Chapter 5

Heart Disease:
Plans for Action

Jean Mayer

Coronary atherosclerosis is the number-one health problem in the United States, with one million Americans killed or permanently disabled every year. In many ways it must be considered a "disease of civilization" brought about in part by our mode of life: a diet overabundant in calories derived from saturated fat (and sucrose) and too high in cholesterol, an almost total lack of physical activity, and heavy cigarette smoking. These have created conditions new to the human race. The United States is particularly hard hit by this new pandemic. The quintupling of our health expenditures in the past 20 years, the results of the most fertile period in medical research ever, have been nullified by the ever-mounting tide of heart disease.

We need not feel impotent before this catastrophe. What we have created, we can reverse. We need

a. to modify our national diet to cut drastically our intake of saturated fat and cholesterol, particularly for middle-aged men;
b. to cut down the unnecessary calories in our diet (Decrease in the sugar content of the diet is an easy way to do so.);
c. to launch a much more vigorous antismoking campaign;

d. to conduct a nationwide campaign of detection and correction of hypertension;

e. to provide universally accessible facilities for adult physical exercise, and reform and extend our physical education programs in schools; plan urban renewal with health problems in mind;

f. to create a network of facilities to give immediate appropriate cardiological treatment to victims of myocardial infarction;

g. to develop systems of information for the public concerning nutrition (including labeling), smoking, hypertension, exercise, and signs of myocardial infarction requiring immediate recourse to appropriate facilities.

Public health must be a component in all aspects of national planning. Let us now examine a number of more detailed points.

The Extent and Nature of the Problem of Heart Disease; Known Factors at Risk

The Size of the Problem   Heart disease is our major cause of death and our major cause of disability. The National Health Examination Survey, in an already outdated survey (1960–62)[1] estimated that 3.1 million American adults age 18 to 79 had definite coronary heart disease ("CHD") and 2.4 million had suspected CHD. They further estimated that 1.8 million Americans under 65 had definite CHD and 1.6 million suspected CHD. Since then, indications are that these numbers have increased. Over 600,000 Americans die every year due to CHD, with a greater toll (three to one) among men than women.

All this means is that an American has one chance in five of developing clinical CHD before the age of 60, most probably in the form of a myocardial infarction. About 25 percent will die within three hours of the onset of symptoms, often before medical care is available or hospitalization takes place. Another

10 percent die within the following few weeks. The life expectancy of survivors is very much abbreviated: they are five times as likely to die within the next five years as their contemporaries without a history of previous coronary. Obviously, if mortality from heart disease is going to be cut down, atherosclerotic diseases must be prevented. This is our major health problem. Now that the elimination of malnutrition due to poverty is well underway, the primary thrust of our nutrition and preventive medicine effort in the next decade must be in this area.

The Nature of Atherosclerosis   Atherosclerosis is the major type of hardening of the arteries (arteriosclerosis). It is accompanied by (or due to) an accumulation of fatty materials (lipids)—in particular, cholesterol—in the wall of large and medium sized arteries. As the walls harden and the internal diameter decreases below a critical size, clinical impairments due to atherosclerotic disease become evident. This means that, by the time any sign can be detected, one is already faced with *severe* atherosclerosis. Interruption of the circulation due to occlusion (*a*) of the coronary vessel, with interruption of the blood supply to part of the heart muscle (myocardial infarction), or (*b*) of an artery irrigating part of the brain, again with interruption of the blood supply (stroke), are the most dramatic examples of consequences of atherosclerosis. (The term thrombotic denotes the occlusion taking place). But the aorta and blood vessels in the kidney and in peripheral locations (notably the feet and the fingers) are also notably susceptible to atherosclerosis.

"Risk Factors" Associated with Atherosclerosis   Epidemiologists are loath to speak of "causes" of disease. The old concept that a single event—e.g., the presence of a microbe—was sufficient to cause a disease has been replaced by the view that diseases arise as a result of the conjunction of many factors, some associated with the host or patient, some with the environment, and some with specific external factors (like bacteria and viruses). In addition, it is not always certain that because an event often or usually precedes another, it is necessarily directly related to it. For these reasons, we shall speak of "risk factors" rather than causal factors. It is nevertheless generally true that if a risk factor is decreased, the risk itself is decreased.

The risk factors that are generally agreed upon by the consensus of medical scientists and all major medical societies in the United States (expressing themselves through the Inter-Society Commission for Heart Disease Resources)[2] are: an habitual diet high in saturated fat, cholesterol, and calories; elevated blood lipids (cholesterol and probably also triglycerides); hypertension; cigarette smoking; obesity; sedentary living; psychosocial tension, and a positive family history of premature atherosclerotic diseases. Let us examine these—with particular attention being given to nutritional factors.

Diet and Serum Lipids. Experimental studies with animals have indicated that arterial lesions cannot be produced without modification of the diet entailing increased intake of cholesterol and fat, leading to elevation of both cholesterol and lipids in blood. Similarly, with few exceptions, human populations consuming diets high in saturated fats and cholesterol have a high cholesterol level in blood ("a high serum cholesterol") and high mortality rates from "premature" (under 65) CHD. Again, with very few exceptions, the risk of developing premature CHD (within a given population group) increases as the serum cholesterol increases. This fact has been abundantly demonstrated within the American male population. Incidentally, the higher the cholesterol level the higher the risk *at any level* (this is not a situation in which risk begins when a magic number—250 milligrams per 100 milliliters or 300 milligrams or what-have-you—is reached).

Detailed data supporting these statements have been obtained, in particular, in the course of the International Atherosclerosis Project,[3] where the degree of atherosclerosis in the aorta and coronary arteries was quantitated in autopsies of over 31,000 persons aged ten to 69 who died in 1960-65 in 15 cities throughout the world. Countries showing a high intake of saturated fat and high serum cholesterol had more severe atherosclerotic lesions than did countries with low saturated fat intake and low serum cholesterol. The subjects from the United States had the highest degree of atherosclerotic involvement. The United States is also near the top in CHD mortality (only little Finland of all countries is higher). Differences even among developed countries are enormous. In 1964, the United States had a mortality rate per 100,000 of 354; Australia with 324, Canada with 311, are also examples of the high-mortality group. Germany (Federal Republic) 132, The Netherlands 162, Czechoslovakia 151, Switzerland 134, are examples of the middle group. Sweden 124, France 74, and Japan 51 are examples of the low-CHD-mortality group. If all the cardiovascular diseases are considered, the differences are less dramatic but still very large: the United States 477, Australia 425, Canada 385 in the high group; Germany 275, The Netherlands 222, Czechoslovakia 263, Switzerland 210 as examples of the middle group; France 202, Japan 251, Sweden 189 in the lower range.

An extensive study of 18 population samples in seven countries (Finland, Greece, Italy, Japan, The Netherlands, the United States and Yugoslavia), totaling 12,000 men age 40-59 confirms the fact that the population groups from the U.S. with a high fat intake had four to five times the rate of CHD mortality shown by low prevalence countries with a low fat intake.

Recently, data obtained by workers in London,[4] as well as some data obtained in this country, have suggested that consumption of sucrose (table sugar) might be a serious risk factor in some individuals in whom it may cause an elevation of triglycerides (another blood lipid). Data obtained in Jerusalem also suggest that high sugar consumption may precipitate the development of disturbances in carbohydrate metabolism, including diabetes in genetically predisposed individuals.[5] It is hardly necessary to point out that sucrose, consumed at the average rate of about 100 pounds per American—man, woman, and child—(up from eight pounds in 1830), and representing close to 500 calories per day, is a prime source of "empty calories," undesirable from the point of view of dental health and general nutrition. From the viewpoint of atherosclerosis, however, the problems raised by the presence of so much sugar in our diet do not decrease the desirability of also reducing saturated fats.

Hypertension. Hypertension aggravates atherosclerosis, particularly in the presence of hyperlipidemia—this statement is supported by considerable clinical data as well as by prospective epidemiological findings (that is, studies in which a population is studied at a given period and the subsequent occurrence of cardiovascular catastrophes is then correlated with individual characteristics). The relationship between blood pressure and CHD, like that between cholesterol and CHD, is continuous: the risk is continuously increased as the blood-pressure levels are increased. There is, fortunately, mounting evidence that antihypertensive treatment (including the use of medication now available, which effectively lowers blood pressure to near normal levels) considerably reduces the risk of hypertension—a fact that dictates the need for a universal detection and correction program.

Cigarette Smoking. The 1964 report of the Surgeon General established that cigarette smoking was a major (average 70 percent additional) risk in the development of CHD.[6] Data obtained since (one study[7] involving over one million men and women, originally ages 40 to 84, for whom data are available after three and six years of followup) show that, for each sex and for every age group, risk increases with the number of cigarettes smoked. The youngest men smoking two or more packs a day were at highest risk; generally, the younger the age group the higher the risk; the risk of CHD (and the risk of strokes) is greater for smokers whatever their serum cholesterol and blood pressure. Cigarette smoking and the other major risks of CHD, hypercholesterolemia, and hypertension, create greatest risks if two or three are present simultaneously.

Obesity. Obesity is a significant risk factor. This has been borne out by a variety of insurance actuarial studies, as well as large-scale studies, particularly those conducted by the Medical Department of the U.S. Army.[8] Risk is a function of the degree of obesity. It must be remembered that obesity is often the result of and is accompanied by sedentary living (lack of "exercise"). There can be no doubt that prevention (or correction) of overweight is a major element in prevention of atherosclerosis.

Sedentary Living (Lack of Physical Exercise). Many authorities assign lack of exercise a lesser role than the evil trinity of hypercholesterolemia, hypertension, and cigarette smoking—and even obesity. This may be because few people have as yet given any thought to (a) the degree to which we have become immobile and (b) the various ways in which different types of physical activity interreact with the factors listed above.

That we have become an extraordinarily inactive population is obvious to travelers to our country; we tend to forget not only how hard our pioneer forebears worked but also how constantly engaged in hard physical labor lumberjacks, miners, farmers, laborers, and factory workers were until labor-saving tools became almost universally available. The advent of mass-transportation systems, and, more recently, the advent of the automobile drastically reduced the amount of walking necessary. In the last few years, occasions for minor and even minuscule physical activity have been eliminated—the electric typewriter, the automatic gearshift, that additional telephone extension in the kitchen being the final dots on the "i's" of inactivity. Surely, in the million-year-old history of man, this completely sedentary mode of life developing in the last 50 years is an entirely new phenomenon, first appearing in all its plenitude in the United States but now speeding to other developing areas (in various degrees depending on local cultural factors).

Yet at the same time, experimental and clinical work have established the following facts:

a. Because, in many individuals, appetite is no longer a reliable guide to need at sedentary levels of activity, habitual lack of physical activity is a major factor in the development of obesity. This was shown to be true in experimental animals, then later in men, women, and children. Inactivity is a particularly important factor in the development of obesity in children; conversely, participation in a daily program (three-quarters of an hour or an hour) of appropriate physical activity is highly effective in reducing obesity in childhood and adolescence. Daily walking of sufficient duration (i.e., at least an hour) has a similar effect.

b. When people engage in several hours of physical labor every day, ingestion of a diet high in saturated fat causes a far lesser rise in blood cholesterol. This has been shown in a comparison between a hardworking, isolated rural Swiss population and a control urban group;[9] similar studies have been conducted in other parts of the world.

c. Work done in Sweden[10] and in the United States[11] indicates that frequent (several times a week) bouts of exercise, which can be brief (20 minutes) but intense (sufficient to bring pulse rate to 100 to 110 per minute) may be instrumental in keeping coronary vessels patent and elastic. Running,

squash, rowing are the type of physical activity involved here.

d. Recent work also suggests that an hour of fairly vigorous daily exercise (e.g., jogging) exerts a favorable effect on blood pressure. Thus, different types of exercise have different roles in preventive medicine.

It is unfortunate that as the need for physical labor decreased in the United States, the opportunities for physical activity did not correspondingly increase. In fact, in the urban areas of our country, facilities for adult exercise are miserably few. Only the very rich can usually afford a reasonable regimen of pleasant exercise. Furthermore, physical-education school programs are deteriorating and are altogether absent in some communities. Where they exist, they tend to favor those youngsters who are highly motivated and would exercise anyway and neglect those who need it most, such as the overweight. Finally the type of sport played by our youngsters does not encourage general participation: high school football is a sport for the heavy, basketball for the unusually tall. While being in good physical shape is a requisite for being a good baseball player, baseball (and baseball instruction) offers very limited opportunities for sustained physical exercise and cardiovascular fitness (as compared, for example, with soccer). The series of presidential assistants for physical fitness appointed by successive administrations have been unable to accomplish anything of significance.

Tension, Fatigue, Lack of Sleep. Emotional crises, fatigue, and a mode of life where sleep is excessively curtailed are known to precipitate catastrophic events (myocardial infarction, stroke) in patients with preexisting severe atherosclerotic disease.

Geography and Pollution. It is known that highly urbanized areas have a higher rate of CHD than rural areas. Lack of exercise, psychological stresses, and a lack of sleep may be factors. It has been hypothesized that certain pollutants may be additional factors. Cadmium is known to promote hypertension under certain conditions. The high concentration in the atmosphere of such pollutants as lead and hydrocarbons from gasoline engines, SO_2 from fuel combustion, rubber chemicals from tire wear is a factor that has been mentioned, though as yet solid evidence is missing.

Other Diseases and Heredity.   A number of diseases are known to promote the development of atherosclerosis, as we have indicated. A family history of premature CHD— or of hypercholesterolemia, hypertension or diabetes—is an additional risk.

Having examined what we know of the problems, what can we do about them?

Prevention of Atherosclerotic Heart Disease and of Sudden Death

Fortunately, a number of the factors that we have examined can be modified by appropriate treatment: prevention or control of hyperlipidemia can be achieved by modification of the diet; weight reduction alone often lowers elevated blood triglycerides, blood pressure, and blood glucose. Drug treatment and diet modification are highly effective in most cases of hypertension; cigarette smoking has been abandoned by many; a number of our citizens are trying to increase their amount of exercise. Greater interest is exhibited now in improving the mode of life of our citizenry. Detailed measures can be taken, some of which can be much facilitated by national collective action (it would be particularly appropriate in these instances for the Senate Select Committee on Nutrition and Other Human Needs to prepare and recommend national legislation).

Medical Measures

Changes in Diet Composition.   Changes from a high-cholesterol to a low-cholesterol diet result in a decrease in the size of lesions in experimental animals. A number of studies suggest that a decrease in the calories, saturated fats, and cholesterol in human diets may also lead to a decrease in the size of atherosclerotic lesions. Certainly, there is evidence from studies in Los Angeles,[12] New York[13] and Helsinki[14] suggesting that reducing the dietary intake of saturated fat and cholesterol (with partial replacement of the saturated fats by polyunsaturated fat) resulted in a significant decrease in CHD mortality. A famous clinical study by Leren in Oslo[10] has demonstrated that in patients who have had a coronary, a similar dietary modification exerts a preventive effect on the occurrence of a secondary coronary. Decrease in sucrose intake is the easiest way to cut down on calories and reduce weight; it may also have a favorable effect on triglyceride levels and abnormalities of carbohydrate metabolism.

Control of Cigarette Smoking.   There is excellent evidence that CHD mortality rates of former cigarette smokers are very much lower than those of smokers and may eventually go down to the levels characteristic of nonsmokers.

Drug Treatment of Hypertension.   Available data show that treatment of hypertension is highly effective in the prevention of congestive heart failure and stroke, and helps to prevent CHD and other atherosclerotic diseases.

Weight Reduction.   There is considerable evidence showing that weight reduction improves the picture of adult-onset diabetes (the form of diabetes typically seen in middle-aged patients) and hypertension. It may also have a favorable effect of its own on CHD, particularly if the weight reduction is sizable. Weight loss is best achieved through a combination of reduction in food intake (with as drastic a reduction in sucrose intake and saturated fat as possible) and daily exercise of sufficient duration.

Exercise. We have already seen that (*a*) daily exercise of moderate intensity and duration keeps the weight down, (*b*) regular exercise of sufficient intensity keeps blood vessels open and patent, (*c*) day-long hard labor keeps cholesterol down, (*d*) regular exercise of sufficient duration and intensity has a favorable effect on the blood pressure and on glucose utilization.

Social Measures

Diet. We need to lower the saturated fat and cholesterol content of the diet to an average of 300 milligrams of cholesterol and to no more than 10 percent saturated fats (roughly a halving of present levels). Note that part of the saturated fats eliminated can be replaced by mono- and poly-unsaturated fat.

Following the recommendation of the Inter-Society Commission, the food industry should be encouraged by the health professions and the government (with a broad campaign of education launched to support this effort) to make available leaner meats and processed meats (a recommendation also of the White House Conference on Food, Nutrition and Health), dairy products, and baked goods reduced in saturated fats, cholesterol, and calories. Visible fats and oils should be manufactured so as to decrease the saturated-fat content and reduce or eliminate the cholesterol content.

Meat could be lower in saturated fat through genetic selection of high-protein, low-fat strains; range feeding with earlier slaughter; and modernization of laws and regulations, in grading in particular. Meat products should be manufactured so as to be as high in protein and as low in fat and cholesterol as possible. Suitably enriched vegetable protein should be allowed as extenders or part-substitutes.

Dairy products, cheeses in particular, should be manufactured so as to minimize the saturated-fat and cholesterol content, as should bakery goods.

Adult men should be encouraged to reduce egg-yolk consumption. The restaurant and catering industries should be encouraged to offer alternative breakfast dishes or low-cholesterol, low-saturated-fat "scrambled eggs" substitutes.

The caloric content of many foodstuffs is enormously increased by the addition of large amounts of sucrose. Baby foods often contain totally unnecessary quantities of sugar. Industry should be encouraged to decrease the large amounts of sugar used in an enormous number of foods (e.g., fruit juices, fruits, wet-pack cereals, and even vegetables). It is to be hoped that if universal labeling of caloric content of household portions is adopted, it would contribute to a decrease in the sugar and calories in a great many foods.

Obviously there must be a gigantic education effort among professionals (college and university home-economics departments; hospital-dietitian instruction programs; schools of medicine, dentistry, and nursing; and teachers' colleges) if these measures are going to be accepted and if numerous individual measures aimed at decreasing saturated fats and cholesterol (and caloric) intake are going to be adopted.

Cigarette Smoking. We need energetic measures to drastically decrease this clear and present danger to the life of tens of millions of Americans: as a first step, the laws presently on the books of almost every state against selling cigarettes to minors should be vigorously enforced, cigarette-vending machines should be removed from medical and public buildings, and smoking should be banned in large meetings and mass-transportation systems.

Detection and Control of Hypertension. We need a national effort to detect and assist all hypertensives; the prevalence is high in the United States (in particular, in the black community). The cost to the individual and to the community of untreated hypertension is horrendous.

Weight Reduction. In addition to a mass-education campaign (which will attempt to correct the many misconceptions propounded by exploiters of the national preoccupation with "dieting" without decreasing caloric intake, we should take advantage of the existence of large, well-organized groups (such as TOPS, Weight Watchers, Diet Workshop) and use public-health resources to improve the quality and effectiveness of their teaching. Special instruction programs for overweight children and adolescents should be supported in schools, colleges, and public summer activities.

Exercise. Although it is obvious that what is advocated here is not sudden violent physical activity in untrained, atherosclerotic middle-aged Americans, we do need a national effort to provide facilities and guidance for physical activity for all Americans, including:

a. Support for construction of facilities and teacher training in physical activities for all schools. Emphasis should be on those activities that will be carried on throughout life and on those activities that entail the maximum amount of cardiovascular training. Swimming and tennis (using indoor as well as outdoor facilities), rowing, and soccer are activities that may be encouraged. It ought to be national policy for every high school in the country to have an Olympic-size swimming pool (indoors in cold climates) and tennis courts. Availability of a sufficient number of well-trained, health-minded physical educators is essential.

b. We need a major effort to provide communities with sufficient exercise facilities and instructors. Every community, every neighborhood of a large city should have exercise facilities: a swimming pool, tennis courts, squash courts, etc. Some facilities can be shared by the schools and the communities; other facilities will have to be developed separately.

c. Urban-renewal plans must be developed with health considerations in mind. By and large, planning of American cities is directed at making walking unnecessary. In most cities, it is neither pleasant nor safe. We need a health input in the planning of our lives, or else all our resources will be insufficient to correct our errors.

d. Low-cost housing must, similarly, offer exercise facilities to young and old.

e. We need additional hiking trails in National and State Parks, as well as the development of hiking trails throughout surroundings of metropolitan areas.

Prevention of Sudden Death. Finally, if prevention of atherosclerosis fails, it is still possible to prevent death from this cause. But we are just beginning to organize ourselves to do so and, with a vigorous national effort, could improve our performance considerably in the years to come.

In recent years, development of coronary-care units (CCU's) has been an effective method of reducing CHD mortality in the major hospitals. Control of arrhythmias in CCU's has shifted the focus from resuscitation to the prevention of the need for resuscitation and has resulted in a 30 percent reduction in mortality of hospitalized patients with acute myocardial infarction.

Immediate further reduction in mortality from acute myocardial infarction should be based on an extension of the experience acquired in the CCU's by bringing the "precoronary care" closer (and earlier) to the patient. The public must be educated to seek immediate hospitalization on mere suspicion of signs of myocardial infarction (which should be taught every adult American), early electrocardiographic monitoring in emergency wards, industrial medical stations, and ambulances. Eventually, we should use our incomparable communication and computer technology to monitor high-risk patients as they go about their daily tasks; we could then "pull them in" the hospital if any premonitory arrhythmia occurs.

Further Research. In the present climate it is necessary to restate that heart-disease re-search must be better supported than it is now. Large-scale prevention studies are expensive but the rewards are enormous. We need research (and training) in all aspects of prevention of atherosclerosis as well as research and training in the prevention of sudden death.

REFERENCES

1. *U.S. National Health Survey Series,* [N.D.]. National Center for Health Statistics, Public Health Service, Department of Health, Education, and Welfare, Washington, D.C.
2. Report of the Inter-Society Commission for Heart Disease Resources-Primary Prevention of Hypertension, Prevention and Early Detection of Peripheral Vascular Disease, Recognition and Prevention of Cardiomyopathy, 1970. *Circulation* 42:A39–A53; Primary Prevention of the Atherosclerotic Diseases, 1970. *Circulation* 42:A55–A95.
3. Keys, A., ed., 1970. Coronary Heart Disease in Seven Countries. *Circulation* 41:Suppl. I.
4. Yudkin, J., 1967. Evolutionary and Historical Changes in Dietary Carbohydrates. *American Journal of Clinical Nutrition* 20:108–115.
5. Cohen, A. M., 1963. Fats and Carbohydrates as Factors in Atherosclerosis and Diabetes in Yemenite Jews. *American Heart Journal* 65:291–293.
6. *Smoking and Health: Report of the Advisory Committee to the Surgeon General of the Public Health Service,* 1964. U.S. Department of Health, Education, and Welfare, Washington, D.C.
7. Hammond, E. C., 1966. Smoking in Relation to the Death Rates of One Million Men and Women. In Haenszel, W., ed., *Epidemiological Approaches to the Study of Cancer and Other Diseases.* National Cancer Institute Monograph Number 19, January.
8. Levy, R. L., White, P. D., and Stroud, W. D., 1946. Overweight: Its Prognostic Significance in Relation to Hypertension and Cardiovascular-Renal Diseases. *Journal of the American Medical Association* 131:951–953.
9. Gsell, D., and Mayer, J., 1962. Low Blood Cholesterol Associated with High Calorie, High Saturated Fat Diets in a Swiss Alpine Village Population. *American Journal of Clinical Nutrition* 10:471–478.
10. Leren, P., 1966. The Effect of a Plasma Cholesterol Lowering Diet in Male Survivors of Myocardial Infarction. A Controlled Clinical Trial. *Acta Medica Scandinavica* 180:Suppl. 466.
11. Frank, C. W., Weinblatt, E., Shapiro, S., and Sager, S. V., 1966. Physical Inactivity as a Lethal Factor in Myocardial Infarction Among Men. *Circulation* 34:1022–1033.
12. Dayton, S., et al., 1969. A Controlled Clinical Trial of a Diet High in Unsaturated Fat in Preventing Complications of Atherosclerosis. *Circulation* 40:Suppl. II.
13. Christakis, G., Rinzler, S. H., Archer, M., and Kraus, A., 1966. Effect of the Anti-Coronary Club Program on Coronary Heart Disease Risk-Factor Status. *Journal of the American Medical Association* 198:597–604.
14. Turpeinen, O., et al., 1968. Dietary Prevention of Coronary Heart Disease: Long-Term Experiment. *American Journal of Clinical Nutrition* 21:255–276.

Chapter 6

The Aged

Donald M. Watkin

National policy on nutrition and aging must be firmly based on recognition of aging as a process beginning at conception and continuing until death. This recognition sets the stage for the consideration of a national policy on nutrition and aging in two parts: (1) the nutrition and health of prospective parents, pregnant women, infants and young children, adolescents, youth and mature adults; and (2) the nutrition and health of those in late maturity and of the aged. There can be no division in real terms of the spectrum of aging between late maturity and old age. In this context, the division is made for purposes of developing a national policy on nutrition and aging with the understanding that the age at which late maturity or old age begins will vary from person to person.

In essence, policy on nutrition and aging must be developed with short- and long-range objectives. The short-range objective is to improve the lot of those who are already old. The long-range objective is to improve nutrition and health among the young with a view toward slowing physiological aging and deferring, to the oldest possible age, the onset of the diseases and disabilities that are manifest among the aged.

Both objectives will be difficult to attain. Improving the lot of those already old by better nutrition requires looking at nutrition activities as a broadly based program area involving far more than the provision of foodstuffs. Nutrition is no panacea for the problems of the aged. Those who dispense nutrition as a panacea bilk aged Americans of hundreds of millions of dollars every year. That food faddism continues to expand despite the forceful efforts of government and professional groups to stamp it out is testimony to the fact that the aged themselves are insufficiently educated in aging as a biological process and nutrition as a quantifiable science. What knowledge and rational interpretation of nutrition and of aging they once had are often dissipated by the weight of their anxieties about old age, leading them to grasp desperately at promises of rejuvenation no matter how absurd or costly these may be. Although it is often said that it is difficult to teach the aged new ideas, it must be acknowledged that no large-scale, concerted effort has yet been made to eliminate undesirable old habits and introduce new and better ones. Herein lies a great challenge for national nutrition policy toward the 20 million Americans who are classified as old.

The young pose no less of a problem. It is difficult to convince any young person that he should follow a certain dietary regimen because it will enable him to survive longer and more happily in his old age. The youth culture permeating society today tends to deny the existence of old age. The young not infrequently proclaim their unconcern for living beyond middle age and often will express desires for an early death. Those who are older recognize that death is rarely welcomed even by the oldest or most disabled. A challenge is to get this point across to those who are young enough to act to prevent premature physiological aging and to defer as long as possible the onset of the diseases and disabilities that often accompany old age.

Education of the Young

Nutrition's role in the deceleration of physiological aging and in the deferment of the onset of disease and disability should be stressed to all, starting in terms of chronological age with the preschool child. Should it be necessary to establish a rank-order priority for the dissemination of this information, top priority should be given to instruction of teenagers who will soon be marrying and becoming parents. Nutrition has its greatest effects on aging as a biological process during pregnancy and the first few years of life. Hence, education of prospective parents regarding proper nutrition during the pregnancy of the mother and during the early life of the newborn child will insure that child of an optimum potential. In addition, education of prospective parents should be directed at preventing the premature onset of diseases and disabilities that may be associated with improper nutrition of teenagers and young adults. Among these conditions are iron-deficiency anemia; obesity; under-nutrition due to improper dieting; osteopenia from dietary calcium deficiency; excessive caries from high carbohydrate diets and lack of fluoride; atherosclerosis from excessive consumption of saturated fats and refined carbohydrates; disorders of the central nervous system and of the gastrointestinal tract from excessive consumption of alcohol; carcinoma of the lung, bronchitis, bronchiectasis and emphysema from smoking; and trauma from preventable accidents.

Education for the young must emphasize the totality of health care. Particular emphasis needs to be placed on the problem of malnutrition secondary to disease. Anemia may afflict the best nourished if he or she is the victim of chronic blood loss, chronic infection, drug sensitivity, undetected neoplasm, parasitism or chronic renal disease. Fat-soluble-vitamin-deficiency syndromes may be present in those with steatorrhea from pancreatic insufficiency or sprue and from misuse of mineral oil as a laxative. Hyperbetalipoproteinemia and hypercholesterolemia with attendant atherosclerosis may be occasioned by diabetes mellitus. Pathologic fractures, nephrolithiasis, and periodontal disease may result from disorders of calcium metabolism accompanying hyperparathyroidism. Angular stomatitis may result from improperly fitting dentures. A variety of health problems may result from excessive family expenditures on food necessitating cutbacks in procurement of preventive and curative health services.

This last item brings up the all important matter of programming, planning, and budgeting for nutrition by families and by individuals. Self-supporting youths rarely have the economic resources of their parents; hence, the nutrition model set by the parental environment is economically inappropriate and must be modified if optimum health is to be achieved by a youth or his young family.

To be meaningful, nutrition education must be delivered in the context of real reference points. Emphasis needs to be placed on the relative prices of comparable nutrient values. Foods need to be labeled so that the potential buyer can evaluate the nutritional value of his purchase. The labeling system should be standardized so that it may play an active role in the process of nutrition education, something present labeling is not doing. (For example, nutrition education now emphasizes the desirability of consuming a variety of items from each of four food groups; however, the labels on most modern foods, particularly those in the so-called convenience category, are not labeled with reference to the four food groups, leaving the person educated by this technique in the position of having been educated in the wrong language.) Furthermore, menus in establishments purveying prepared meals should also identify the nutrient value of the food served in terms meaningful to the consumer. Not only should the consumer be able to select the main entree but he should also have choice in the amount of the main entree that he wishes to consume, just as he would have if serving a meal in his own home. A choice of this kind would obviate the necessity of having separate menus for adults and children and would permit those who wished to limit their food intake or to expand it to do so rationally and in a manner eliminating personal embarrassment and economic waste.

Education for the young must keep abreast of developments in communication. The mass media have successfully been used to establish market preferences and even to promote health measures like the avoidance or abandonment of smoking. The food industry has long used the mass media for promoting specific products.

So far, this discussion has dealt primarily with problems in the field of nutrition education. Obviously, aging education must also be an important element in the total educational package. Aging is a program area that has had relatively few productive thinkers, investigators, implementers, and educators. Many highly skilled nutrition educators know virtually nothing about aging and have themselves contributed to much of the misinformation of the impact of nutrition on aging. In view of the long life span of man, definitive studies on the effect of nutrition on aging as a life-long biological process have not been completed. Transposing the results of studies in lower animals to man has obvious disadvantages. An education vacuum, therefore, has existed, with the result that food faddists and well-meaning professional nutritionists have treated the public to a shower of misinformation. Fortunately, the aging process is similar in all species, suggesting that much of what is learned in lower animals can be translated directly to man. In addition, epidemiologic techniques can be applied to study of this problem, although little has been done in this field to the present time.

Far more is known about the pathogenesis of diseases and disabilities that harrass the aged. Here health educators need to emphasize the importance of nutrition in the development of these diseases and disabilities. To do so these educators need to know more about nutrition, but they also need to know more about the early onset of diseases and disabilities of which they speak.

Finally, education must bring to the young the realization that no problem is insoluble. In this country today, no one need go hungry, no one need be malnourished, no one need go without medical care. Nonetheless, millions are hungry, malnourished, and ill. This is indeed an indictment of our educational system. This indictment justifies placing education of the young at the top of priorities in establishing a national policy with respect to nutrition and aging.

Education for Late Maturity

The needs for nutrition and health education in late maturity will depend on the assimilation and application of information previously acquired by those now in this age category. The effectiveness of previous exposure, if any, during childhood, youth, and middle age, to nutrition and health education is not a function of social or economic class, as demonstrated in some of the national nutrition program health surveys, which revealed that biochemical parameters compatible with malnutrition were not confined to low income levels. At present, thousands of examples of good nutrition and health during late maturity may be found in the American population. Many leaders in government, industry, labor, the professions, and volunteer organizations are living testimonials of this observation. Even so, the percentage enjoying good nutritional status and health in the total population of adults in their late maturity is extremely small and may well represent the influence of an elite genetic endowment that characterizes not only intellect and physique but also nutritional habitus and resistance to disease and disability.

The real objectives of nutrition and health education in late maturity are the nonelite majority whose genetic endowment has not bestowed upon them the benefits of a desirable nutritional habitus or built-in resistance to disease and disability. Fortunately, by the onset of late maturity the entire die has not been cast. By careful attention to nutrition and by supervision of existing health problems, the impact of disease and disability can be minimized. In addition, since most persons in late maturity are still employed, they may take advantage of the preretirement education programs now being offered by many industries, labor unions, and professional organizations. While much of the educational material in these preretirement programs concerns matters that may seem far removed from nutrition and health, it is important to remember that economics, housing, transportation, mental hygiene, and vocational readjustments all have their impact on nutrition and on health. The success of many group-activity programs in helping control obesity, a major problem in late maturity, suggests that group approaches to nutrition and health education would be a desirable component in any preretirement-education program. As with the young, the use of nutrition and health-education messages over mass media needs further development. Particularly, education in late maturity needs to stress modern information on the biology of aging and the pathogenesis of chronic diseases and disabilities. Such education will provide the basis for a rational attack on the dangers of food faddism, whose hucksters lie in wait for unwary victims of the ennui and anxiety associated with old age. As with the young, education in nutrition and health during late maturity needs support if it is to succeed. This support includes the availability and utilization not only of properly labeled and appropriately priced foodstuffs of high nutritional quality but also of health services stressing preventive as well as curative medicine.

By late maturity, many persons have already acquired a disability or a chronic disease. For some of these, the onset of the disease or disability is the signal to pay more attention to their nutrition in the hope of improving their health. For others, it is the beginning of a period of fear, anxiety, uncertainty, and unbearable suspense—during which friends and relatives offer condolences and advice based on folklore, and health professionals treat them as pathologic diagnoses rather than whole persons. These persons in late maturity need education to enable them to find an appropriate *modus vivendi*, as well as requisite foodstuffs and health services.

By late maturity, the full impact of lifelong dental neglect is evident. Dental care must be included in the health services available to and utilized by persons in late maturity. Without adequate dentition, either endogenous or exogenous, the person is a dental cripple and a nutritional cripple as well. A major role of dental personnel is the education of those in late maturity on the importance of maintaining their dentition and using this dentition properly for the ingestion of appropriate foodstuffs.

The nutrition and health education of those in late maturity must include instruction in and practice of daily strenuous physical work to a level tempered only by medical contraindications. Nutrition education must emphasize the balance between energy intake and energy expenditure; health education must stress the potential of daily strenuous physical work for the maintenance of suitable body composition, excellence of cardiovascular responses, emotional stability, and freedom from lassitude and fatigue. The combination of restriction of calories with daily strenuous physical work as the only sensible method for the control of obesity needs reiteration to reinforce the information available to all which is now recognized mainly in the breach.

Nutrition and health educators of those in late maturity looking forward to retirement could well follow the examples set by bankers and attorneys who advise clients to plan ahead by preparing wills, making funeral arrangements, and, in general, anticipating the inevitable. Fortunately, in nutrition and health education, the task is planning for life, not death. It should include plans to live on less income and to live in dwellings modified for the family size, built for the convenience of the aged, and located near low-cost, readily accessible transportation. Equally important, this education should include didactic and problem-solving sessions designed to teach the aged how to find for themselves the best and most appropriate systems for the delivery of nutrition and health services.

Attention should be paid, in the case of married couples, to such contingencies as the death of one spouse. In preretirement education, instruction in homemaking should be given to the man who survives after the death of his wife, but who has had no previous experience in preparation of meals. Contrariwise, the wife, who also must participate in the postretirement education, should be trained in methods of coping with dietary practices appropriate to a single person living alone. Instruction in attitudes toward living alone after the death of a companion of many years is an essential part of health education for those in late maturity. For those who have never married, education to correct undesirable practices developed earlier in life, to manage on reduced income, and to substitute other vocational or avocational activities for those experienced during working life is an indispensible part of retirement education.

Education for the Aged

In the United States over 20 million persons fall into the age group over 65. Since the time of Bismarck, 65 has been the designated retirement age in the vast majority of public- and private-sector operations. For practical if not for scientific reasons, 65 seems to be an age acceptable for retirement at present and one that will not change until very significant progress has been made in increasing the average age at death, which may in turn be dependent upon increasing the life span of man. While some may argue that those ready for retirement should not necessarily be called aged, most nutritional and health problems of the aged are those directly linked with the economic, psychological, social, and health needs stemming from the transition from working life to retirement. For purposes of this discussion, therefore, the aged will be assumed to be those over 65 years of age and particularly those who are in retirement. Since many of the persons over 65 who are still engaged in active vocational or professional life are characterized by a unique genetic background and may need little in the way of education in nutrition or health, this distinction is probably justified.

The major problem of the aged today is the fact that they have limited income. The latest statistics from the Administration on Aging of the Department of Health, Education, and Welfare indicate that 25 percent of those over 65 are living below the Orshansky Index, which marks the borderline between poverty and nonpoverty. This restricted income limits the availability of foodstuffs, the quality of the housing, the character of food storage and preparation facilities, and, in general terms, the adequacy of nutrition. At the White House Conference on Food, Nutrition and Health, a recommendation was unanimously approved by the Panel on Aging suggesting that the minimum Social Security benefit available to the aged should be increased to $120 a month within the next two years and that the benefits available to the aged should be increased by 50 percent in addition to the revision of the minimum benefit. It was also recommended that the aged who had contributed to Social Security should never receive less than the minimum awarded to welfare recipients under any new legislation that might be passed by the Congress and approved by the administration. Furthermore, the Panel on Aging recommended that every effort be made by the Congress to improve the food stamp distribution program as a means of providing better nutrition to the aged until such time as cash income adequate for all needs of the aged could be assured.

Since the White House Conference on Food, Nutrition and Health in December, 1969, improvements have been made in the Social Security payments, although these fell short of the recommendations. Substantial changes have been achieved in the food stamp program, so that this mode of providing better nutrition to the aged is now generally available. Pilot projects sponsored by the Administration on Aging have been testing various methods for delivery of whole meals to aged persons unable to procure and prepare food for their own consumption. In isolated instances, special housing for the aged has been developed that includes meal preparation and serving facilities designed for those who are unable or who do not care to prepare food in their own facilities. Special research projects have examined various methods of educating aged persons in the value of appropriate nutrition and have attempted to provide in some instances health services to complement the nutrition program.

In the two years preceding 1970, substantial numbers of nursing homes were constructed to provide long-term care for aged unable to care for themselves. The stimuli for this development were the Medicare and Medicaid programs, which guaranteed federal funding to support part of the cost of nursing-home care. In 1970, some of the more ambitious schemes for developing chains of nursing homes have collapsed for lack of fiscal planning. Furthermore, other nursing homes have refused to accept patients sponsored under Medicaid because of uncertainties of state payments delayed because of suspected irregularities in charges submitted by some proprietary and voluntary establishments. Even setting aside the fiscal problems, nursing homes in general have been plagued by their inability to provide adequate nutrition and adequate health services to their clients. Complaints from aged persons and from their families have been manifold. In large measure, these are due to the lack of supervisors in nutrition and lack of sufficient personnel willing to work for the remuneration offered in nutrition and in all aspects of the delivery of health services.

The Panel on Aging of the White House Conference on Food, Nutrition and Health acknowledged the gravity of these problems by recommending that persons and agencies providing residential or home health care for any number of the aged be required to supply adequate nutrition and health services for their clientele. Recognizing the

administrative and fiscal difficulties encountered by the states in implementing this recommendation, the Panel on Aging also recommended that the federal government establish a national code of health, nutrition, and personnel standards and use all of its fiscal powers of persuasion to encourage each state to adopt and enforce this code.

Obviously, the costs of providing adequate nutrition and health services to all potential clients in the over-65 age category is so great that the client himself cannot be expected to foot the bill, nor can the client be supported by insurance or by tax dollars. In other words, a new approach to the provision of nutrition and health services to the aged must be found that will care for those in all categories of physical and mental health.

The process of developing these new methods must begin with a campaign of carefully designed education. One of the keys of this education will be the organizations of senior citizens. The leadership of these groups often has been derived from those with an elite genetic background whose nutrition and whose health has left little to be desired. They are active, vigorous, and talented and need to be recruited for the task of educating those whose genetic background is less elite and who have suffered from malnutrition and inadequate use of health services during their lifetimes. Research studies in the education of the aged have suggested that the aged are much more receptive to education presented by members of their own generation than by those from younger age groups. Hence, identifying, recruiting, and training the leaders of the elderly in nutrition and health education techniques is an essential first step toward bringing about improvements in what is admittedly a bad situation.

As noted earlier, dramatic changes in the nutritional or health status of someone who is already aged cannot be based upon any change in genetic programming nor can it be based on the prevention of disease and disability that began during intrauterine life, childhood, youth, and maturity. What can be accomplished by means of appropriate nutritional measures and health services is the prevention of any further worsening of already bad situations and the prevention of the development of new complications.

For example, many elderly persons have been committed to mental institutions not because they were truly insane but rather because their mental faculties had been distorted by lack of appropriate B-complex vitamens in their diet. Even among residents of institutions for the aged, nutritional deficiency diseases have been produced by vitamin losses from perfectly acceptable dietary ingredients occasioned by improper cooking and from inadequate ingestion of proper foods because of inability of the aged to feed themselves and inadequate staff to assist in the feeding process. These circumstances lead to vicious cycles in which the nutritional deficiency itself increases the degree of disability for which the aged person was originally institutionalized. Education in behalf of the aged must be directed, if this problem is to be resolved, not at the aged themselves but at those who are in charge of the nursing homes and other extended care facilities into which the aged are placed or committed. This requires more funds for support of nutrition and health services in institutions and the training of many more nutrition and health service personnel to fill this need.

For the vast majority of the aged who live outside of institutions, education, for the time being, must be concentrated on assisting them in obtaining the best nutritional and health services available within the limits of their resources. Planning meals, budgeting resources, procuring the best nutrition for the least cost, preparing food to provide optimum nutrition, extending limited cash income through the use of food stamps, utiliz-

ing community sponsored meal-delivery systems, and recognizing the importance of physical activity in the maintenance of health —all of these subjects form the basis of the education curriculum in nutrition and health for the aged. Nutrition education for the aged should be planned by professionals and carried out by appropriate mixes of professional and subprofessional personnel remunerated by the health-care systems.

While the young and those in late maturity may be approached through the mass media with considerable success, this method should not be relied upon to the exclusion of person-to-person contacts among the aged. Mass-media approaches reinforced by person-to-person contacts and discussion groups have succeeded in demonstration settings. Institutional meals and home-delivered meals lacking the personal touch, although higher in mechanical efficiency, have been deficient in social, psychological, and health benefits. A vast increase in the number of persons of all ages engaging in person-to-person contact with present-day aged is essential to the improvement of nutrition and health education for the aged. Such an increase would also expand the education of those making the effort and provide a source of hope that, through the education of physiologically younger segments of society, for them the unfortunate circumstances of many present-day aged may be deferred to a much older age or avoided completely.

Conclusion

This statement of nutrition policy for aging has centered on education to give emphasis to the preeminent role education must play in a rational approach to the universal phenomenon of aging. It has stressed the need for interest early in life in the roles of nutrition and health in decelerating physiological aging and in deferring to the oldest possible age the onset of diseases and disabilities manifest among the aged. It has suggested that the needs of today's aged and the aged of the future can be met by existing mechanisms or by mechanisms yet to be developed, provided the persons experiencing the needs understand the nature of their problems.

Obviously education without food or the income to purchase food would be meaningless. However, food or income for food without education would delay for decades society's progress in understanding the importance of nutrition—nutrition is the one environmental factor directly under man's control that can be used effectively in the maintenance of health, the prevention of disease and disability, and the deceleration of physiological aging. The temptation to pour all resources into the provision of food is great, especially considering the pressures generated by farm and food-processing interests who would benefit directly by government food subsidies. This temptation should be resisted. A substantial proportion of resources devoted to aging should be invested in nutrition and health education.

Similarly, the temptation is great to concentrate all available resources on implementing programs based on presently available knowledge, bypassing the need for basic and applied research on the influence of nutrition on the aging process and on the diseases and disabilities of old age. Since few quantifiable data are presently available on the optimum nutrition to decelerate aging and to prevent disease and disability in man, research supported by a substantial proportion of resources devoted to aging is essential.

Food faddism survives because knowledge is so fragmentary that a comprehensive, logical, data-quoting assault on offenders is difficult to mount. Through education, through the development of new, low-cost, highly nutritious food lines, an assault on food faddism can be effective. If possible,

these efforts should be matched by strengthening existing law-enforcement agencies and passing new, more stringent legislation protecting all persons and especially the aged from food fad frauds.

Legislation has been suggested that would substitute for food stamps cash increments in allotments to low-income individuals and families. Such a change, if passed by Congress, would justify even more the allocation of substantial resources devoted to aging to education in nutrition and to research on the interrelation between nutrition and aging and the diseases prevalent in old age. The aging and the aged must be convinced by education that nutrition offers a major means of avoiding or minimizing health problems of old age and is worthy of investment of their cash income. They must also be persuaded by quantifiable data developed through research and by law enforcement by adequately staffed agencies that cash income should not be squandered on food fads.

Policy regarding housing, institutional construction, and other physical facilities (such as social centers) must include considerations of the nutrition of those using the facilities. Specifically, all new housing should be required to provide not only intrahousehold meal-preparation facilities but also meal-service facilities and markets where food can be purchased. Optimum nutrition in intrahousehold feeding depends (a) upon procurement of food and meal preparation by persons sufficiently motivated to undertake these chores or (b) upon the delivery to the household of meals prepared elsewhere by caterers remunerated by fee for service payments, by philanthropic donations or by tax dollars. Socialization under these two circumstances is sporadic or rudimentary, respectively. Since the vast majority of the aged are rarely home bound, an arrangement whereby major meals would be prepared in a central kitchen and consumed in a communal dining area is feasible. In such a setting, socialization at major meals becomes a reality. Socialization with those living near but not in new housing complexes also would become feasible, offering solutions to the nutrition problems of those living in older, unrenovated structures near new construction. The new central meal preparation facilities would also serve those unable to reach the communal dining area because of proven personal health or environmental conditions.

While physical facilities are essential, their utilization is dependent again on the major theme of this presentation: education for the aging and the aged. For the aged, a well-planned presentation of the economic and social values of communal dining must be followed by nutrition and health education built into the act of dining. For the aging, acceptance of communal dining after retirement must be a goal whose achievement will depend on developing throughout life an understanding of modification in life styles appropriate to postretirement years.

Identification of the aged in need of assistance in nutrition and health is a major unsolved problem. Poverty, enfeeblement, and fear have led many aged people to withdraw from society into a life of loneliness characterized by malnutrition leading to additional physical and emotional disturbances. Younger age groups and physically and emotionally fit aged people should be organized to find these unfortunates and to persuade them to participate in the nutrition and health delivery systems now available and being developed.

These find-and-change-through-persuasion agents must be recruited, trained, and evaluated as they pursue their assignment. So must the persons who staff the delivery systems for nutrition and health services. These needs imply the necessity of education for professionals and for sub-professional community-based aides as well as for education of the participating aged themselves.

The criticism that such programs in government hands are inefficient to the point of being wasteful is valid and itself implies the need for strict evaluation of performance and prompt management decisions to correct deficiencies. The same criticism is valid for voluntary agencies that become involved in training and service programs. A sound solution is the development in advance of specific standardized objectives and the rigid application of strict evaluation and decisive management to achieve the desired objectives. This solution will depend in large measure on its acceptance by the aged and their lobbying organizations. No solution will be found if positions are awarded indiscriminately without regard to an individual's ability to contribute effectively to the desired end result.

Finally, a quantifiable policy on society's obligation to provide nutrition and health services must be defined. Responsibility must be apportioned among the government, voluntary associations, family and the individual person. Quantification requires a choice between the full Recommended Daily Allowance of the Food and Nutrition Board and some fraction of that full allowance. The provision of health services affords a range of choices from completely open-ended to fee-for-service only. Making these choices for the aged of today constitutes a national emergency requiring action of such magnitude that it can be mounted only by a dedicated federal government using its powers to evoke equally concerted action by state, county, and municipal authorities.

In 1971, the White House Conference on Aging was the occasion for community and state conferences leading up to the national conference beginning November 28. Not only were the aged represented but also those in late maturity, middle age, and youth. The pattern of this White House conference suggests that federal initiative can stimulate concern and action at all levels in public and private sectors and among persons of all ages.[1]

While it would be unwise to prejudge the policies developed in 1971, it is reasonable to refer back to policies recommended by the 1969 White House Conference on Food, Nutrition and Health[2,3] and to note recommendations of the Panel on Aging that the federal government assume the obligations of providing the opportunity for optimum nutrition and health to every aged person. Since the resources to achieve this objective are available, no policy falling short of this objective seems valid. The challenge lies in developing programs to implement such a policy and to encourage through education the participation of the aging (of all ages) in the development process.

REFERENCES

1. *Final Report: White House Conference on Aging.* U.S. Government Printing Office, Washington, D.C. To be published.
2. *Final Report: White House Conference on Food, Nutrition and Health*, 1970. U.S. Government Printing Office, Washington, D.C.
3. *Addendum to Final Report: White House Conference on Food, Nutrition and Health*, 1970. U.S. Government Printing Office, Washington, D.C.

Suggested Supplemental Reading

Watkin, D. M., 1970. A Year of Developments in Nutrition and Aging. *Medical Clinics of North America* 54:1589–1597.

Watkin, D. M., 1968. Nutritional Problems Today in the Elderly in the United States. In Exton-Smith, A. N., and Scott, D. L., eds., *Vitamins for the Elderly: Report of the Proceedings of a Symposium held at the Royal College of Physicians, London.* John Wright and Sons, Bristol; Williams and Wilkins, Baltimore.

Watkin, D. M., 1968. Nutrition for the Aging and the Aged. In Wohl, M. G., and Goodhart, R. S., eds., *Modern Nutrition in Health and Disease*, Fourth Edition, Chap. 41. Lea and Febiger, Philadelphia.

Watkin, D. M., 1966. Nutrition and Aging. In McHenry, E. W., and Beaton, G. H., eds., *Nutrition: A Comprehensive Treatise*, Vol. 3, Chap. 4. Academic Press, New York.

Watkin, D. M., 1966. The Impact of Nutrition on the Biochemistry of Aging in Man. *World Review of Nutrition and Dietetics* 6:124–164.

Watkin, D. M., 1965. New Findings in Nutrition of Older People. *Journal of the American Public Health Association* 55:548–553.

Watkin, D. M., 1964. Protein Metabolism and Requirements in the Elderly. In Munro, H. N., and Allison, J. B., eds., *Mammalian Protein Metabolism*, Vol. 2, Chap. 17. Academic Press, New York.

Chapter 7

Indians, Eskimos, and Other Groups for Whom the Government has Special Responsibility

Michael C. Latham

The largest single panel at the White House Conference on Food, Nutrition and Health was that which considered problems of, and made recommendations concerning, the groups for whom the federal government has special responsibilities. These groups included inhabitants of the District of Columbia, military personnel, migrant and seasonal farm workers, the Indians, Eskimos and other Alaska natives, the natives of the U.S. Caribbean islands (Puerto Rico and the Virgin Islands), and, finally, inhabitants of the Pacific group of U.S. islands (Guam, American Samoa, and the U.S. Trust Territories). This chapter attempts to describe the nutritional problems of these disparate groups of people.

The District of Columbia

The citizens of the nation's capital deserve to have political representation in Congress and to have a similar say concerning their own services as do the citizens of the 50 states. There is no good reason why Wyoming, with a population of less than half a million, should have two senators and one representative in Congress when the 850,000 people of the District of Columbia have no voting congressional representatives.

If, and when, Washington, D.C. is granted the required degree of autonomy and representation, then the nutritional problems of the District will be open to the same solutions as those of the 50 states. The other chapters in this book dealing with nutrition problems for children, for pregnant women, for the aging and so on will have equal impact on the citizens of Washington, D.C. as they will on any other group of citizens. The recommendations of the White House Conference that deal with the District of Columbia are important because they will provide early relief for a disgracefully deprived population, but the nutrition recommendations are only a stopgap measure prior to increased self-determination and do not therefore constitute nutrition policy for the nineteen-seventies.

Poverty is prevalent in the district, and is accompanied by a host of urban health and nutrition problems. The infant-mortality rate in the poor areas of the district is about 44 per 1,000 live births, compared with a national average of 24.7 per 1,000. Iron-deficiency anemia has been found to be a major problem of the district's children; a recent study[1] has revealed that 65 percent of children below 18 months of age in the poor areas suffer from anemia. These are a few examples of the district's nutrition problems, which are essentially similar to those of poor ghetto areas across the country.

The Military

Military Poor   It is perhaps surprising to discover that undernutrition is a problem in the American military establishment; however, the lower ranks of the military and their families do in some cases have nutritional problems related to poverty. Secretary of Defense Laird said in 1969 that there are at least 50,000 soldiers, sailors, and airmen whose military salaries fall below the poverty line. These are mostly enlisted men of low rank who have sizable families to support, so that the total number of military poor may be 250,000.

Since malnutriton and hunger among military families are related mainly to poverty, it would be preferable simply to raise military pay rather than to devise special food and nutrition programs for those affected. There is evidence that the executive and legislative branches of the government are aware of this problem; the seventies should see an end to poverty among military families. In the meantime, as a result of recommendations of the White House Conference, commissaries on military bases have been authorized to accept food stamps.

Increased pay in the lower ranks of the services would also lead to greater ease of recruitment, could make it much easier to end the draft, and could finally make possible an all-volunteer peacetime army, such as those maintained by many other industrialized nations.

Nutrition Research   The Department of Defense has supported nutrition research in the past and currently has excellent and productive nutrition laboratories and other facilities. These establishments have made important contributions in the development of rations, in survival techniques, in nutrition surveys and in several spheres only marginally related to military nutrition.

Assistance in Disasters   The armed services are in an excellent position to provide nutritional and medical aid in the case of national and international disasters. This is a humanitarian task that the military should continue to perform. At the present time the Department of Defense lacks sufficient highly experienced staff to deal with famines and other disasters leading to starvation. They should where necessary call in civilian consultants to advise on or even to direct their relief efforts in other countries.

The United States, probably for political rather than military reasons, has provided less skilled relief than it should have in the major famines of the last two decades. Although American food has been furnished in vast quantities, there has been a very limited use of professional personnel and of skilled teams of relief workers.

Negative Actions by the Department of Defense   It is unfortunately true that the Department of Defense has contributed to hunger and malnutrition. Although international policies are outside the scope of this volume, let us consider one international example: the use of herbicides in Vietnam for the destruction of rice and other food crops. The extensive destruction of food crops has substantially contributed to hunger and malnutrition (and to death and disease) among civilians in Vietnam. Yet it has been shown that, historically, crop destruction or food interdiction is militarily ineffective and grossly discriminates against nutritionally vulnerable groups among noncombatants in its effects.[2,3] The proposal has been made that starvation be banned as a weapon of war by international agreement.[4]

Use of Purchasing Power   On the domestic scene, there is evidence to show that the Department of Defense greatly increased its purchases of grapes during the long strike of California grape pickers. Cesar Chavez, a leader of the United Farmworkers Organizing Committee, who has long fought for a decent wage for those who harvest the crops, has charged that the Department of Defense has also used its purchasing power to thwart farmworkers' demands by deliberately increasing its purchases of lettuce from producers not recognizing his union during the lettuce strike. Similar charges were made by Congressman William Ryan of New York,

who stated that he intended to introduce legislation that would prohibit the military from increasing its purchases from growers involved in the labor dispute.

The grape and lettuce strikes are now over, but the problems of farmworkers are not. What is regrettable is that a branch of the government, and one to which a high percentage of each tax dollar goes, has been charged with contributing to poverty and malnutrition among farmworkers and has not satisfactorily answered these accusations concerning its purchasing practices. The Department of Defense should be directed to use its purchasing power in a positive fashion to assist the efforts of people to help themselves and in a manner that will reduce, not increase, the extent of poverty.

Migrant and Seasonal Farmworkers

The Basic Problems of Migrants   At present migrancy is a way of life for over two-and-a-half million farmworkers and their dependents in America. These workers are an essential feature of the agricultural economy of this most productive of nations. Their labor subsidizes the American public and the food industry, because seasonal farmworkers perform essential menial agricultural tasks at substandard wages.

The government has provided billions of dollars in agricultural subsidies while largely ignoring the social and economic problems of those who harvest the crops. Today, we are faced by the paradox of an efficient, highly productive, and profitable system of agriculture that includes gross inequities and appalling conditions for farmworkers.

Malnutrition and hunger among migrants and their families are a result of low wages, seasonal employment, geographic migration, social deprivation, government inaction and insensitivity, and a lack of coverage in the legislation that protects other workers. The unique cultural and economic problems of migrant farmworkers have not been addressed. Existing programs designed to alleviate the problems of the poor in the United States have not involved farmworkers in their planning and operation.

Farm mechanization is reducing the need for agricultural labor and has displaced many farmworkers. Despite this, the need for labor in agriculture has not disappeared, and will not. There is a need now to train workers in new farm skills. Such training could stabilize the family, cultural, and economic life of farmworkers by providing them with more permanent jobs; it would assist them by upgrading their status, by meeting their social and health needs, and by allowing them to participate fully in community activities.

Of all the occupational groups in the United States, migrant farmworkers have the lowest mean annual income. In 1968 this was $1,018 per worker for those who did only farm work. In their home base, migrants are impoverished and accordingly they live in the poor housing that is all too characteristic of forgotten Americans. On the farms they are often crowded together in camps consisting usually of substandard buildings with poor sanitation. Housing regulations that do exist are seldom stringently enforced; regulatory officials are usually sympathetic to, and sometimes influenced by, the growers.

In many farm operations a large percentage of the seasonal farmworkers are children. The Western world many years ago got rid of the scourge of child labor, which allowed children to work long hours in coal pits and factories, but the American system of agriculture still permits thousands of children, sometimes as young as ten years old, to work hard and long in hazardous agricultural tasks. Twenty-six percent of all migrant workers are said to be children.

Migrant and seasonal farmworkers are largely deprived of the benefits of most social, economic, and related legislation designed to protect the rights of other workers. They are in many respects treated as second-class citizens. They are partially disenfranchised because they are so often away from their home states during elections; due to registration restrictions, they cannot vote in the counties in which they work.

Nutrition and Health Problems   There have been rather few comprehensive health- and nutrition-status studies conducted on migrants and their families. Enough work has been done, however, to show that they often have serious health and nutritional problems. A study of 111 black migrants in camps at King Ferry in New York showed low biochemical levels of thiamine in 36.5 percent, of riboflavin in 33.3 percent, and of ascorbic acid in 14 percent of subjects.[5] An investigation in Palm Beach County in Florida revealed one case of kwashiorkor, several children with nutritional marasmus, and a high percentage of children whose growth is stunted.[6]

Further evidence concerning the health of the children of migrant workers comes from reports of Dr. H. Peter Chase of the University of Colorado Medical Center. Before the U.S. Senate Select Committee on Nutrition and Human Needs, he reported severe cases of kwashiorkor and nutritional marasmus reminiscent of the malnutrition seen in Biafra, of malnutrition severe enough to stunt growth and jeopardize mental development, and of an infant-mortality rate of 63 per 1,000, which is three times the national average. In the New England Journal of Medicine, he reported on 19 children less than a year of age with generalized malnutrition who had been admitted to Denver General Hospital between 1962 and 1967. These children were given intelligence tests some years later. The mean development quotient of the 19 previously malnourished children was 82, while that of 16 children chosen on the basis of age, sex, and birth weight was 99.[7] Dr. Jean Mayer has stated that in the year following the White House Conference, the University of Colorado Medical Center has admitted seven children with kwashiorkor and literally dozens with nutritional marasmus.[8] Factors contributing to this malnutrition include (a) the need for infants to travel with their parents, (b) the fact that migrant families are not, in practice, in the Medicare-Medicaid hospitalization programs, (c) the frequency with which they are refused admission to private hospitals, and (d) the fact that the families cannot benefit from food-stamp and similar programs while travelling.

There is a tendency to blame large-farm operators for the condition of migrant workers. Certainly many of the operators have often been callous; they have political muscle whereas the workers do not, thus allowing them to ignore laws and regulations; and they have put the increase of profit before human welfare and social justice. Among the guilty farm operators have been all sorts of individuals and institutions normally regarded as respectable and humane. It recently came to light that Cornell University's College of Agriculture owned and operated a farm that had a migrant workers' camp with substandard housing and sanitation. Shortly after the matter came to public attention, the University, rather than correct the situation, decided to bulldoze the camp and to mechanize the farm. This was despite pleas from the student-dominated University Senate to have the migrant camp improved and operated as a model facility. It took student pressure to ensure that arrangements would be made for the migrant workers, nearly all of whom are blacks from Florida, who the same year would return hoping to find their old jobs. This incident clearly showed that at least one college of agriculture regards its mission as being solely to assist the farm operator.

Solutions to Problems of Migrants If the position of migrant workers is to improve, then the government will have to take a stand on their behalf; it seems unlikely that the government will act unless the public and the media push for reform. With cries for "law

and order" ringing in our ears, it can surely be hoped that the government can override objections by employers and by local bodies, when necessary, to obtain compliance with federal programs and standards in relation to conditions of housing and work for migrants. There should also be a presidential review to examine and recommend changes in federal, state, and local legislation and related policy regulations that limit the benefits available to farmworkers. This should lead to the unequivocal removal of the barriers that prevent migrant workers from enjoying the full benefits available to other workers and citizens, including the food program and unemployment compensation.

Adequate funding should be allocated to provide education, training, orientation, and counseling to assist migrant workers to enter the labor force in agriculture and in other occupations, on a year-round basis. The necessary social services to help families adjust to a normal, stable life in the community should be provided. The best way to solve the nutritional and related health problems of migrants is to end migrancy as a way of life. Until such time as this goal has been achieved, some sort of national registration is necessary to permit migrant workers to participate in Medicaid, Food Stamp and Food Commodity programs, and other programs throughout the country. If United States agriculture is dependent on seasonal work, then U.S. food, nutrition, and health services must be geared to give agricultural workers full benefits. Farm workers must be permitted, and encouraged, to organize and to bargain. Their exclusion from the National Labor Relations Act is discriminatory and is an indication of the political influence of farm owners.

In 1951 President Truman's Commission on Migratory Labor wrote:

Migratory farm laborers move restlessly over the face of the land but they neither belong to the land nor does the land belong to them. They pass through community after community but they neither claim the community nor does the community claim them. As crops ripen farmers anxiously await their coming; as the harvest closes, the community with equal anxiety awaits their going.[9]

This quotation clearly shows that in 20 years—despite commissions, despite White House conferences, despite improved wages in all other industries, despite general concern for minorities and for the deprived—there has been little change in the conditions of, nor the attitude of the nation towards, migrant farmworkers. Two decades later the description of their way of life and of their plight is still essentially accurate.

American Indians and Alaska Natives

Basic Problems   Another group of neglected Americans is made up of the Indians and the natives of Alaska. It is especially shameful that these people, whose land was taken from them, should now, of all Americans, see least hope for a life for themselves that includes dignity, cultural pride, and decent living conditions. One, among many, of the problems faced by American Indians and Alaska natives is that of poor nutrition. But as with other deprived populations, malnutrition is a symptom and a part of the poverty to which this group of Americans has been condemned. Food and nutrition programs are important, but they can only have a full impact if they are part of a broad program that will raise the level of living of these people.

In round figures there are 600,000 Indians in the 48 mainland states, and 360,000 of these are under federal jurisdiction. There are, in Alaska, 50,000 Eskimos, Indians, and Aleuts. The mean age of Indians is 17 years and of the Alaska natives 16 years, whereas that of the U.S. population as a whole is 30

years. The figures for the Indians and native Alaskans are reminiscent of some of the poorest countries in Africa and Asia, yet these people are citizens of the world's most productive and wealthy nation.

Infant-mortality rates per 1,000 live births in 1967 were 30.1 for Indians, 55.6 for Alaska natives, and 22.4 for Americans generally. In 1967 about 15 percent of Indian and Alaska native deaths were due to infective and parasitic diseases. These figures are a reflection of a life lived in an environment where poverty rules, where many basic elements of public health are lacking, and where medical treatment is minimal.

In about half the houses where Indians live, there is no running water and only inadequate means of waste disposal. The majority of six-person families have fewer than two bedrooms. Over half these families have incomes below $2,000 annually and approximately 65 percent earn less than $3,000 per year. The poverty line has been set at various levels in the United States but is frequently quoted as $3,500 for a family of four. Therefore, by far the majority of Indians live below the poverty line. While many think a crisis exists when national unemployment figures reach 6 percent, there has been no murmur of alarm about the unemployment figure for Indians, which has hovered for years around 40 percent.

These are just a few figures that illustrate the living conditions of a people who have been passed by, who have been largely ignored by successive administrations, and who have not developed the militancy of other minority groups. Because of their relative isolation and passivity, their plight has failed to prick the conscience of most Americans.

Indians and Ecology   For many years the Indian was depicted as incompetent, and the view was held that land needed to be taken from him so that it could be properly utilized for the benefit of mankind. Now that the white man has brought matters to the point of ecological crisis through his reckless exploitation of the land, we might ponder whether there was not more than a little wisdom in the Indian view of what land means.

The recent return of 48,000 acres of mountain land around Blue Lake to the Tao Indians in New Mexico constituted a small gesture. The U.S. House of Representatives twice passed legislation to return this land but twice the Senate balked. Perhaps Senators feared the Indian Claims Commission estimate that 90 percent of the land in the United States could on similar grounds (through "aboriginal title") be claimed by various tribes.

But there is special ecological significance in the restoration of the Blue Lake land to those Indians who have inhabited it for centuries. A statement by Paul Bernal, the Tao secretary to the Pueblo Council, quoted in a *New York Times* article by Winthrop Griffiths illustrates this point.

> That land—the 48,000 acres which we now control—is our church and our school. It is filled with life, given by God. God makes a determination of what you will be even before you are a human being. And that's the way it is with the evergreens—a fir, or an aspen or some other pine—and with the animals up there—the deer and elk, blue grouse and squirrels, the black bear and wild turkey.

> All these are like people, we do not discriminate about life, in our prayers and action.

> I am sorry, but we cannot let other people in, non-Indians. I have seen what the United States Government does to the land, with its so-called multiple-use policy for conservation, commercial development and recreation. It is desecrated, ruined. We will conduct a survey of all 48,000 acres, train some of our own people in forest management and then fence it all. We'll use natural materials for the fence,

fallen timbers, to keep the land private and sacred.

> The new law prohibits us from any commercial gain from the land. That is fine with us. We will hunt a bit on it, taking only what is necessary. We are responsible, really, for the shelter of all the wildlife. That's the reason we don't believe in cutting the trees. We are responsible to help let nature take its own course, to follow its own purposes. We must let the place be fertile.

> We are trying to make this place as holy as possible . . . .

The land of the Taos, and their adobe housing, have probably changed very little in the past 500 years, while much of the country has been blighted by pollution and man-made ugliness. Unlike other Americans, many Indian people have their religion and their culture rooted in their land, with its water and rocks and sand, its vegetation and its animal life. Perhaps it is significant that most Americans call earth "dirt"—a word with connotations of filth and lack of hygiene. Americans might have cause to wonder whether there would not be great good in returning much more land to its original inhabitants.

Malnutrition among Indians and Alaska natives is linked with an overall socio-economic and physical environment characterized by poverty, inadequate housing, overcrowding, poor sanitation, and social instability. Isolation leads to difficulties in purchasing food, to increased costs of food and other necessities, and to exploitation by traders who have a near monopoly of retail business. A harsh climate and often arid land make agriculture difficult. Over two-thirds of the Indian population live on land that has only marginal economic potential and where other employment opportunities are extremely limited.

The federal government has a special responsibility for those Indians who live on the reservations, and it has failed to meet its obligations to them. If America really means to banish hunger and malnutrition, as the President has stated, then greatly increased efforts will have to be made to assure an adequate diet for Indians and Alaska natives. Action will have to be taken not only to ensure that they are well-nourished but also that they receive adequate education and are provided with a greatly expanded program of preventive medicine and medical care.

Off-Reservation Indians   The one-third of American Indians who do not live on reservations have lost their right to most special federal services. In most instances urban Indians can return to the reservations, establish residence, and after a period of time become eligible again for the services provided by the Bureau of Indian Affairs. The controversial question is whether Indians should or should not have special federally provided services when they do not live on the reservations. The urban Indians as a group have specific health problems; they often lack education and industrial skills; they start urban life from a base of extreme poverty. They have these problems as a result of federal neglect.

The government argues that it would be discriminatory to provide urban Indians with special health and other services that were not available to other minority groups. However, the government provides special education allowances to ex-servicemen and maintains very expensive medical facilities in urban areas for veterans who spent only a few years in the military. If veterans can, in this sense, remain wards of the federal government, a case can surely be made for providing certain federal services to Indians who move from the reservations.

The Indian Health Service could provide medical facilities and services in urban areas with large Indian populations. Ways could be found to allow early participation in federally supported food programs for Indians moving off the reservations. There should also be job training, educational programs, and special social services for Indians living in urban areas.

Nutritional and Health Problems   Serious nutritional problems among Indians and Alaska natives have been found in the few studies that have been conducted. In 1961 a comprehensive nutrition survey was carried out on the Belknap Reservation in Montana.[10] The results showed evidence of deficient caloric intake in a significant percentage of adults, low dietary intake of iron in women and adolescents, low calcium intakes in all age groups, markedly low intakes of vitamin A and its precursor carotene in nearly all subjects; intakes of vitamin C were commonly only 25 percent of the recommended dietary allowances. Much of this dietary information was corroborated by biochemical assays of urine and blood. For example, anemia was prevalent in women and preschool children; almost half the subjects had a urinary excretion of riboflavin in the "low" range; blood levels of vitamin A were very low in nearly all age and sex groups, but the serum levels of vitamin C were in most cases satisfactory. Slight or moderate thyroid enlargements in women indicated a deficiency of iodine.

In 1958 a nutrition survey was conducted in Alaska. The conclusions of that survey were that the "Alaskan aboriginal people have had and continue to have a remarkably successful adaptation to their rigorous and unique food supply. This adaptation is imperiled in the cultural transition they are now undergoing." In this survey serious nutritional problems were not very frequently found. However, vitamin C intakes were very often deficient, plasma levels of vitamin A were low, dental disease was rampant, and infectious diseases constituted a major problem.[11]

Recently Dr. Jean van Duzen has reported many cases of kwashiorkor and nutritional marasmus among Navajos treated in the Tuba City Hospital.[12] These are severe cases of protein-calorie malnutrition, and even in hospital there is a high mortality rate.

From what is known it seems clear that the Indian and Alaska-native populations have certain disease and health problems that are different in magnitude from those of the average American. Life expectancy is shorter; the infant and child morbidity and mortality rates are higher. Nutritional anemia is widespread among Indians and Alaska natives with a particularly high incidence among infants and women of childbearing age. Significant underweight on the one hand and significant obesity on the other are common. Retarded physical growth is a frequent occurrence in the preschool child. Diabetes mellitus is reported to be as much as five times as prevalent among Indians as among the general population, and the frequency of gall bladder disease is also high; both may be influenced by diet.

Most illnesses requiring hospital or outpatient care of Indian and Alaska natives are due to infectious diseases and their residuals (including gastroenteric and respiratory infections, tuberculosis, and ear infections). Approximately one-third of Indian children are partially deaf due to the effects of otitis media. The synergistic relationship between nutrition and infection is well established and is of particular concern in this population whose diets are poor. The frequent occurrence and serious effects of gastroenteric infection, tuberculosis and other respiratory infections, and parasitosis in the Indian and Alaska native populations are intimately related to malnutrition.

In addition to important infectious diseases, a wide variety of other conditions and diseases are related to nutrition, either because they affect nutritional status or impair the individual's or family's diet. Poor oral hygiene and dental disease, eye and visual problems, alcoholism and mental, emotional, and behavioral diseases are widespread among the Indians and Alaska natives. Inadequate attention has been given to these health problems among the Indians and Alaska natives.

Deficiency diseases occur per se, but malnutrition also contributes substantially to many other health problems, such as infectious disease, retarded physical and possibly mental development, high rates of infant morbidity and mortality, anemias, obesity, and many chronic diseases.

There have been rather limited dietary, clinical, and biochemical nutrition surveys conducted on Indian reservations. There is a need therefore for the federal government to undertake detailed nutrition status surveys, to base remedial action programs on the findings, and to provide for continuing surveillance.

Solutions for their Nutritional Problems
Finances should be made available to support longitudinal studies of growth and development of native Alaskan and Indian children. These should be combined with health and nutrition programs. The latter should include nutrition education activities; comprehensive applied programs for the preschool child, perhaps including "under-5" clinics and nutrition rehabilitation centers; immunization programs; and day-care centers with proper facilities for feeding and for intellectual stimulation of children. The effects of these programs on physical growth and intellectual development of the children should be carefully evaluated; the government might be wise to contract out such work to universities. Adequate guarantees would be necessary to make certain of the

full participation of Indians and Alaska natives in the running of the services and to ensure that local people were trained to take over the services after a very few years.

In order to solve the nutritional and health-related problems of American Indians and Alaska natives, they themselves must not only participate in the activities but they must learn to direct the planning and implementation of the programs.

Food programs of all kinds that are financed by the federal government should be available on Indian reservations. A good argument exists for continuing the food-commodity distribution program in remote areas of Alaska and on reservations even when the food-stamp program is introduced into these areas. It would also be sound policy to introduce free school lunches to all children and to make available school breakfasts as well.

Special government attention needs to be directed to agricultural productivity. While Washington pours millions of dollars into farm subsidies for wealthy farmers, there has been too little spent to improve agriculture in those areas where Indians and Alaskan natives try to eke out a living by farming land that is often arid and that is subject to harsh climatic conditions. Financial credit for farm improvement, for mechanization and for irrigation, and farm subsidies for seeds and fertilizers should be made more freely available.

Indian water rights have too often been ignored. It is incumbent on the Department of Justice to take vigorous legal action to enforce these rights and on the Department of the Interior to help develop Indian water resources.

People living in remote areas such as Alaska and on Indian reservations often pay excessively high prices for the food they purchase. Frequently this is because they must rely on a single merchant or trading post. A near monopoly, combined with frequent abuses, leads Indians and Alaska natives to get less food per dollar than is the case for most other Americans. This limits the quantity of their diet and is a factor in the causation of their malnutriton. The trading-post operator often is disliked because he is known to overcharge, and yet he must be befriended because he is the only source of credit for many Indians.

The enactment of new laws and the enforcement of existing statutes to regulate prices and profits of traders would be helpful, provided it does not result in the closing of trading posts without the establishment of alternative retail markets. Federal assistance should be provided to encourage the development of consumer cooperatives managed and operated by Indians and Alaska natives in their own communities.

Finally it should be realized that health and nutrition programs alone cannot solve the problems of disease and malnutrition that are prevalent among Indians and Alaska natives. The basic solution lies in ending poverty among them through education, training, improved housing, legal protection, removal of discrimination, and a number of other means. Until such time as conditions have been improved, Indians and Alaska natives need to be assured of a minimum income, in the same manner as is proposed for other Americans.

Guam, American Samoa, and the U.S. Pacific Trust Territory

Common Background and Shared Problems

The three U.S.-controlled Pacific territories—namely, Guam, American Samoa, and the U.S. Pacific Trust Territory—although geographically, ethnically, and politically separate, share certain economic and social problems affecting health, nutrition, and welfare. Despite marked differences between them, they are nevertheless all more similar to each other than they are to the mainland United States.

Some of the shared features are:

a. An isolated tropic island environment, thousands of miles from the United States, from world markets, and from sources of supply of certain commodities.

b. An uneven economy based on a declining agricultural industry, with copra still one of the most important cash crops. There is the promise of economic gains from tourism and from commercial fishing. Some areas, notably Guam, are highly dependent economically on expenditures by the Department of Defense.

c. Despite the agricultural economy, 30 percent of the inhabitants now live in towns. Yet production is characterized by a pattern of subsistence farming and fishing.

d. A scarcity of capital for developmental investment in industry and agriculture.

e. Levels of unemployment that are much higher and levels of income that are much lower than in the United States.

f. A high rate of emigration from the islands. This is a serious problem, because it is usually the better educated and those with the most technical training who tend to leave.

g. A rather low percentage of the population who have completed high school education and an even lower proportion of people who receive any professional or technical education.

h. Problems related to food and nutrition are linked with physical difficulties of transporting food between and to the islands and are also adversely affected by laws and regulations which limit the movement of food.

i. Much of the commerce and industry of the islands is in the hands of nonislanders, who appear to be concerned more with profit than with the long-term interests of the islands or their people.

j. Federal food and other programs are applied in a seemingly haphazard and uncoordinated fashion in the three territories. Many programs available in the United States are not available to all or to any of the Pacific area territories. Their introduction, or nonintroduction, appears to be dictated by political expediency or on whims of the Secretary of the Interior. Local wishes have seldom been consulted, and local people have been too little involved in planning and implementation of programs.

Nutritional Status   There has been no comprehensive nutrition survey (of the ICNND* type) carried out in the islands. There have been a few surveys investigating specific problems. Health records are available from government institutions.

Cases of kwashiorkor, a form of malnutrition commonly seen in developing countries, are seldom encountered in the islands. This may be due to the availability of fish. However, there is evidence of poor growth in children and of other signs of mild or moderate protein-calorie malnutrition in the weaning and post-weaning period. This is due in part to the consumption by preschool children of poor diets consisting largely of starchy local staples such as taro, breadfruit, bananas, and of imported cereals. Other closely related factors are the high prevalence of common infections such as gastroenteritis and the frequent infestation of children with a variety of parasites.

Although statistical proof is lacking, there is a strongly held local belief that in many areas the nutritional status of both children and adults has declined in recent years as a result of changes in food practices and in the way of life due mainly to European and U.S. influence. This may well be true, for when people abandon their life as farmers and fishermen they move to the towns where unemployment rates are high and where traditionally eaten foods are replaced by imported foods, which are often more ex-

*Interdepartmental Committee on Nutrition for National Defense.

pensive and in some cases are nutritionally inferior.

There is evidence that dental caries is much more prevalent now than in past decades and this is almost certainly due in part to new food practices.

Nutrition Policy Recommendations   The subpanel of the White House Conference on Food, Nutrition and Health that made preliminary recommendations concerning the three Pacific areas included among its members persons from all three areas—physicians, health workers, educators, social scientists, politicians, and others. The subpanel considered in some detail the root causes of poor nutrition among the people in the islands, and then in a constructive manner suggested practical solutions, ones that could be realized given sufficient good will, hard work, and financial support. What follows is largely based on their recommendations.

Coordinating Nutrition Committee.   Highest priority should be given to the coordination of existing services and of all work relating to nutrition. The present lack of coordination of nutrition-related activities within each island group and among the island territories needs to be remedied. There is at present little coordination of the nutrition work of agricultural, health, educational and community development staff. There is a paucity of research, and the few existing services designed to improve nutrition have not been evaluated.

The populations of Guam, of Samoa, and of the Trust Territory are each too small and the financial resources too limited to suggest the establishment of three nutrition units or institutes, one for each territory. A coordinating nutrition committee for the three areas is needed and a physician well trained in nutrition should then be appointed as executive director. The responsibility of this director and the committee would be to initiate and coordinate food and nutrition activities; to

undertake the evaluation of nutrition programs; when necessary, to direct dietary and nutrition surveys. A sum of perhaps $200,000 annually would suffice for this purpose. In placing high priority on this recommendation, the subpanel was aware that coordination was one of the most important and basic needs in improving the nutritional status of peoples in developing regions and that WHO and FAO had successfully encouraged other countries to establish such coordinating mechanisms.[13]

An early responsibility of the director and his committee should be to collect together and review published material and reports of previous surveys and committees, and to implement where feasible recommendations emanating from these. After this initial review the prime function of the director and his committee would be in training and in education relating to nutrition.

Recognizing the diversity of the needs of Guam, Samoa, and the Trust Territory, the subpanel also suggested that the legislatures of each should consider establishing local nutrition committees.

Food Production, Transportation, and Preservation.   Food production, transportation, marketing, and preservation are important topics related to nutrition. In the Pacific Islands, the high consumption of imported as opposed to locally produced foodstuffs is a major economic and nutritional problem. Statistics showing the rapidly increasing rate of importation of food into a predominantly agricultural and nonindustrial region give genuine cause for economic concern. The result of this trend is an increased cost of food and frequently also a nutritionally inferior diet. A remedy to this problem lies in stimulating local production; reducing transportation costs; removing barriers that limit the movement of food in the Pacific area; encouraging new or improved methods of preservation, processing, and marketing of local foods. The Departments of the Interior and of Agriculture should assign a group to study and then take the necessary steps to improve the marketing, transportation, and preservation of indigenous food products. In regard to food preservation, there is a need for food canning facilities and for improvements in other methods of food preservation. Another major problem to be dealt with is poor transportation between and on the islands.

In order to stimulate both agricultural production and food processing, there is a need for the establishment of a scheme to provide low-interest loans to farmers and groups of farmers for mechanization and improvement of farming, and for establishment of small industries related to food preservation. The setting up of farming and marketing cooperatives could be an important integral part of a plan to stimulate food production and preservation.

An examination of available indigenous foods reveals that there is a shortage of animal protein in the diets of some sections of the population. Yet there exists in some areas an excellent potential for greatly increased livestock production for both meat and milk. Existing government regulations, often made in Washington, are frequently a deterrent to fulfilling this potential. For example, regulations forbid the free movement of meat among the islands. The government insists on the inspection of meat and on USDA standards being met. Yet in most of the islands, facilities for inspection do not exist and are not provided. In this instance it does more harm than good to insist that stringent regulations designed for cattle production in the United States apply also to remote Pacific islands.

Apart from beef and milk production, there could be a great increase in the quantity of poultry and fish produced locally. Specific recommendations were made that could help increase the supply of protein-rich foods of animal origin.

Institutional Feeding. Nutritional benefits would accrue from improvement of the meals served in residential institutions (such as boarding schools and hospitals) and by the provision of free school lunches to all school children. Though not ideal, the diets in hospitals and schools could be used as a basis for nutrition education of the public. They should include mainly indigenous foods, and the dishes prepared should always take local customs into account.

Money is needed to provide facilities for preparation of lunches in the schools that do not now have them; once these have been established, then the practice adopted in Puerto Rico, the U.S. Virgin Islands, and in many progressive countries of providing a free nutritious lunch for all school children should be adopted in Guam, Samoa, and the Trust Territory. Furthermore, a free breakfast should be available for those children with special needs. Finally, school teachers require additional training so as to equip them to provide nutrition education to their pupils.

Dental Caries. A specific nutrition-related health problem in the Pacific area is dental caries. Medical and dental workers believe the situation is deteriorating due mainly to an increased consumption of carbonated drinks, candy, and other refined carbohydrate foods. The problem is aggravated by the shortage of dental workers to provide curative care, let alone to introduce adequate preventive measures. In several industrialized countries, notably New Zealand and the U.S.S.R., and in many developing countries, a cadre of dental workers has been trained to undertake simple dental procedures, including filling tooth cavities, and thus to relieve dentists of a huge burden of work. These persons need a much shorter period of training than do dentists, and they are less costly to employ. They are taught to recognize more serious dental problems, which they refer to dentists; to undertake simple dental procedures themselves; and to provide preventive dental care in the communities where they work.

Even if more dentists were available, small remote islands could not hope to attract or to support a fully trained dentist. In such areas, an auxilliary dental worker would have a very important role to play.

Recommendations were made for an investigation of the extent and reasons for the recent increase in dental caries, for the necessary steps to be taken to alleviate the problem of dental caries by providing more dentists and dental hygienists, but above all for the local training of a new cadre of dental workers to be known as dental assistants.

The problem of the overall need for more trained medical and public health workers was considered. An increased use of the training facilities available in Suva, Fiji, by persons from Guam, Samoa and the U.S. Trust Territory is desirable. The South Pacific Commission should be asked to make more places available in the medical and dental school, and the federal government would need to make available the funds to support this.

Getting physicians and dentists to work away from large towns is a universal problem in the Pacific area. Realistic financial inducements and other innovations should be adopted to encourage medical and dental staff to work in more remote areas.

Puerto Rico and U.S. Virgin Islands

Although the mean per capita income in these U.S. island possessions is considerably higher than in other areas of the Caribbean, nevertheless important nutrition problems related to poverty do exist both in Puerto Rico and in the Virgin Islands. The problems of poverty in both places are intensified by very high birth rates.

In Puerto Rico, poverty, unemployment, and lack of opportunity lead to a large emigration of people to the United States and principally to New York City. During the last ten years the population of the U.S. Virgin Islands has more than doubled, due in part to the number of births exceeding deaths, but also because of immigration from neighboring Caribbean islands.

Nutrition Surveys   There have been reasonably comprehensive nutrition-status surveys conducted in Puerto Rico, but no similar surveys have been undertaken in the Virgin Islands.

In 1966 a nutrition survey was undertaken using a stratified sample of the Puerto Rican population. A total of 870 families were interviewed in their homes, information concerning income, educational levels, family size, occupation, and waste disposal was obtained. Records were made concerning dietary patterns, frequency of consumption of various food items, and facilities available for preparation of food. A subsample of about 600 subjects were clinically examined and had blood and urine taken for biochemical determinations. Unlike studies elsewhere, the findings showed evidence of malnutrition among those with relatively high incomes as well as among the poor. The survey also indicated that those living in isolated rural areas were often better fed than slum dwellers.[12]

An earlier rural study in the remote village of Dona Elena showed that 76 percent of children were below the third percentile for height and 74 percent below the third percentile for weight using United States standards. Sixty-five percent had angular stomatitis probably due to riboflavin deficiency; 52 percent had marginal swellings of the gums perhaps associated with vitamin C deficiency; 18 percent had enlargement of the thyroid gland; the average child had 3.8 carious teeth.

The average family size was 7.3; 55 percent of persons were under 16 years of age; 24 percent of persons over 11 years of age had never been to school (45 percent had had less than three years of schooling); the income of about half the families was below $500 for the previous year. This village was probably quite typical of rural Puerto Rico.

An intensive applied nutrition program in Dona Elena led to considerable improvement in living conditions and in the nutritional status of children when the village was resurveyed five years later.[13] This shows that the conditions are remediable.

Food Production   In Puerto Rico local production of fruits and vegetables that are good sources of vitamins A and C is rather low for a subtropical agricultural island. Some fruits and vegetables are even imported. In the U.S. Virgin Islands things are much worse; most fresh foods, including meat, are imported.

In both Puerto Rico and the Virgin Islands the people are becoming increasingly aware that milk is a nutritious food, especially for children. However, milk is priced too high to be regularly consumed by low-income families. This situation could be alleviated if government incentives and perhaps subsidies encouraged the local production of filled milk with taste, color, texture, and nutritive value similar to fresh milk.

Malnutrition Related to Poverty   Many of the nutrition problems of Puerto Rico and the Virgin Islands are intimately related to poverty. Whether these islands are to remain under the protection of the U.S. Government or move towards statehood, it is important that their inhabitants be allowed to benefit fully from national nutrition programs and other measures aimed at reducing the effects of poverty. For example, if the Family Assistance Plan becomes a reality, its benefits should extend to cover Puerto Rico and the Virgin Islands.

REFERENCES

1. **Gutelius, M. F.,**   1968. Iron Deficiency Anemia Among Negro Preschoolers. Account of 1965 study given to APHA Conference, 1967. *Public Health Reports* 83:213.

2. **Mayer, J.,**   1965. Famine, *Postgraduate Medicine* 38(5):A117–A122.

3. **Mayer, J.,**   1967. Starvation as a Weapon, *Scientist and Citizen* 9:115–121.

4. **Mayer, J.,**   1970. Famine Relief. In *Famine,* Swedish Nutrition Foundation Symposium. Almquist and Wiksell, Stockholm.

5. **Thiele, V. F., Brin, M., and Dibble, M. V.,**   1968. Preliminary Biochemical Findings in Negro Migrant Workers at King Ferry, New York, *American Journal of Clinical Nutrition* 21:1229–1238.

6. **Kelsay, J. L.,**   1969. A Compendium of Nutritional Status Studies and Dietary Evaluation Studies Conducted in the United States, 1957–1967. *Journal of Nutrition* 99, Suppl. 1, Part II: 123–142.

7. **Chase, H. P., and Martin, H. P.,**   1970. Undernutrition and Child Development. *New England Journal of Medicine* 282:933–939.

8. **Mayer, J.,**   1971. In speech at Follow-up White House Conference, Williamsburg, Virginia.

9. **Nelkin, D.,**   1970. In *On the Season,* Published by Cornell School of Industrial and Labor Relations. (This publication was used extensively for the material on migrant workers.)

10. *Fort Belknap Indian Reservation Nutrition Survey,* 1964. Interdepartmental Committee on Nutrition for National Defense, Washington.

11. **Mann, G. V. et al.,** 1962. The Health and Nutritional Status of Alaskan Eskimos: A Survey for the Interdepartmental Committee on Nutrition for National Defense, 1958. *American Journal of Clinical Nutrition* 11:31–76.

12. **van Duzen, J.,** 1968. In CBS Report: "Hunger in America." See *Congressional Record,* 90th Congress, 2nd Session, Hunger in America: Chronology and Selected Background Materials, October 1968, pp. 127–129. U.S. Government Printing Office, Washington, D.C.

13. **Latham, M. C.,** 1967. Some Observations Relating to Applied Nutrition Programs Supported by the U.N. Agencies. *Nutrition Reviews* 25:193–197.

Chapter 8

A National Surveillance System

D. Mark Hegsted

There have been relatively few studies of the nutritional status of groups within the United States in recent years. With the exception of the National Food Consumption Survey of the U.S. Department of Agriculture (USDA) which has been done each ten years for the past several decades, the only data available are from scattered studies, most of which have been undertaken by university groups in their own localities.[1] In retrospect, these studies should have served to alert the medical and public-health professions to some major problems but obviously did not. Also, it is apparent that the effectiveness of various programs (such as the Commodity Distribution Program) in solving nutrition problems has never been measured. Thus, the panels of the White House Conference concerned with surveillance readily agreed that efforts must be made to develop an adequate surveillance system.

We apparently do not have sufficient experience to outline an effective system in detail, however the general characteristics of a surveillance system appear fairly clear. Nutritional problems, whatever they may be, are obviously dependent upon the foods consumed; these will depend upon income, food habits, availability of foods, and so forth. These are to a greater or lesser degree, local problems. These problems and their solutions must be measured at the local level. The inadequacy of the statement "food stamps or food commodity programs are available in every county" is clear to everyone. If we are to do the job adequately, we must be able to identify specific high-risk groups, evaluate their nutritional status, and inform the local group concerned with specific solutions.

Broad national surveys, even though statistically accurate, may have little utility. Suppose, for example, that such a survey concludes that 1 percent of the total population of the United States is suffering from a certain nutritional deficiency. This small figure will probably be of doubtful statistical significance, although it would represent some two million individuals. Unless data are available concerning the age, sex, and geographic distribution of those suffering, it is doubtful whether action can be taken. Similarly, in evaluating the success or failure of ameliorative programs, we can predict that this will vary from area to area. Only the evaluation of local programs will provide the kind of information needed to spot successful or unsuccessful programs and indicate the modifications necessary. Therefore, the panel concluded that broad national surveys of nutritional status should be given a very low priority.

In general, it is clear that nutritional deficiency must develop in the following manner: first, there is an inadequate intake of the nutrient; second, the tissue reserves of the nutrient fall; third, after the tissues are depleted, clinically evident disease develops. The objective of any adequate nutrition program must be to *prevent* the disease from developing—not to cure the disease after it develops. Thus, if there is any appreciable amount of clinically evident disease in a population, the surveillance system has failed. Clearly, a system that relies largely on counting the numbers of malnourished persons is inadequate. The system must identify "high-risk groups" and call for programs that will reduce the risk. This is an extremely important point and one that is usually not appreciated. Those in the medical profession, by and large, are trained to identify and cure disease.

Methods

Offhand, it might appear that the most sensitive method of surveillance would be to evaluate nutrient intake, especially since the objective of a nutrition program is to assure that intakes of all nutrients are adequate. There are clear difficulties with this approach, however. It must be remembered that the nutritional status of an individual is related only to the average nutrient intake over a considerable period of time. The question then, is, how does one determine the average intake? The usual procedure is to ask people what they have eaten—yesterday, for the past week, or what they usually eat. Clearly, the result depends upon the skill of the interviewer and the memory and cooperativeness of the person being interviewed. Even when a person can accurately remember what he eats, it is difficult to ascertain how much has been eaten. Recipes vary and food composition varies. Another method—the inventory method—calls for recording all foods that are in a household and all foods that enter the household during the test period; this method ignores which persons in the household eat what or how much they eat. Another method is to have the housewife or subject or another person weigh all of the foods eaten. This is expensive and requires a great deal of cooperation from the subjects.

It is clear that one cannot easily determine with accuracy what anyone usually eats. We do not know how great the errors actually are in any of the proposed methods. When this uncertainty is combined with the fact that people's dietary requirements vary, and some require more of a nutrient than others, it can be seen why dietary history alone seems an inadequate method for the evaluation of nutritional status. If a particular study indicates that on the day the study was done 10 or 50 percent of the diets were inadequate in a specific nutrient, a large proportion of this percentage may represent error (for instance, perhaps the day chosen was not typical), and it cannot be concluded that 10 or 50 percent were malnourished.

On the other hand, dietary surveys do provide some useful information. They allow comparisons of one *group* with another: one group may have many more diets that are inadequate than does another, or the average intake of one group may be different from another group's. These are meaningful statistics. Dietary surveys also supply information for those designing ameliorative programs; such programs must be based upon knowledge of what foods will be eaten by the population they serve. It is thus clear that dietary surveys are an essential part of a surveillance program; however, it is also clear that they are insufficient for evaluating the extent and severity of malnutrition.

Another way to evaluate nutritional status is to measure the biochemical or physiological parameters that indicate (*a*) nutrient stores in the body or (*b*) early functional changes that precede nutritional disease. Such methods hold the most promise for adequate surveillance. There are many difficulties, however. The best methods require a blood sample, some of them a rather large blood sample. For certain groups in the population, young children, for example, this makes them unacceptable. Thus, there is great need for the development of many more methods that can be done with a single drop of blood obtained from a finger prick; some are available but not nearly enough.

Some of the methods now available are rather complex chemical determinations and are not well suited for use in routine clinical laboratories. We must develop local facilities so that samples can be analyzed and the results can be made readily available.

Many of the methods are not sufficiently accurate. Some of the methods in current use are based upon the nutrient content of urine. These are much less satisfactory than those based upon blood or serum content or upon physiological tests. There must be a search for better methodology.

Methods are available only for a limited number of nutrients; the ordinary battery of biochemical tests includes those related to seven or eight nutrients, those that have been our concern for many years. Continual attention should be paid to the development of new methods because we may find that, with our changing food supply, other nutrients will become critical. Today, the nutritional status of the United States population with regard to many nutrients is unknown.

Finally, there is the interpretation of these kinds of tests. Since the purpose of dietary and biochemical tests is to anticipate problems rather than identify disease, there will always be argument over what standards should be applied. If they are set high, to assure an absolute minimum of risk, they become unconvincing to some people; if they are set low, near the level where clinical disease becomes apparent, they do not serve their function adequately. Only continued research will lead to a reasonable concensus.

As has been mentioned, physical examination by a physician is considered a relatively insensitive method of surveillance. However, this must always be included in a surveillance system, since it is important that any deficiency disease that exists be detected. Anthropological measurements and x-rays should be included. The latter to detect rickets and retarded bone growth, the former for measurement of obesity and retarded growth in children. Dental problems are directly and indirectly related to the diet, and provision should be made for dental examination in the surveillance system.

The Sample to be Studied

When most people speak of surveillance, they conjure up the idea of a rather elaborate system in which (a) appropriate samples of the population are studied and (b) the resulting data are fed into a central organization. As has been indicated, the majority of the panel found such surveys to be of interest but of less importance at this time than the strengthening of local efforts to identify and solve nutrition problems.

There are many types of programs already in existence, such as maternal and child-health programs, head start programs, comprehensive-health-care programs, and so forth, which are to a greater or lesser degree concerned with solutions of nutrition problems at this time. Undoubtedly, these programs will be expanded and other types of programs with similar concerns will be developed. It cannot be expected that all of these various programs can or should develop the laboratory facilities and acquire the technical personnel required to monitor the success of the programs or to conduct nutritional surveillance of the populations they serve. Rather, a beginning should be made to provide these services through area nutrition-service centers. Such regional centers would not only provide technical backup for operating state programs but would strengthen and coordinate programs for the delivery of nutrition services. The centers should also develop more effective means of monitoring nutritional status. The panel emphasized that if such programs are to be really useful, they must not be simply re-search institutes or repositories of information but must develop means for a rapid exchange of information to and from the operative programs. Effective operating examples of such programs do not appear to be available. It is important that support be provided for experimental trials by various groups who appear to be capable of developing the kinds of model programs that may eventually lead to an adequate surveillance system.

It should be noted that unbiased monitoring of action programs can rarely be done by those responsible for the program itself. We should search for means to provide independent evaluation aimed, of course, toward the provision of more efficient and effective solutions.

Concern with undernutrition and poverty, although of primary interest, should not be allowed entirely to dominate nutrition programs or surveillance systems. It is known, for example, that iron deficiency is not limited to poverty groups; that obesity is a general problem as is teenage nutrition; that coronary artery disease may be influenced favorably by appropriate nutritional practice. Thus, surveillance programs should be broad enough to be concerned with the entire range of nutritional problems in the community they serve.

Conclusion

There is great need, then, to develop systems for the surveillance of nutritional status and to monitor the effects of nutrition programs. However, if these are to be maximally useful, they must not be simply data collection centers, but should provide technical support and other assistance for local efforts directed toward (a) the identification of high-risk groups and (b) the operation of ameliorative programs. Local efforts to develop such programs should be vigorously supported.

It is apparent that surveillance programs must include the collection of data on (*a*) food and nutrient intake, (*b*) biochemical and physiological parameters, and (*c*) physical and anthropological measures. It should be recognized that most available methods have rather serious limitations. Efforts must be directed toward the development of more specific and simpler methods, field testing, and the collection of the basic information required for the interpretation of the data collected.

REFERENCE

1. **Kelsay, J. L.,**   1969.. A Compendium of Nutritional Status Studies and Dietary Evaluation Studies Conducted in the United States, 1957–1967. *Journal of Nutrition* 99, Suppl. 1, Part II: 123–142.

PART 2

Monitoring the Wholesomeness and Nutritional Value of Our Foods

Chapter 9

Food Manufacturing

V. D. Ludington

In the seventies, food—its supply and its quality—will become of increasing concern to all of us. Food-manufacturing companies will have an increasing responsibility for the quality and, most importantly, the safety and the nutritive value of the foods they produce. The government will place additional requirements on industry to provide safety and nutrition, and consumers will come to expect this.

As our society has changed from an agricultural society to an industrial society to a postindustrial society, our population has shifted from rural to urban, with less than 5 percent of our population remaining on the farm today. The typical consumer no longer purchases food from the farmer or the independent neighborhood grocer but from a highly complex food-production-and-delivery system. The foods he or she buys are of greater variety and include many processed foods with labor-saving features.

With food far removed from its farm source and highly modified to offer the modern consumer variety and convenience, the consumer must increasingly rely on the food-delivery system to control the freshness or nutritive value of what he or she buys. For this reason there is a clear trend in the seventies for the government to set additional requirements in regard to the safety and nutrition of food. Requirements concerning safety and nutrients will be stringent, since the consumer has no way to evaluate them. They are hidden factors and not measurable by the consumer as are other regulated qualities, such as flavor, texture, and color or appearance.

Thus, anyone in the food-manufacturing business in the seventies must be prepared to produce a product that meets high standards of safety and nutritive value as well as of flavor, color, and texture. These standards will be a part of the rules of the game, and the cost of achieving them must be factored into the cost of goods. Many manufacturers have found this additional cost to be considerable.

Good Manufacturing Practices

This trend toward greater governmental regulation of quality increases the responsibilities of the operations manager, whose three chief concerns—inseparable but not necessarily always compatible—are cost of goods, quality of product, and production schedule. Quality control will be as important as cost control or inventory control and will override all other considerations when nutrition or safety are in question. The trend toward increased quality control is evident in the increasing use of the term "quality assurance." There is widespread concern now with the total environment in which the product is produced as well as with the raw materials, as GMP's (good manufacturing practices) issued by the Food and Drug Administration indicate. And there is increasing use of modern statistical methods and computers to assure quality. It is significant that the quality-assurance people report not to production departments but to higher echelons of management.

Nutritive Value

Safety and nutrition, both hidden qualities of food, have been mentioned together because they are closely related. We cannot obtain nourishment from unsafe food.

As the manufacturer prepares to produce a food, his thinking must encompass nutritive value as well as cost, quantity, and quality. Whether the subject be raw material type or source, plant facility, process, packaging material, or product shelf-life, each must be considered in terms of many factors, including nutritive value.

The standards for nutritive value are going to become increasingly difficult to define as more highly processed, less natural foods are produced. An important question is how to distribute nutrients in our food supply to ensure that the individual food consumer will be well nourished. This will require a continuing surveillance of food-consumption patterns so as to fortify the foods people are eating. It will also be necessary for the population to have a better understanding of nutrition. In addition to knowing that foods are important to them as a supply of nutrients, they must have some knowledge of what these nutrients are.

There are three bases that may be employed in determining the nutritive value a food product should have; they are:

1. comparing it with a natural food product it may replace,
2. comparing it with the raw material that was used in making the product,
3. choosing a standard and fortifying the product so that its caloric density and nutritive density bear some constant relationship.

In developing the specifications for nutritive value of a product, we can look forward to another trend. That trend is toward a better understanding of nutritive requirements and, probably, an increasing number of nutrients with which to be concerned. For instance, it is becoming clear that very small amounts of trace minerals are needed by man and that an oversupply can be as harmful as a shortage. Thus, standards will have to identify both a minimum and a maximum intake.

There will also be important questions raised in the future concerning small quantities of toxins that threaten the safety of food. The mycotoxins, produced by certain bacteria and viruses, will be of growing concern.

Nutrition Guidelines

Increasingly, manufacturers will follow guidelines from government to determine the nutritive value of products that are to be offered for sale. Here the manufacturer's tendency will be to consider competitive products, the economics of preserving or restoring nutrients, and consumer demand for nutrient content. The most important factor in determining the nutrient content of a product is in determining how it will be consumed, what it might replace in the diet, and, therefore, what contribution it might be expected to make to the nourishment of an individual. One must also consider whether this product is one to be consumed broadly or by a particular age group or ethnic group.

Having determined the nutrient specifications for a product, the next consideration is how the specifications are to be met. The raw material or raw materials are the first source of nutrients and the least expensive. The question usually is: Are they present uniformly in quality and quantity so as to be a dependable source? Considering the economics of nutrients, it may be less expensive

to pay a premium for a uniform raw material than to pay for nutrient fortification.

The Ingredients

Protein   Protein, because of the large daily requirement, is the most expensive nutrient. Its quality varies widely according to source and prior processing. The blending of proteins from a number of sources (e.g., corn, soya and wheat; fish and wheat) can improve total protein quality substantially. In many cases, the protein quality of grains and legumes can be improved by relatively light processing. However, generally, the application of heat in high-temperature drying or toasting will substantially reduce the value of the protein. Very careful forethought in regard to the selection and processing of raw materials can result in a product with a good level of protein with good quality and at very low costs.

Supplementation can usually be employed to improve both quality and quantity of protein. However, this is usually at an added cost of goods and may also introduce problems in flavor or texture to the product. Milk protein (casein or whey proteins), soy protein, fish flour, yeast protein, and cottonseed protein are some of the proteins that are commercially available for supplementation. Each must be considered in the light of its protein quantity and quality, flavor, cost, and functional properties (dispersibility, film forming, emulsifying, or water binding).

Vitamins and Minerals   Vitamins and minerals can usually be added to supplement a product: because of the small quantities needed, they are not expensive. It may be more expensive to maintain control over additions and, through quality-control procedures, maintain the levels within pre-scribed specifications. There are instances where flavor problems are encountered, such as with thiamine and potassium. In these instances, it is advisable to maintain the quantities present in raw materials rather than to supplement them. Most of these nutrients are stable under normal processing conditions, and only extremes of heat or leaching would remove them.

When vitamins and minerals are being added to a food product, careful considera-tion must also be given to how the product is packaged and distributed and how the prod-uct is handled and consumed in the home. The ideal is to be able to guarantee a level of nutrient fortification to the consumer as the product is eaten. For instance, in the case of a dry-mixed product, vitamin-and-mineral supplementation can be lost (or the level altered) in storage bins, airveyor systems, filling machines or in bulk containers in transit to stores and homes. These factors, plus storage on pantry shelves and reconsti-tution and measurement in the home, should be considered in developing standards of supplementation.

If vitamins and minerals are sprayed on a product such as rice, then consideration must be given to the home preparation. Are the vitamins and minerals lost in a rinsing or presoaking step? If this is the case, another form of fortification must be developed.

Other Food Additives Nutrients are, of course, only one of the classes of food addi-tives. Closely associated and often essential to satisfactory addition of nutrients are these other additives (with examples from each class):

1. *nonnutritive sweeteners* (saccharin)
2. *flavoring agents* (vanilla)
3. *coloring agents* (FDA-certified colors)
4. *emulsifiers and stabilizers* (vegetable gums)
5. *acids and bases* (fruit acids)
6. *preservatives* (BHA, BHT)
7. *improving and bleaching agents* (flour-bleaching agents)
8. *miscellaneous* (chelating agents, anti-caking agents, and texturizers)

All of these additives have come into use because they improve food products in some respect. A great many of them come or came from natural sources, and certainly there are examples of all classes found in natural foods.

One hears concern today about "chemi-cals" added to our foods. It is often over-looked that all foods are combinations of chemical compounds. The natural flavor of strawberries, for example, is produced by some 80 chemical compounds. And what are carbohydrates, fats, and proteins but chemical compounds? The fact that particu-lar chemicals are synthesized and used in place of natural compounds does not alter their utility or safety.

The safety of our food supply has also come under much discussion, and examples of hazardous substances have been identi-fied. It is true that there are substances "toxic to man" in many of our everyday foods; however, the level at which they are harmful is far beyond any reasonable level of con-sumption. So one might say there are no safe or unsafe foods or food additives; there is, rather, safe and unsafe use of foods or food additives. Any chemical or chemical compound, even water, can be hazardous to man if consumed in large excess.

Summary

The clear trend of the seventies is for more government regulation of the safety and nu-tritive value of our food supply. This trend will be paralleled by a rise in consumer expectation. The food manufacturer must convince both parties that he accepts this growing responsibility. The only basis the manufacturer has for a viable business is a satisfied customer.

At the same time, the consumer must develop a better understanding of the science of nutrition or the value of food and nutrients. Food is the only source of nutrients that are required by the body for its normal function. Eating the proper foods has a major effect on how one looks and acts and feels. The development of the understanding on the part of the consumer or the education of the consumer, the influencing of consumer attitudes about foods and nutrition, are big jobs for either the government or industry. However, government and industry, supported by our public-education system, can accomplish this education job. Therefore, it is essential that all concerned lend their efforts toward this end. At the same time, it is well to remember that foods suited to our life styles that are attractively presented, that have good flavor, color, and texture, are more readily accepted by all consumers and, thus, are the best vehicles for the proper nourishment of the individual.

Chapter 10

New Foods

Richard Gordon

A policy for new foods must take into account not only technological, but also consumer trends. One of the most significant is the rapid movement in the United States away from the so-called classic "four" or "seven" foods in favor of increasing dependence on foodstuffs that have been processed and, to an ever-growing extent, reconstituted for consumption. As a result, there seem to be several ways of defining new foods: (1) food that is new in the eye of the user; (2) food that contains components or ingredients not in common use; (3) food that has been processed by a new technique; (4) food that is "new" in the eyes of present law.

If one focuses on the need to develop and distribute new foods at lowest possible cost, with greatest wholesomeness and attractiveness, then any policy dealing with new foods in the seventies would, besides stimulating development of foods to help overcome malnutrition, also have to take into account the following: (1) the increasing trend towards consumption of "fast foods" away from the home; (2) the increasing percentage of preprepared meals being eaten in the home; (3) the increasing percentage of foodstuffs, food components, and even complete dishes that can be prepared from a very narrow range of basic ingredients.

If one sets as the primary goal the eradication of hunger and malnutrition in this country and adopts as a corollary that the full fruits of modern technology be utilized to achieve this goal, the question might be asked: Would such a policy also benefit the more affluent consumer sectors? The consensus appears to be "yes."

In examining case histories, however, it quickly becomes apparent that the primary barrier to utilization of modern technology in product innovation is a small number of regulatory policies that ". . . unduly restrict innovation and competition in the food industry." In short, after a great deal of deliberation, it seems clear to a majority of persons, and was virtually the unanimous opinion of the Panel on New Foods at the White House Conference, that present regulatory procedures reflect both a social climate and a technological base that no longer exist. Regulatory practices, in many cases, no longer seem to be in the best interest of consumers. In short, examination of the technological options involved in supplying, most attractively and at lowest cost, total nutrient needs no matter what the source, shows convincingly that a considerable amount of refinement and improvement is needed in the present food regulatory system "to make the system more responsive and realistic to consumer needs and demands." Most people do not realize how much flexibility exists in the present law; many of the bars to innovation are more the result of 20 to 30 years of administrative practice and could be modified by the Secreaty of HEW, the Food and Drug Administration or the U.S. Department of Agriculture, with very little need for major congressional reform.

As a consequence, it appears appropriate, in describing any policy that will foster the introduction and use of new foods in the next decade, to start with the following as a definition of new foods: (1) traditional foods nutriously upgraded beyond present standards; (2) foods that simulate traditional foods; (3) wholly new classes and types of foods.

In order to define a policy for new foods, one must be clear about the goals that the policies will bring about. These new national goals are:

1. more nutritious, appealing, and lowercost food for all consumers;
2. closer cooperation among consumers, industry, government;
3. competition based on quality (reflecting technological improvement and nutritional benefit) and price, instead of competition based on packaging, advertising, games and give-aways;
4. creation of a system to survey the nutritional status of the U.S. population and to take remedial action with minimum changes in food habits.

In our society there has been a great lack of communication and cooperation among various interests. Issues have not always been faced, and many times responsibilities have been overlooked.

It is necessary, first of all, that there be a desire to change. The incentive of corporate profits provides this in part, but public pressure and government support could increase the rate at which change occurs.

Industry must have the freedom to experiment and innovate; however, it must not be overlooked that industry has often resisted legitimate government regulation, has often been unresponsive to consumer inquiry, and, particularly, has neglected to inform consumers as to the value and content of its products.

On the other hand, consumer organizations have in general failed to gather information systematically and to study issues long enough to become knowledgeable and effective. Rather, they have relied too often on snap judgments and sloganeering.

In addition, the government often fails to use the flexibility built into many of our existing laws to cope with situations that have not appeared before. Government has not adequately accepted the joint responsibility both of protecting consumers and of stimulating innovations at reduced costs to consumers.

So, if the three sectors—industry, consumers, and government—are to move quickly into developing meaningful and synergistic relationships aimed at bringing better food at lower cost to the American public, the price of freedom to move where there is need requires acceptance by each sector of new responsibilities.

Freedom for industry to experiment and innovate means that industry must become responsive to consumer inquiry and to government regulation.

Freedom for consumers to exercise choice in the marketplace based on knowledge, as well as to petition and inquire, requires the consumers to become knowledgeable, able to communicate intelligently to the other sectors.

If the government is to encourage innovation through flexible use of its regulatory power, then it must act and it must explain its actions, even though complex, as the best course to protect consumers. Within this proposed climate, existing consumer-protection laws, such as the prohibitions against economic adulteration or misleading promotions, and the requirement that functionality and safety be proved for food additives, should remain applicable and be rigorously enforced.

The Present Laws   The Federal Food, Drug, and Cosmetic Act (the FD&C Act), the Federal Trade Commission Act (the FTC Act), the Fair Packaging and Labeling Act (the FPLA), and the Federal Meat and Poultry Inspection Acts, together with their numerous amendments and implementing regulations, provide more than sufficient regulatory authority to assure the public of safe and nutritious foods, that are accurately and truthfully labeled and advertised. The adulteration provisions of the FD&C Act prohibit deleterious or unsanitary substances in food. They also provide that a food product is "economically adulterated," and therefore illegal, if any valuable constituent has been omitted, or if a cheaper ingredient has surreptitiously been substituted for a more expensive one, or if damage or inferiority has been concealed, or if an ingredient has been added to increase bulk or weight, or reduce quality or strength, or otherwise make the product appear better or of greater value than it is.

The food-additive provisions of the FD&C Act provide that no ingredient may be added to food unless it is generally recognized as safe, or the Food and Drug Administration has approved it on the basis of adequate safety and functionality data. The FDA's regulations specifically require submission of proof not just that the proposed use of the ingredient is safe but that it will accomplish the intended physical or technical effect that the manufacturer states it will accomplish in the food.

Both the FD&C Act and the FTC Act prohibit any false or misleading claims on the package, in labeling material included with the package, or in advertising of any type. Under these provisions, the agencies are charged with stopping promotional claims that cannot be substantiated, whether they relate to economic questions such as size and weight, to the nutritional value of the product or to any other matters. The FPLA provides additional authority to require full disclosure of the net quantity of contents in a food product, to reduce the number of sizes in which foods are available, to prohibit slack fill, and to regulate other potentially confusing practices in the marketing of foods. In general, the U.S. Department of Agriculture has the same authority over meat and poultry products as FDA has over all other food items.

Thus, the question is not one of legal authority, but rather one of prompt and full enforcement of the law.

An obstacle to establishment of consumer-sector responsibility is that although university, government, and industrial sectors tend to create a corpus of organized knowledge and action, the consumer sector is, almost by definition, unorganized. Further, there is an acute need for increased nutrition education for consumers at all income levels. Finally, the interaction between food, nutrition, and health needs re-stressing as a part of any national policy for new foods.

Nutrition and Public Health

With life expectancy little changed in recent years in the United States and with sectors of our society demonstrably disadvantaged as a result of poor nutrition, even in the middle-class suburbs, nutritional well-being becomes one of the chief means of improving the public health.

Therefore, the need to make sure that any food consumed in significant quantities has nutritional value becomes an issue of the highest national priority. Yet, almost in every case, when foods are fortified, they become, in the eyes of the law, new food. Most believe, however, such fortification should become a major objective of any national policy on new foods. In short, whether a common ingredient or a total prepackaged meal, a substance that constitutes a significant portion of the human diet should make a proportionately significant contribution to nutritional well-being.

Furthermore, a society that can provide an adequate diet for sailors at sea or in a submarine under the sea for a year, or for passengers in airplanes, can surely provide adequate diets for every citizen in its schools or in remote rural areas. Therefore, the development of new delivery systems becomes an-other consequence of an aggressive new-foods policy. It is worth reiterating that a consequence of more efficient distributive systems is the availability of complete pre-processed and prepackaged meals. Let us first begin, however, at the staple level.

The nutritional requirements of submariner or airline passenger reflect a sharp break from tradition and from everyday life. Consequently, our society has felt free to do whatever is necessary to meet such requirements. In the case of the consumer at one end of the food chain, and the grower, processor, manufacturer, distributor, and retailer at the other end of the chain, however, the diffuse nature of the marketplace and the evolutionary nature of the changes have kept us unaware of the gaps that have appeared in the distribution process.

Let us highlight two discontinuities: (1) the old grocery store versus the supermarket; (2) the distribution of "surplus" grains to the poor.

The Old-time Grocery and the Supermarket
There is a great discontinuity between the earlier preoccupation of the grocer with buying and moving largely perishable basic commodities, and the goal of the modern supermarket chains to bring the most popular foods to the greatest number of people possible. There is today very little communication between those individuals who study nutritional requirements (either with laboratory animals or humans) and those concerned with trying to make the most popular foods not only attractive and desirable, but also the most nutritious.

The Distribution of Surplus Foods The history of the surplus-grain-distribution program in the United States usually shows that we have given people with the greatest need and the greatest nutritional deficit products that were largely unusable; those very people would seem to be the least able to formulate or compound such surplus grains into recognizable foods. (The problem is compounded by the fact that poor people are bombarded through the media with appealing pictures of foods and dishes into which most surplus commodities just cannot be transformed.)

In fact, in a society where rich and poor are given freedom of choice, very few have stopped to think through what people prefer to eat and then to consider how to upgrade such preferences for greatest nutritional impact per food dollar. Americans in particular, have been accustomed to sending missionaries and aid overseas to help those less fortunate than themselves. This philanthropy—in fact, the preoccupation with raising money to send abroad—has allowed many Americans to ignore what was going on in their own country. Accordingly, it has come as a great shock to the average citizen that there are people in this country ill-housed, ill-fed, with various debilitating diseases.

On a broader scale, it is only within the last five years that the public has become aware that, despite billions spent on medical research, life expectancy in this country has not changed appreciably in the last 20 years. Then we ranked in the top five nations; today America is twentieth to twenty-fifth, and slipping all the time, as other nations improve the life expectancy of their citizens.

Nobel Prizes testify to the fact that health-oriented research in this country has achieved outstanding successes. Certainly, despite the worrisome appearance of trace pollutants, which at very high concentrations might have the potential for doing harm, never have foods been more wholesome, more uniform, and safe for the consumer. Where, then, have we failed if people are in fact starving and malnourished in this country? It appears that we have failed to develop a delivery system that brings the benefits of the research, of all the new knowledge, to people who have the greatest need. As revolutionary as the new

biology has seemed, it is clear that the means of delivering its fruits must also be revolutionary or at least require radical alteration.

One of the tragedies, therefore, of the present lack of effective delivery systems is that the interdependent sectors of our society behave in ways that increase their isolation from each other rather than build new bridges that reflect interdependence. A common example, often cited by spokesmen for the poor, is that chickens and pigs in this country are better fed and better housed than are most low-income families. To one of the spokesmen of the poor on the New Foods Panel, the government-industrial food system for man, as compared with that for animals, seemed "musclebound." Most hungry people are not impressed with long arguments that rage in academic circles over whether a particular foodstuff should have one-third or one-quarter of a minimum daily requirement. In fact, description of the lengthy hearings concerning FDA's proposed regulation for special dietary supplements is heard by them with great disbelief.

One of the most beneficial results of the White House Conference was agreement by spokesmen for various interests concerning the need to apply available knowledge now to alleviate malnutrition. While nutritional requirements for man may not be precisely known, the order-of-magnitude requirement for nearly all nutrients by age or sex is certainly at hand. Further, statutory authority already exists that could permit rapid translation of principles, successfully used in supplementing animal foods, to meet human nutritional need in this country.

Meeting Nutritional Need: An Immediate Priority is Complete Supplementation of Foodstuffs

The best short-term answer to nutritional needs appears to be an immediate food-fortification program that will provide nutritionally complete foods to the public rather than a program that simply supplies foods that are not nutritionally adequate (as in the distribution of surplus commodities). The key change in outlook for the professional nutrition worker is to agree to make supplementation proportionate to caloric intake rather than to some absolute or "theoretic" standard of daily requirement. Based on the preponderance of data from modern nutritional research, man, as well as animals, tends to eat to satisfy caloric requirements. In the case of many target populations in this country (e.g., Indians on a reservation who may consume 60 percent of their diet as wheat), there should be no reason why if 60 percent of their calories are eaten as wheat, such wheat should not also contain 60 percent of vitamins, minerals, protein and other essential nutrients required. As for designing new foods to meet the urgent needs of the starving and severely malnourished, this is less appropriate than raising their income.

Role of Staples There are a small number of staple foods that could be fortified with all nutrients needed for meeting complete daily human requirements, which could have an immediate and major impact. Each of these basic foods should be fortified with nutrients. In coming to this particular conclusion, the White House New Foods Panel said:

"Each of these basic foods should be fortified with the nutrients selected to a level such that if it were consumed as the sole source of an adequate caloric intake, it would supply complete daily nutrient needs. Since consumption of food is controlled by caloric intake, this concept would prevent either excessive or deficient intake of critical nutrients. These nutrient requirements should be based upon the general population, recognizing that such special groups as infants, preschool children, and expectant mothers have special needs requiring additional nutrients beyond those

furnished by the fortified foods. Subject only to processing and handling limitations, industry should be urged to make such products broadly available in the regular commercial distribution channels. If any particular nutrients present a special processing or handling problem, industry may omit such nutrients until the problem is overcome. Such fortification should require the use of proteins, amino acids, vitamins, and minerals in ways that will employ the full range of nutritional knowledge and technology. Alternative sources of any nutrient should be permitted, to encourage development of nutritious foods at lowest possible cost."

In the present law, the temporary-permit authority of the FDA to allow a temporary variation from a published standard (including fortification) in order to demonstrate the feasibility of a proposed new product is apparently not sufficient legal authority to allow the type of widespread marketing contemplated in the preceding paragraph. A proper *new food policy* would give the Secretaries of Agriculture and Health, Education, and Welfare powers in this area so they could initiate regulatory action resulting in publication of a list of important foods, whether they be standardized or not (such as flour, bread, noodles, rice, processed meats, corn meal, etc.), that could be immediately fortified with appropriate nutrients. The technological goal, which could either be left to industry or which the secretaries could specify for each product, would then be to establish a level of fortification to make each food as nutritionally complete as possible without altering its acceptability to the customer through major changes in flavor, appearance or use characteristics.

There are a great number of malnourished persons in this country who could be reached by present governmental distribution of institutional food programs. Therefore, another element of a new food policy is that, in as short a time as possible, such enriched staples be used mandatorily in all government-funded or managed food-distribution or feeding programs. The question remains: Is the system so "musclebound" that it cannot already apply what is everyday practice for animals to the continued distribution of foods for the poor and/or malnourished? Certainly, a great deal depends on unifying divergent points of view with respect to this goal—this leads us to the next recommendation for food policy.

The Ability to Survey Nutritional Status of the U.S. Population and to Take Remedial Action Without Requiring Major Changes in Food Habits

If one accepts the continuing need to update knowledge concerning the nutritional status of the American population, particularly as newer knowledge comes to the fore, then the remaining problem is to make the needed change in the food supply once a consensus is reached in collaborative discussions between government, health, and nutrition professionals; industry; and consumers. Example of such a discussion now taking place is that being stimulated by the Inter-Society Commission for Heart Disease Resources. The commission believes there is a need to replace saturated fats with more unsaturated fats in the human diet. If this view prevails over present objections, then there are two ways available to accomplish such a substitution: (1) change foods eaten by changing food habits; (2) change the chemical constitution of foods presently eaten.

It has been repeatedly documented that it takes a relatively long time to change the food habits of a population. Therefore, as a practical alternative, modern chemistry and food technology afford the option of upgrading the composition of present foods. A new food may be an old food with a different chemical constitution. In essence, the prob-

lem becomes how to manipulate the diet for health reasons in a manner both consonant with present law and with establishing a consensus of purpose, giving manufacturers the freedom to try different ways and approaches. To be operative a national policy for the enrichment of staples or changing fatty-acid or caloric composition requires agreement concerning interlocking guidelines for regulatory policy, development of nutritional standards, labeling, etc.

The Federal Role: Regulatory and Continuing Definition of Priorities and Approaches

A Common Regulatory Policy Food products now derived from or utilizing inspected meat and poultry are presently subjected to regulation under separate federal laws administered by the Department of Agriculture. Virtually all other food products are regulated by the Department of Health, Education, and Welfare under the various sections of the Federal Food, Drug, and Cosmetic Act. There are significant differences in the ways the two departments administer these programs, as well as redundant efforts. There is also a large discrepancy in the way Congress appropriates money: the meat-inspection division of the USDA receives something like double the entire FDA budget.

President Nixon, in his State of the Union message to Congress in 1971, proposed federal department reorganization that would implement the recommendation made over 20 years ago by the Hoover Commission that a single federal agency regulate all foods. In view of the vested interests of the bureaucracies and their constituencies, it will probably be difficult to achieve this reorganization quickly.

As an interim step, however, the President could establish by executive order an interdepartmental coordinating committee on federal food regulatory policy. Such a committee could be comprised of representatives of all federal departments and agencies having jurisdiction with respect to safety, sanitation, identity, and labeling of any food.

In particular, the committee should also deal with inspection procedures and other practices protecting the public health and welfare. Certainly, there should be one place in the government below the President where food policy, food requirements, and a regulatory point of view are thrashed out.

A Separate Administration for Nutrition Science

There is considerable agreement that except for the occasional force of personality of an FDA commissioner or deputy commissioner, the regulatory mind is not liable to be concerned with matters other than enforcing the law. Further, regulatory agencies usually are neither intended nor equipped to undertake broad investigations that would lead to enunciation of broad new goals. Further, as nutritional knowledge increases, there is ample evidence to indicate that regulatory agencies find it difficult to keep abreast of current developments.

Therefore, while the language varies, many panels of the White House Conference felt there should be an independent federal agency that would devote primary attention to developing and promulgating a national nutrition policy that also would have an important input to any top-level coordinating committee.

Although there are compelling reasons for consideration of placing such an administration in either the Department of Agriculture or in HEW, the New Foods Panel felt "because of the health related and surveillance activities of HEW . . . such an Administration for nutrition science and technology is best assigned to HEW."

In any case, for an administration to carry out the action envisioned, it must embrace the idea of a food system: from production to delivery. No matter where such an administration is finally located, USDA and HEW must continue their close collaboration. In any case, an independent federal agency that stimulates and supports detailed scientific investigation concerning exact nutritional requirements, and so forth, should become another key part of any interdepartmental food coordinating committee on food policy and regulation.

To avoid confusion and to make the administration for nutrition science and technology clearly different from the Food and Drug Administration, such an administration's primary role in dealing effectively with hunger and malnutrition in the nation might be considered to comprise the following responsibilities:

a. maintain surveillance of the nutrition status of the nation and of methods being used to eliminate hunger and malnutrition;

b. develop new approaches to the eradication of hunger and malnutrition wherever it occurs in the United States;

c. develop and review broad national nutrition policy and propose laws and regulations consistent with health and food goals;

d. consult with federal regulatory agencies to develop and implement national nutritional policies;

e. encourage and accelerate the development of new foods designed to improve the nutrition status of the nation;

f. coordinate knowledge and carry out research on the development of food science and technology relating to nutrition;

g. promote widespread nutritional knowledge and demonstrate, through government purchases, sound nutrition practices;

h. conduct, and encourage others to engage in, basic and applied nutrition research.

Uniform Applications

It goes without saying that a final objective of nutritional policy in the seventies is that all federal regulations with respect to new foods must have uniform application throughout the nation, and must be enforceable not only by federal, but by state and local officials. As pointed out in the report of the New Foods Panel:

> Under present Federal, state and local law, different and often inconsistent regulatory requirements for the sanitation, labeling and marketing of new foods prevail throughout the nation. These inconsistent and different requirements result in artificial trade barriers that impede the orderly marketing of foods, hinder sound nutrition, raise the cost of new foods to consumers, and directly interfere with the public interest.

Further, restrictive regulations and practices hinder the development of new foods, and some have the unexpected effect of preventing the adaptation of traditional foods, through the use of modern food technology, in order to meet nutritional needs. Every food should be permitted in the marketplace, provided only that it is truthfully labeled, safe for consumption, prepared under sanitary conditions, and nutritious.

Certainly, one might say then that one key to a successful nutrition policy, particularly one where new foods could become an important vehicle for delivering results of new technology to the public, is uniform governmental treatment at all levels, but involving points of view considerably broader than the regulatory. Presumably, a federal interdepartmental coordinating committee would be able to rise above the more parochial concerns of big government departments in thinking through what is truly best for the public and the industries that serve the public.

Informing the Consumer

It is clear that it is time to develop a national policy that would have as its aim the provision of "accurate, complete and helpful label information to consumers and (which) would ensure that foods are truthfully named and that such foods meet appropriate nutritional standards."

It was interesting that during the conference, representatives of militant consumer groups, "hard-line" regulatory officials, and food manufacturers' associations—all were able to come to a consensus, although, when persons who had negotiated with the panel returned home, they were often unable to convey the sense of this consensus. In particular, some of the leaders of several consumer groups became convinced after the conference, that any attempt to make the system more flexible and open constituted a direct attack on the present FDA.

It is important that leaders of various consumer groups be encouraged to become more informed as to how flexible the present laws are, and that they can and should make recommendations to the Secretaries of HEW and USDA. In any case, such postconference reflections were regrettable, but given the present climate, predictable. In brief, any national nutrition policy must make it incumbent on the manufacturer to provide proper labeling and any other information required by consumers as long as we believe that it is the manufacturer's responsibility to take the initiative. This labeling and information should not only conform to the letter of the law, but should follow the spirit of the law and of any administrative guidelines established by governmental authorities.

The national budget cannot afford the kind of medicine for all that is practiced in research hospitals nor can it afford the kind of food-inspection system that virtually requires the equivalent of a state trooper for every automobile driver. This view has been attacked not only by members of consumer groups, but also by the food industry because of the recommendations (below) to tighten up labeling and to make the information required more precise.

The panel on new foods, upon licking its wounds, took some comfort from the fact that it was attacked from both sides, feeling that the middle position it had adopted was probably the most satisfactory. Fortunately, most of the following provisions can be implemented by the Secretary of HEW, if he chooses, and do not require a major clash of sensationalist charges and counter-charges in front of the Congress, only to arrive at the same position in five or ten years.

Names Foods are known to the public usually by both a brand name and a generic name, i.e., a common or usual name or a statement of identity as to what the food is. Many new foods are often required by government policy to be called "imitation"; in truth, the "imitation" label has been required whether a new product is inferior to the old or whether it is superior. The New Foods Panel felt quite strongly that foods should be labeled for what they are rather than for what they are not, with the generic or common name accurately describing, in as simple and direct terms as possible, "the basic nature of the food or its characterizing properties or ingredients."

Label The important point of the use of a name on the label is that whatever information is important to consumers with respect to composition and nutritional properties should be used. The great problem is how to know how much information should be put on the label. Clearly, there is little point in inundating the consumer with long lists of chemical names or material that could well be put in a package-inclusion folder (as is the practice for some drugs).

Certainly, the maze of present laws and regulations leads to confusing or incomplete information as foods are now purchased. For example, the label of an unstandardized food bears a full statement of the ingredients, whereas because of the standards, bread, being defined by standard as "bread," does not disclose the mandatory ingredients. Consumers are entitled to more meaningful and useful information than now provided.

General statements are relatively easy to agree upon until one gets specific (i.e., how many cherries must a pie contain before it can be called a "cherry pie"?). If I buy a spinach souffle, what am I really receiving besides calories—how much protein? How much vitamin C? While the cyclamates were still on the market, a "dietary beverage" meant one that had no sugar and no calories. Yet, many "dietary beverages" now sold contain sugar and make a significant caloric contribution. How *does* one become informed?

The answer seems to be a "standard of characterization" for foods that should move away from the present recipe base to consideration of options built around a characterizing ingredient (cherries in a cherry pie). The FDA, in the standard for breaded shrimp, has created a fairly workable model of what might be possible to do with other foods in the future. One should be clear that present law prohibits adulteration of food with cheap fillers or nonfunctional ingredients, and requires proof of both safety and functionality for any food additive. Yet, from the economic point of view, if one were to make a peanut butter with less than 95 percent peanuts, say 50 percent soy butter, which would, say, be half the price of peanut butter but equally nutritious, how would one label it? Is "peanut-flavored soy spread" meaningful to consumers? Do people know what is now in peanut butter?

In general, there is a consensus that, if a new product is designed to *look* like an established product, it should still be called what it actually is, and characterized for what it actually contains, but that minimum nutritional qualities must also be ensured whether: (*a*) the new food represents or is intended to substitute for or replace a well-established food or (*b*) it is, notwithstanding what it looks like, consumed in a significant portion of the diet.

(NOTE: Such decisions should be based on actual rather than potential consumption patterns since it is clear that some foods, intended to be ancillary, can be eaten by various faddists as 100 percent of their diet. There seems to be no satisfactory way to provide for such persons.)

The net effect of the above, to be incorporated in a nutrition policy, is

> to permit the utilization of new food technology in the development of new foods that are not only variations of traditional products, that may be wholly new foods that resemble traditional products, but not tied to traditional ingredients, or to totally new foods themselves. It is clear that whatever standards are adopted (must) be sufficiently flexible to permit alternative safe ingredients within the limits of the basic nature of the food.

Review of Actions of Manufacturers by Consumers and Government

Once the conference adjourned and members returned home, the consensus that seems to have survived the least concerned creating broad-enough guidelines in the seventies to give a manufacturer the privilege of innovating, to give consumers the right to ask at any point for more information, and for the government to create a better means of inquiry. The agreed-upon purpose, using the conference as a model, is to create a system wherein all sectors are consulted in the establishment of regulatory requirements for new foods or in basic design and distribution of a food to meet new needs. The underlying idea is to create a climate in which administrative procedures and inquiry are fair and impartial and not conducted under adversary conditions.

There was also a consensus that regulation by arbitrary fiat regardless of whether such a fiat is promulgated by government, industry, or consumers, was not acceptable.

"Discussion among consumer, industry, government and other interested groups must be utilized to develop policies, resolve issues, and minimize the need for formal and protracted public hearings." There was a strong consensus that the present standard-making machinery is cumbersome, time-consuming, and requires manufacturers to develop a defensive, adversary position because changes are so slow in being approved; that those whose foods are "standardized" in general resist requests of those who seek modifications; that rarely are alternative solutions or approaches to a food allowed to compete in the marketplace.

The effect on consumer prices is already well known. The breads, which are all standardized, can only compete through advertising, not through nutritional quality or by technological improvements, and in our haste to prevent people from making claims concerning relative levels of vitamins or other nutrients, the net effect is that foods that could easily be supplemented so that per calorie they are nutritionally complete, are not. Certainly, any national nutrition policy dealing with new foods as defined above must come to grips with these issues through some fair proceedings that deal with actual and realistic use and consumption rather than fancied or improbable conditions.

Conclusion

Overall, if a receptive climate for new foods is to be established in the seventies, it requires an attitude of cooperation not really manifest today. The experience of the White House Conference was that, by and large, representatives from all sectors could meet and iron out specific approaches possible under present legislation and administrative practice or, through their deliberations, recommend legislation to the extent necessary to implement their recommendations. It is clear that the prime elements of a policy for new foods consist of the following:

1. immediate fortification of certain staple ingredients, wherever possible, so that, per calorie consumed, the staple represents a complete food;
2. establishment of uniform regulatory policies at the federal, state, and local levels;
3. establishment of an independent administration for nutrition science and technology, which devotes its primary attention to national nutrition and food policy and problems;
4. development of explicit naming and labeling of foods so that the consumer understands what is being purchased, yet the manufacturer is not hamstrung by specific recipes and has the freedom to use optional ingredients to insure that a new food will provide the minimum nutritional qualities of the food it replaces, or furnish those necessary if it is to be consumed as a significant portion of the diet;
5. much greater use of task forces and conferences to establish policies and regulatory requirements for new foods, with government, consumer, industry, and university sectors represented, so that on any given subject, they can take account of all that is known and establish both action and further studies, as required, or propose legislation to the extent required, to avoid the present formal protracted and largely adversary proceedings.

These recommendations, of course, presume that all of us, no matter what our employment or profession, are ultimately consumers. We all share the same concerns in developing a nutrition policy as one arm of a broad health policy that aims at preventing disease and improving the quality of life rather than relying on drugs and hospitalization. They presume too, freedom to develop new systems for the delivery of foods and possibly to change the historic role of the grocer. The supermarket can become more of an "educational enterprise," increasingly free of the tyranny of spoilage and variability of fresh produce, with the manufacturer constantly searching for the most economical, reliable—and safe—sources of ingredients and foodstuffs.

Chapter 11

Safety of Foods

Julius M. Coon and John C. Ayres

Man's food constitutes by far the most complex part of his chemical environment and is much less understood chemically than are the air he breathes and the water he drinks. No natural food product has ever been as fully characterized chemically as have air and water. Several times in every day of his life, a man consumes many chemical substances that are still unknown. Nearly 150 distinct chemicals have been identified as natural components of one of our simplest foods, the potato. This number, in itself, signifies the incompleteness of the analysis.

In addition to the myriad chemical substances that constitute natural food products, three major categories of agents that may be present in foods should be taken into account in any comprehensive consideration of potential hazards. These are: (a) micro- or macro-organisms or their metabolic products, (b) chemicals used by man to aid in the production or processing of foods, and (c) chemicals that contaminate foods as a result of carelessness, ignorance, inadvertence or accident.

The following list presents a skeleton outline of the general types of potentially harmful substances in foods, and cites selected examples of things that have proved to be harmful or can potentially be harmful. This outline is far from complete in respect to the specific types of agents listed under each major category, but it provides an adequate perspective for viewing the whole problem of food safety.

Among the groups of agents listed here, the greatest known injury to man has been produced by groups 1, 2, 8, and 3, in that order. Group 3 is currently a very minor factor in the United States. Agents listed in groups 4 to 7 are not known to have produced significant damage to health when good agricultural or manufacturing practices

in food production are adhered to in their use. Despite comparisons of the extent of the known adverse effects of these different groups of agents on human health, the greatest amount of research, publicity and governmental regulatory attention in the decade 1961 to 1970 was directed toward the safety of pesticides and food additives in our food supply (groups 4 and 5). On the other hand, proportionately less attention in the last decade was focused on the problem of contamination of foods by the toxins of

Potential Hazards Associated with Foods

Natural Origin

1. *Infections*
   Viral
   Bacterial
   Protozoan
   Parasitic (helminths)

2. *Toxins*
   Bacterial toxins
   Mycotoxins
   Seafood toxins

3. *Normal chemical components of natural food products*

Essential nutrients	Nitrates
Trace elements	Solanine
Goitrogens, other	alkaloids
sulfur compounds	Plant phenolics
Estrogens	Enzyme
Carcinogens	inhibitors
Cyanogenetic glycosides	Photo-
Colors and flavors	sensitizing
Lathyrogens	agents
Oxalates	

Man-made Origin

4. *Agricultural chemicals*

Insecticides	Animal feed
Herbicides	additives
Fungicides	Plant growth
Rodenticides	regulators
Fertilizers	

5. *Food additives*

Essential nutrients	Stabilizers and
Preservatives	thickeners
Colors	Emulsifiers
Flavors	Buffers and
Oxidizing and	neutralizing
bleaching agents	agents

6. *Materials used in packaging foods*

Synthetic films	Adhesives
Treated papers, wood,	Printing inks
cloth	
Paraffins and waxes	

7. *Chemical changes induced by food processing*
   Heat
   Ionizing radiation

8. *Accidental or inadvertent contamination*

Food-holding utensils	Household
Environmental	accidents
pollution	Miscellaneous

microorganisms and by the organisms that produce infections, which have been by far the most common causes of injury to health due to food consumption.

This apparent reversal of priorities may be considered, in the mind of some, to be related to two factors. First, the food-borne illnesses caused by toxins and organisms are largely acute, self-limiting in nature (with some exceptions), and fairly well characterized as to cause and effect, whereas the potential or suspected adverse effects of pesticide residues and food additives are chronic, progressive, more serious in nature, may affect larger segments of the population, and are as yet mostly unknown as to cause and effect. Second, in a large proportion of cases the presence of disease-producing toxins and organisms in food results from carelessness or ignorance at the stages of distribution of prepared meals to the consumer and is thereby relatively difficult to regulate. On the other hand, food distributors and the population at large can do little to avoid consumption of pesticides and additives that enter foods at the production and processing level, yet the use of such substances is relatively susceptible to regulatory control.

These factors are not sufficient to justify the imbalance of the attention focused upon these two aspects of food safety. The fact remains that there is much that can and must be done in research, development, and regulation to minimize the excessive incidence of food-borne illness due to toxins and infective organisms. In the coming decade this aspect of food safety should have the consideration it deserves in proportion to its importance to the public health.

Toxins and Infectious Agents

The Epidemiological Picture In regard to acute illness, man's food supply probably is safer today than at any time in recorded history. The risk for reported food illnesses in the U.S. is about one illness for seven million meals consumed. During the past several years, fewer than 400 outbreaks of food illness per year have been recorded by the National Center for Disease Control (NCDC). During 1970 there were 366 outbreaks as compared with 371 in 1969 and 345 in 1968. A total of 23,448 individuals developed food poisoning during 1970; in 1969, 28,563 persons were ill; in 1968, 17,567 had food-borne disease.

Public-health investigators insist that food-borne diseases are grossly underreported and that the true incidence may be many times larger than that shown by the data submitted to the NCDC. This point is well illustrated by comparing U.S. data with those from countries where food-poisoning surveillance has been well developed. In 1967 when only 345 outbreaks were reported to NCDC, there were 705 incidents of food poisoning in England and Wales. If one assumed proportionate numbers of outbreaks on a population basis, the number of such episodes in the U.S. would exceed 2,800.

In about three-fourths of reported outbreaks less than 50 individuals have been involved. However, at least one large food poisoning incident (over 100 ill) occurs almost every month. In 1970, bacteria were responsible for about 63 percent of all food-borne outbreaks and caused about 84 percent of all food illnesses. No causative agent has been identified for 27 percent of the outbreaks. The remaining 10 percent has been attributed to chemicals, parasites, and viruses. Combined, these latter agents affect less than 2 percent of those who suffer from foodborne illnesses.

During the five-year period from 1963 to 1967, salmonellae were the organisms most commonly involved in massive incidents of food-borne illness. In 1963, *Salmonella derby* was incriminated in a very widespread hospital-acquired infection in the Mid-Atlantic

States. An episode of international interest attributed to *S. typhi* occurred in 1964 in Aberdeen, Scotland when about 450 patients were hospitalized after consuming contaminated imported canned beef that had been sliced in a large food shop. The following year (1965), one of the largest outbreaks of gastroenteritis due to *S. typhimurium* occurred in Riverside, California; 18,000 symptomatic cases of salmonellosis were thought to have occurred.

The isolation of an exotic salmonella serotype species, *S. new brunswick*, from instant nonfat dry milk in 1966 prompted the federal government to investigate and remove large quantities of dry milk from the market and to institute a rigorous surveillance program throughout the food industry. This effort notwithstanding, there were two massive salmonella outbreaks in 1967. The first and largest was traced to improperly pasteurized frozen egg yolks used by a New York City firm to make kosher imitation ice cream. This ice cream was served to about 18,000 persons attending at least 14 banquets; about 9,000 of these developed salmonellosis. The second episode involved a turkey barbecue in Oxford, Nebraska. It was estimated that 1,350 of 5,000 attending the barbecue suffered food illness.

After 1967 the picture began to change. While salmonellae remained prominent as a source of food illness, there was only one outbreak in 1968 wherein at least 100 persons suffered from salmonellosis. *Clostridium perfringens* and staphylococci were the major sources of large-scale food-borne outbreaks. There were 14 outbreaks in which over 100 persons became ill as a result of poisoning by *C. perfringens*, six in which *Staphylococcus aureus* was involved and two wherein streptococci were found to be the toxic agents. In every instance, these illnesses were attributed to food service sources such as school lunches, restaurants, catered meals, cafeterias, meals served at military bases, and banquets.

In 1969 one episode of *C. perfringens* poisoning placed 67,188 school children at risk and, of these, 13,500 became ill. In addition, there were three outbreaks involving 153, 550, and 750 school children, respectively, and three others wherein food served in a cafeteria or hospital, or was catered, accounted for 200, 175, and 250 cases of *C. perfringens* poisoning. Two outbreaks of shigellosis, four of salmonellosis, one *Escherichia coli* infection and seven staphylococcal poisonings involving more than 100 persons also were reported. As in 1968, all but one of these were attributed to food service agencies (schools, church suppers, caterers, restaurants, camps, military bases). The only exception was an *S. typhimurium* outbreak traced to custard cake prepared by a bakery.

Of the 23,448 individuals who developed food illnesses during 1970,[1] about 30 percent had *C. perfringens* food poisoning, 20 percent had salmonellosis, and approximately the same number suffered with staphylococcal enterotoxin. Thirteen large-scale outbreaks (over 100 ill) were caused by salmonellae, nine by *C. perfringens*, five by shigellae. In 1970 the last-named organisms were responsible for 7 percent of food illnesses, *E. coli* for 5.5 percent, *Bacillus cereus* and other bacteria, trichinae, viruses and chemicals for 2.9 percent, and 14.6 percent of the illnesses were of unknown origin. These illnesses emanated from foods served by restaurants, cafeterias, schools, churches, delicatessens, caterers, airlines, clubs, armed-forces bases, factories, camps, picnics, and in the home.

Today, scores of illnesses are attributed to shigellae, *Escherichia coli*, and *Vibrio parahemolyticus*. Occasionally, trichinae, viruses, toxic fish and shellfish, mushrooms, residues of toxic metals, insecticides and other chemicals are implicated.

Though there has been an increased awareness on the part of public health officials and the lay public of the hazards in the food supply, epidemiological information is far from uniform. Five of the States did not report in 1970, ten had no reports in 1969, eight in 1968. During the entire three-year period, no food illnesses were reported in Wyoming, one each were reported in Nevada, New Hampshire and South Dakota, two each in Delaware and Maine, three each in Arizona, Mississippi, and Nebraska and four to seven each in Alabama, Rhode Island, North Dakota, Vermont, Iowa, Utah, Massachusetts, Wisconsin, Kentucky, and Oklahoma. During this same period Washington (164), California (117), New York City (114), New Jersey (49), South Carolina (40), Florida (33), Tennessee (33), Illinois (29) and Michigan (26) reported 605 such episodes—about 56 percent of the nation's total.

A long-range program is needed for the seventies that will provide improved information concerning the detection, investigation, and reporting of infections, toxemias, and harmful chemicals in foods. In addition to coordination at federal, state, and local levels, a mechanism is essential that will enlist the participation of practicing physicians and individual citizens in reporting such illnesses. It is probable that a fiscal incentive will be required so that states, cities, and practitioners can and will participate in a satisfactory and uniform manner.

Characteristics of Food-borne Illnesses Ordinarily, public-health workers characterize food-borne illnesses according to their action on the host organism. Using such criteria these illnesses can be segregated into three categories: (1) those wherein the agent is transferred via food to man in whom it multiplies, causing an infection, (2) those in which a living agent may contain, produce or elaborate a toxic substance in the food and (3) those nonliving entities which may contain residues that are poisonous when consumed by man. Salmonellae, E. Coli, Shigellae, Entamoeba histolytica, V. parahemolyticus, viruses (infectious hepatitis), and trichinae cause infections; staphylococci, streptococci (?), C. botulinum, Clostridium perfringens, B. cereus, and certain mushrooms (Amanita spp.) dinoflagellates (Gymnodinium spp., Gonyaulax spp., etc.), and fish (puffers and other reef fish) produce biological toxins. Metals and metal compounds (copper, cadmium, mercury, etc.), insecticides (parathion, organic phosphates), and a miscellany of chemical residues occasionally may be present in foods.

Conceivably, mycotoxins (aflatoxins, orchratoxins, islanditoxin, rubratoxin, zearalenone, etc.) eventually may be added to group 2, but until conclusive evidence is presented to show that any of these agents is present in food in sufficient amounts to be hazardous to health, their inclusion is premature.

Food-borne Infections Despite concerted efforts on the part of the Food and Drug Administration and the Department of Agriculture and an evaluation of the salmonella problem by the National Academy of Sciences in 1969, the number of reported human isolations of salmonellae in the U.S. has remained relatively constant. It is generally recognized that some serotype species have specific host requirements and that others do not. However, much remains to be learned regarding the milieu that results in infection.

As was indicated earlier, there has been a shift in primary foci from which the organisms are disseminated, that is, food service organizations are entering into the picture more prominently than previously. Despite the fact that these organisms are commonplace in many raw foods and especially those of animal origin, tests for their detection and identification are cumbersome and time consuming. Simpler and more convenient techniques need to be developed.

The role of enteropathogenic E. coli as a food-borne illness has only recently been recognized. Ordinarily E. coli, found universally in the intestinal tract of man and animals, has been considered merely to be an index of pollution, but recent investigations have demonstrated that certain strains of *E. coli* cause infantile diarrhea and gastroenteritis. In 1969 these organisms were responsible for food illnesses associated with turkey served in a factory cafeteria and with raw oysters served in a restaurant, and in 1970 with hamburger served to school children. Exploration of the genetic behavior of escherichia, salmonella, and other enterics may reveal interesting phenomena concerning spontaneous or induced hybridization patterns within the family.

There is no indication that shigellosis is increasing; yet the occurrence of bacillary dysentery remains alarmingly high. As in the past, shigellae continue to be spread by drinking polluted water or eating contaminated food. In the United States, most of the illnesses have been traced to cafeterias, caterers, hospitals, camps, picnics, and banquets.

Amoebic dysentery is spread in the same manner as are the intestinal bacteria. The most important means by which these protozoa are introduced into foods are water, food handlers, and house flies. The incidence of infection by these organisms is higher in the tropics than in the temperate zones. Investigators in 1968 estimated a general infection rate in the United States of 4 to 10 percent and cited human carriers as the only important source. Yet little is known concerning how resistance to amoebiasis is acquired by the carriers. Such information is essential for diagnosing and preventing the disease.

It was recently reported from Japan that 1,500 to 2,000 outbreaks of *V. parahemolyticus* food poisoning occur annually, with about 30,000 to 40,000 cases. In that country, where it is a custom for the people to eat raw fish, 60 to 65 percent of food-borne outbreaks implicate fish and fish products. Until recently, these bacteria have not been identified from food illnesses in the United States, but in 1969 and 1970 (in two camps, a restaurant, and a country club in the state of Washing-

tion), four outbreaks attributed to these organisms have occurred when contaminated shellfish were served. Episodes involving *V. parahemolyticus* are of the infectious type with gastroenteritis appearing about 12 to 14 hours after ingestion of the infected food. Abdominal pain and diarrhea, often accompanied by headache, fever, and prostration with recovery in two to five days usually characterize the illness. The organisms are facultatively anaerobic halophiles growing best at pH 7.5 to 8.5 and at 37°C. They are sensitive to furylfuramide and to most antibiotics except polymixin B and colisten. Only the hemolytic cultures are considered enteropathogenic, but to date no relation has been demonstrated between the organism's biochemical and serological properties and its hemolytic activity. It is quite likely that illnesses in the United States attributed to marine fish and shellfish will reveal an increased number caused by *V. parahemolyticus*.

Except for the knowledge that the viruses associated with infectious hepatitis are present in feces and that infection is contracted through ingestion of contaminated water or food, little other information concerning enteroviruses is certain. Symptoms generally appear three to four weeks after exposure and may be abrupt or gradual. Gastrointestinal discomfort, headache, fever, anorexia, lassitude, and jaundice are common, and there is often liver damage. The liver and spleen are palpable and tender. Water is the common vehicle and even when the organisms are food-borne, the water incorporated in the food seems to have been the source. Shellfish (clams and oysters) are often offenders since their gastrointestinal tracts and contents are often eaten with the rest of the soft tissue with little or no cooking. However, raw milk, pastries, salads, sandwiches and beverages and other foods can become contaminated.

Adequate techniques for the detection of viruses that can cause infectious hepatitis need to be developed to show the importance of food as a transmitting vehicle. It is likely that a number of food-borne illnesses would be traced to these organisms if clinicians were properly informed as to typical symptoms and had reliable tests to define the source. The development of a suitable laboratory host or hosts would prove invaluable to the further exploration in this area. Knowledge is needed concerning how many and what types of hepatitis viruses exist.

Government meat inspection has been fairly successful in reducing the amount of infection caused by tapeworms (*Taenia*) but such inspection does not attempt to detect *Trichinella*. Protection from trichinal infections depends upon the thorough cooking of pork products and hamburger of unknown composition. Except for 1966, 1967, and 1968, when the rates were respectively 115, 66, and 77, about 200 cases of trichinosis have been reported each year over the past decade. In almost every instance these infections have originated in the home or from products that were prepared without inspection. Adequate programs need to be evolved to prevent trichinosis and other parasitic diseases in such food products. The major stumbling block seems to be lack of education on the part of lay people concerning the manner by which these infections are transmitted.

Food Toxemias In 1968, 1969, and 1970 staphylococci accounted for about one-fourth of all food-borne outbreaks; this organism was second only to *C. perfringens* in the number of individuals affected. Since staphylococci are able to multiply and elaborate sufficient enterotoxin the cause illness within a few hours when foods are held at room temperature, strict attention must be paid to sanitation and cleanliness, to the danger of working with food while having a skin infection, and to prompt refrigeration of chopped meats, salads, and filled pastries until sale or use. When enterotoxin is present in an offending food, the interval between the time of consumption and the onset of abrupt and severe nausea, cramps, vomiting, diarrhea, and prostration is usually two to four hours. Authorities differ concerning the use of certain media and testing procedures to detect those strains that are responsible for food poisoning; also, work must be undertaken as soon as possible to provide a reliable test for the identification of staphylococcal enterotoxins. As with many of the other leading food-borne illnesses, the majority of toxemias have been traced to food-service establishments and to homes, and there is every indication that such attacks will continue almost unabated in the years ahead.

The organism is a nonspecific pathogen—at times being responsible for mastitis, osteomyelitis, pneumonia, meningitis, abscesses, pimples, boils, carbuncles, etc. Staphylococci possess a wide array of biologically active substances, including alpha-toxin or alpha-hemolysin, beta-toxin or hot, cold hemolysin, delta-toxin, leukocidin, fibrinolysin (staphylokinase), hyaluronidase, penicillinase, DNase, coagulase, exotoxin, and enterotoxin. Of these toxic moieties, only enterotoxin produces emesis. A, B, C, D and E enterotoxins have been characterized. While early work[2] indicated enterotoxin to be resistant to heat, more recent findings show that the various enterotoxins vary somewhat in heat resistance. Less than 50 percent of enterotoxin-B activity was destroyed by heating at 100° C for five minutes; enterotoxin A was inactivated in one minute at that temperature.[3]

Since staphylococci are always present on the skin, particularly that of the hands and forearms, they are readily transferred to meats, milks, salads, pastries, custards, and cream fillings. It is estimated that from one-third to one-half of the population are carriers of toxin-producing staphylococci; yet factors leading to the establishment of the carrier state are unknown. Techniques for the detection of carriers are of only limited value owing to the widespread occurrence of infected fingers and skin, abscesses and nasal secretions among food handlers.

C. perfringens outbreaks have increased at and alarming rate, but only in the past few years have any meaningful data been tabulated. Before 1967 the usual attitude concerning this illness was that it was a relatively mild disease of short duration and, therefore, that it would not be possible to secure any useful or accurate information. However, when data were amassed, it soon became evident that C. perfringens poisoning was our most common food-borne disease. In 1967 about 3,500 persons suffered from this illness, in 1968 about 6,000, and in 1969 over 18,500 became ill. Outbreaks are generally associated with a lapse in food-service sanitation when certain cooking practices are employed. Often food handlers fail to serve foods immediately, and when meat dishes or stews are prepared in bulk and inadequately heated or cooled, the anaerobes have an opportunity to multiply and produce the toxic enzyme lecithinase. The intestinal disorder caused by the organism is characterized by a sudden onset of abdominal colic and diarrhea about ten to 12 hours after the consumption of the offending food, followed by recovery in a day or less.

Of the major types of C. perfringens, only type A has been associated with food poisoning. Type A produces alpha, kappa, mu, nu, and theta toxins. Of the components that occur in filtrates for type A, those strains causing food poisoning produce smaller amounts of alpha-toxin, more nu-toxin, and no theta-toxin. The alpha component is thermostable and lethal for mice, guinea pigs, rabbits, pigeons, and sheep and, when given intradermally, produces a necrotic lesion. It is hemolytic for red blood cells of most animals except the horse and the goat. Kappa is a collagenase or lethal, necrotizing gelatinase, mu is a hyaluronidase, and nu is a deoxyribonuclease. The alpha-toxin of type A is a lecithinase—lecithinase C or phosphorylase

C—whose action is proportionate to the rate at which it hydrolyzes or splits the lecithin present in food to phosphorylcholine and diglyceride. Phosphorylcholine is suggested to be the toxic principle.

B. cereus has been identified as the etiological agent for several human and animal infections. Normally it is not considered a pathogenic species although at one time it was suggested[4] that B. anthracis might be a pathogenic variant of B. cereus. Although there is marked similarity between the two species, they differ in biological activity, molecular composition, and immunological characteristics.[5] The toxin of B. cereus is a simple protein that acts very rapidly on mice, whereas anthrax toxin consists of three components (lethal, edema, and protective antigen). Also, the skin lesion produced by B. cereus toxin differs markedly from the edematous reaction caused by B. anthracis toxin.[6]

In 1968, one outbreak of food poisoning was attributed to B. cereus; in 1969, there were two outbreaks; in 1970, the organism was associated with three outbreaks. In all instances the patients had nausea, cramps, abdominal pain, vomiting, and diarrhea; in one case there also was fever. Two episodes were traced to meat dishes or gravy served at camp, two were related with foods served in restaurants, and the remaining two were attributed to foods prepared for a church social or eaten at home.

Despite the biological and biochemical similarities between B. cereus extracellular products and C. perfringens alpha-toxin, they are unrelated. Antisera prepared against purified B. cereus phospholipase C and toxin did not cross-react with phospholipase C and lethal activities of C. perfringens alpha-toxin.[7] Similarly, anti-alpha-toxin had no neutralizing effect on B. cereus phospholipase or toxin. Introduction of chelating agents at the time of administering B. cereus toxin did not prevent it from being active while C. perfringens alpha-toxin was cation dependent. The toxigenic abilities of *B. cereus* are still not known, and this organism's contribution to foodborne illnesses remains to be determined.

The National Center for Disease Control has attributed several food-poisoning outbreaks to streptococci. The number of these outbreaks and the variety of foods incriminated (meat dishes, sausage, milk, pudding, and so forth) strongly support epidemiological findings involving *Streptococcus faecalis* and *S. faecium* as the etiological agents of a mild food-borne illness (nausea, abdominal pain, diarrhea) occurring within six to 12 hours after ingesting the offending food. However, the accuracy of diagnoses that rely only on the presence in the food involved of large populations of these streptococci has been questioned. This is a valid criticism. Yet sizeable outbreaks have been reported in the past few years of episodes of streptococcal food poisoning in schools, restaurants, catered and store foods, as well as in homes. The true role of enterococci or other streptococci in food-borne disease certainly needs clarification in the near future.

Except for 1963 to 1964 there have been fewer than 20 cases of botulism reported in the U.S. each year after 1957. Until the early sixties *C. botulinum* A and B generally were the strains implicated in sporadic outbreaks occurring in the home, at camp or other outings, or at small gatherings. In 1963, however, a botulinum E strain grew and produced toxin in commercially canned tuna and in packaged smoked fish. This organism grew and sporulated even when held at low temperatures (40° C or below). In addition, further investigation in 1967 revealed that a strain of *C. botulinum* B was able to grow at low temperature. These observations caused concern among scientists that dangerous types of botulism existed about which there was insufficient information and that food-processing procedures were inadequate to eliminate these types. Very extensive studies

from 1965 through 1970 have helped to allay these fears, but surveillance must continue so that adequate precautions are followed in the safe and sanitary processing of foods. Within these guidelines the industry must evolve satisfactory procedures for the newer foods such as meat analogs, fortified foods, semidried foods, mildly processed packaged foods, precooked chilled or frozen foods, and other ready-to-eat foods. In all probability, the seventies will witness a dramatic increase in partly or wholly prepared food dishes, and great care will be necessary to avoid hazardous or foolhardy processing innovations or service inadequacies or errors.

Normal Components of Natural Food Products   In the preceding list of potential hazards are several groups of substances and specific chemicals that occur normally in natural food products. The list could be much extended.[8,9]

Any evaluation of the hazards of foods should include a consideration of the chemical substances that constitute their natural composition. All foods in their natural, uncontaminated, "pure" state are composed *only* of chemical substances. Many of these are important for the body economy, provide attractive colors and flavors or determine form and consistency. But the largest number have no recognized importance or function whatever as far as the consumer is concerned. Thousands of specific substances in natural food products have been identified chemically, but it is likely that even a larger number have not. Whether or not a certain food component has a desirable function or has been identified chemically, it is toxicologically axiomatic that it can cause harmful effects in man if consumed in sufficiently large quantity. The toxicity of each of the multitude of the natural chemical components of foods varies to such an extent that some can cause injury under certain unusual circumstances in the amount normally present; others cannot be harmful because their intrinsic toxicities or their concentrations in the foods are so low.

Throughout history man has learned by experience what natural products he can include in his diet with safety, or what precautions or steps he should take to render them safe for consumption. There is still a substantial incidence of illness throughout the world resulting from ignorance or the preponderance, by necessity, of single food products in the diet. Much of this illness is due to nutritional inadequacy or imbalance, but an important contribution is made by the toxic natural components of foods, especially when one kind of food constitutes a large proportion of the diet. For instance, the "macrobiotic" diet, which is practiced by some food cultists, places heavy emphasis on one or two natural products, such as brown rice and seaweed. Diets such as this are potentially hazardous to health because they provide an inadequate amount or balance of essential nutrients or an excessive amount of some natural chemical component. In this instance, the nutritional inadequacy may lead to an increased sensitivity to the toxicity of some natural component.

Many of the chemical substances with recognized toxic properties that are naturally present in our foods have never been known to cause injury in man through his consumption of foods which contain normal levels. Among these may be listed the elements arsenic, mercury, lead, cadmium, cobalt, copper, iron, fluorine, and iodine; and compounds such as vitamin D, tannic acid, safrole, nitrates, and various estrogenic isoflavones. Many foods containing such agents have long been considered safe in spite of the now recognized fact that most of these substances, even some that are nutritionally essential, are present at levels much closer to the known toxic levels than would now be permitted for food additives or pesticide residues. Furthermore, many substances na-

turally present in food products would not be permitted in any amount as food additives because of their suspected carcinogenic, mutagenic or teratogenic properties. This would be notably true for the goitrogenic and estrogenic substances, with known tumorgenic activities, that are widely dispersed in many common items of our diet.

Most of our common natural food products have never been scientifically evaluated for their safety for chronic consumption. They have been accepted as safe because throughout a long history of use they have not produced evident injury when consumed in reasonable amounts by millions of people at frequent intervals over a long period of time. Yet current toxicological philosophy does not accept this as adequate proof of safety. It is recognized that a long delayed harmful effect of a substance consumed with many others may be extremely difficult to relate to that specific substance as its cause. The question persists, therefore, whether any of the natural components of our diet such as the goitrogens, estrogens, cholesterol, arsenic, cadmium, sodium chloride, etc., are responsible for, or contribute to, the ultimate development of chronic degenerative diseases or a shortened life span.

In the light of our present knowledge this question cannot be answered for any single substance or for all the known natural toxic components of foods together. Also, it is not conceivable that any grand research program could be designed that would provide a reliable answer. It seems more reasonable, in the absence of evidence of any insidious long-term effects of the chemical substances naturally present in our diet, to consider our foods safe when consumed in a sensible quantity and variety. Intake of a variety of foods is obviously the best insurance against absorption of toxic amounts of any single food component.

Though much is known about the chemical composition of natural food products and about the toxicology of specific substances in them, our information in these respects is far from complete. Further investigation is necessary to provide full knowledge of the amounts of toxic substances present, and of the quantitative relationship between these amounts and those that might be deleterious. Such information is important to the food industry, which has the obligation to avoid concentrating toxic substances in its processing of foods or in its production of new foods from materials derived from natural products. Similarly plant geneticists and breeders, in their attempts to improve certain aspects of the quality of plant food products, must be alert to the changes that might occur in the content of toxic components in any new plant variety they may develop. An example of what can happen in this respect was seen in 1970 when a new variety of potato was developed in which the level of toxic solanine alkaloids was substantially increased. As a result of this finding, the U.S. Department of Agriculture terminated further development of the new product. Use of breeding methods to produce plant varieties with lower levels of toxic substances of course suggests itself; however, unless a hazard is detected or suspected from the natural presence of a toxic component in a food plant, there would be little urgency in this approach.

An important further reason to have definitive knowledge of the natural levels of toxic substances in foods is to provide a base upon which to assess the significance of man's addition of the same or related substances through his efforts to improve our foods or through his pollution of the environment. The food industry must avoid oversupplementation of its processed foods with those essential nutrients, such as some of the vitamins, minerals and amino acids, that have toxic properties in excessive amounts. In the area of pollution we are currently confronted with the question of how

much of the mercury in our food supply is derived from natural unavoidable sources and how much from man's industrial processes. Similar questions are now being asked in regard to lead, cadmium, and other metals.

Another matter of justifiable concern is the possibility of adverse toxicologic interactions between the natural components of foods and chemicals that are added to foods or gain access in other ways. It is apparent, of course, that all the subliminal toxicities of all the chemicals consumed in our diet are not additive. If they were we would certainly consume a lethal quantity of the aggregate in a short time. A current active field of investigation involves toxicologic interactions between drugs, between pesticides, between drugs and pesticides, and between both these types of agents and other chemicals. But little or no attention in this regard has been given the natural chemical components of foods. Selective exploration in this area may well reveal interactions of interest, if not of potential toxicologic significance.

In spite of these considerations there is no known reason for alarm in regard to the natural chemical components of our foods, though there is a certain element of uncertainty concerning the long range toxicologic significance of some of them. A reasonably diversified diet provides so many different substances that each is consumed in apparently harmless amounts. Grossly abnormal patterns of consumption are necessary to reveal the toxic manifestations of any single agent. At the present time it would not seem reasonable to expect the food and agricultural industries or the regulatory agencies to make any effort to remove or impose limits on, for example, the oxalates in spinach and rhubarb, goitrogens in cabbage or the turnip, estrogens in the carrot, safrole in nutmeg, lycopene in the tomato, or cyanogenetic glycosides in the lima bean. Such things should be known and kept in mind, however, by those involved in food production and food safety, who should remain alert to the potential significance of such substances in relation to food production and processing methods.

Food Chemicals of Man-made Origin

Of the various categories of chemicals listed in the preceding list that enter into foods as a result of man's activities, pesticides and food additives have provoked by far the most controversy and general concern in recent years. Of the other categories, food packaging materials as a potential source of chemicals in foods, and chemical changes induced in foods by processing methods, have hardly achieved public notice. However, in the area of accidental or inadvertent contamination of foods by toxic chemicals, a problem of perennial importance, episodes of variable nature and public-health importance continue to crop up intermittently and unexpectedly, sometimes gaining much public and official regulatory attention. It would be expedient now to look briefly at these latter problems of food toxicology before returning to a general consideration of pesticides and food additives.

Food Packaging Materials More than 500 chemical substances are used in the manufacture of various types of food wrappers or containers. They include prepared papers, parchment, cellophane, acetate films, polyethylene, polyvinyl chloride and acetate, polystyrene, saran, pliofilm, paraffins and other waxes, cloth, wood, cork, metal and metal foils. In these materials, chemicals function as coatings and sizes, pulping agents, germicides, fungicides, plasticizers, stabilizers, antioxidants, adhesives, printing inks, etc.

The technology of the production of packaging materials and of the methods for testing them (*a*) for extent of migration of their chemical components into foods or (*b*) for their interactions with the chemical ingredients of foods have become highly developed and well controlled by law. Any new synthetic film (or paper or other material prepared in a new way) must be tested thoroughly, under a wide range of practical conditions, with all the food products for which it is proposed to be used as a wrapper or container. As a result of established precautions and practices, there is no evidence that toxicologically significant amounts of chemicals are gaining access to our foods from this source.

Heat Processing The safety of the application of heat to cook and preserve foods has never been seriously questioned. On a strictly scientific basis, however, its safety has never been proved by direct testing. However, many of the advantages and benefits of heating or cooking foods have been well demonstrated scientifically, such as killing or destruction of microorganisms or their toxic products and destruction of various natural toxic components of foods such as the goitrogenic substances and the cyanogenetic glycosides in various vegetables, not to mention the improvement in consumer acceptability of flavor, variety, and digestibility. Cooking and some of its attendant processes, of course, are known to reduce the nutrient quality of foods through destruction of vitamins or leaching out of essential minerals. This can be adequately compensated for, however, by supplementation of foods with the required nutrients. Certainly the benefits of cooking or heating foods far outweigh its disadvantages. Indeed, the serious hazard of inadequate use of heat in a commercial process was recently demonstrated by a fatality due to the botulinum toxin in canned potato soup. Insufficient use of heat in home canning has often been the cause of death or illness from this toxin.

Ionizing Radiation　After two decades of intensive studies, fluctuating fortunes and many frustrations, use of ionizing radiation for preservation of foods is still in the throes of development as far as the safety of irradiated food products is concerned. Many chemical changes in foods have been found to result from their exposure to ionizing radiation, including destruction of some vitamins, just as in heat treatment. The significance of some of these changes to the health of experimental animals fed certain irradiated foods throughout their lives has not been clarified.

The technology of the irradiation process, its effectiveness as a preservation measure, its commerical feasibility and its effect on consumer acceptability of irradiated food products, have become well established. The safety of irradiated foods for human consumption, however, has not yet been adequately proved to the satisfaction of government food-safety officials. In 1968, regulations for perviously approved irradiated ham and bacon were withdrawn on the basis of a reexamination of the results of earlier tests on experimental animals and a reevaluation of the data in the light of newly developing criteria of safety. This was a severe setback of the food-irradiation program and led to a renewed attempt to put it on a firm footing as a commercial food-processing method. Now the U.S. Army has launched a comprehensive long-term laboratory test of the safety of irradiated beef. The detailed procedures involved in this test have been approved by committees of qualified scientists and by experts in the Food and Drug Administration. Observations for possible carcinogenic, reproductive, mutagenic, and teratogenic effects in several species of animals will be made, in addition to complete histopathologic and extensive biochemical examinations. These studies and a full evaluation of the results should be completed by 1975.

If it can be proved safe, irradiation of foods would be of inestimable value. It would permit meat, fish, and poultry products, for example, to be stored or transported without refrigeration for long periods of time. It can substantially prolong the shelf life of fresh fruits and vegetables. The advantages in civilian life and in the delivery of foods to nutritionally needy areas of this country and the world, and to the military in the field, is abundantly self-evident. It is to be hoped that in this decade the usefulness of the irradiation of foods will be finally evaluated.

Accidental or Inadvertent Contamination　The intrusion of toxic chemicals into foods through carelessness or error has always been a frequent cause of serious poisoning in man. The different ways in which adventitious chemicals can gain access to foods are so numerous that only a few illustrations can be provided here.

Food-holding Utensils.　Of much current concern is the contamination of foods by lead and other metals from the glazing of ceramic products used as food or drink containers. Severe lead poisoning of a California family of five was recently reported to have been caused by use for several years of a Mexican earthenware pitcher to hold orange juice. There is nothing new, however, in this hazardous association between foods and their containers. It is thought that the Romans suffered from chronic lead poisoning when they drank wine from pewter mugs. Thirty years ago numerous cases of acute cadmium poisoning occurred from acid foods kept in cadmium-galvanized containers. Antimony and zinc from kitchen utensils have also been the cause of illness. Use of toxic materials in the manufacture of all types of products for holding foods can be controlled by government regulation, but this control could not be expected to reach every conceivable article any individual might use out of his ingenuity. One could hardly blame government laxity for illness that might result when someone finds a flower pot to be a handy receptacle for lemonade.

Environmental Pollution. A considerable stir was created in mid-1970 by the finding of unexpected levels of mercury in canned tuna and swordfish and later also in fresh specimens of these and other fish. Though part of this contamination is assumed to have reached the fish through industrial pollution of their environment, undoubtedly a natural background of mercury in the water has made a contribution. Surprisingly high levels have been found in waters in localities where industrial waste is obviously not a factor. Thus mercury might be considered a normal and natural chemical component of fish. The situation is complicated, however, by the wide variability in the mercury content of natural unpolluted waters and the variable tendencies of different kinds of fish to accumulate a body load, depending on their comparative metabolic rates and the duration of their lives.

A beneficial result of the finding of the hazards of lead in ceramic glazes and of mercury in fish has been a flurry of analytical work to determine the levels and distribution of these and other toxic metals in foods and in other aspects of our environment. Since the nature of the compound in which the metal exists may be an important factor in the hazards involved, attention is also being paid to this problem. The compound methyl mercury, for example, is considered the primary hazard in fish. In the meantime, a limit of 0.5 part per million, officially set as a temporary guideline for mercury in fish, is estimated to permit safe consumption of three pounds of fish per week. Thus, only a person on a diet inordinately high in fish is thought to be at risk. Guidelines have also been set for permissible levels of lead and cadmium in earthenware products.

It is hoped and expected that in the next few years knowledge of the toxic metals and their compounds in our environment will lead to satisfactory evaluations of their hazards to public health and to conclusions as to what should be done to avoid undue exposure to these agents.

For the last 20 years there has been some anxiety about contamination of food sources by radioactive fallout following testing of nuclear weapons or from other applications of atomic energy. Of the radionuclides resulting from early above-ground weapons testing the most important were strontium 90, cesium 137 and iodine 131. Strontium 90 was considered the most hazardous because of its long half-life, its tendency to concentrate in the bones, and its effective transmission through the food chain. Surveys in the United States following the tests of the early sixties revealed trace amounts of these agents as contaminants in milk, vegetables, wheat and other cereals, fruits, meats, and eggs. At no time, however, did radioactivity in foods reach a level considered significant to the public health, and the level has declined in recent years because of the cessation of the type of weapons testing that gives rise to fallout. At present a concern is expressed by some in regard to the possibility of radioactive contamination in the neighborhood of nuclear power plants. There is as yet no good evidence that the food supply is endangered in such areas.

Chemical and Food Transport. Some of the largest and most serious outbreaks of poisoning have been caused by contamination of foods being shipped with toxic chemicals. The insecticide parathion shipped in liquid form has been most often implicated. In India in 1958 more than 100 persons were killed by grain contaminated by parathion that had leaked from its containers during shipment. In Wales 59 people were severely poisoned by bread made from flour transported in a freight car that had just previously carried a cargo of the highly toxic insecticide endrin. In 1967 in Tijuana, Mexico, 17 children died and 250 other children and adults were made ill from bread baked with flour that had been stored near parathion in a warehouse. Similar needless tragedies have been reported from other countries.

This type of accidental contamination of foods could be readily prevented by strict enforcement of regulations requiring adequate separation of food products and toxic chemicals during shipping and storage.

Household Accidents. Occasionally poisoning has been reported to result from a housewife mistaking, for example, sodium fluoride cockroach powder for baking powder, barium carbonate rat poison for flour, or boric acid for sugar. In Korea in 1954, 14 persons became ill and two died when they ate food to which warfarin had been added as a rat poison. In 1964 five deaths and six other cases of poisoning in infants resulted in a hospital nursery from the use of a boric acid solution instead of distilled water in preparation of a milk formula. The kitchen is a common site of storage for highly toxic household chemicals that might be placed alongside packaged foods or materials to be used in cooking. Under these conditions an occasional slip might be expected of a careless, absent-minded, nearsighted or tipsy housewife. Children "playing around" at cooking might also cause contamination of edibles.

Episodes of this kind are difficult to prevent by official regulatory mechanisms. Enforced precautionary labeling of hazardous chemicals for domestic use is an approach to the problem but this offsets the causes of human error only to a small degree. Characteristically shaped containers for such substances, with special mechanisms for opening, may make some contribution to safety. Public-education programs are notably ineffective because they reach only a few and many of those reached soon forget their lessons. Perhaps a presidential proclamation of a food-safety week would be of some added benefit if it was attended by sufficient "noise" through the public-communications media.

Miscellaneous. In Turkey thousands of people were poisoned in 1960 when seed grain treated with benzene hexachloride as a fungicide was diverted in error into human food channels. A fatal misuse of seed grain treated with a mercurial fungicide occurred recently in the U.S. when a farmer fed his hogs the grain and later butchered the animals for consumption by his family. Lead poisoning has resulted from bread baked in ovens in which lead-painted wood was used as fuel. More than 300 Australian soldiers became ill from meat cooked on skewers cut from oleander bushes, which contained a potent heart poison as a natural constituent. In 1964 an outbreak of strammonium poisoning occurred in Tennessee when a tomato grower grafted tomato plants to jimson weeds to produce a hardier tomato plant; the toxic strammonium, similar to the drug atropine, appeared in the tomatoes that went to market. The tyramine content of certain cheeses, as in aged cheddars, Stilton, Brie, and Camembert, has been responsible for serious hypertensive reactions in patients under therapy with various drugs classed as monoamine-oxidase inhibitors; these drugs suppress the normally rapid detoxication of tyramine. Outbreaks of honey poisoning have occurred in the U.S. and Europe when bees collect nectar from mountain laurel, oleander, rhododendron or azalea; these plants contain glycosides that are potent heart stimulants.

This short miscellany of examples illustrates how unexpected hazards might arise from unfortunate combinations of circumstances in which only man is at fault or in which nature plays a role over which man has no control until after he has learned by experience.

Agricultural Chemical Residues and Food Additives

Those aspects of food safety that have received the most persistent attention from government officials and the public in the past 15 years involve chemical substances that man has employed in his well-intentioned efforts to produce more and better foods: the pesticides used in agriculture and the additives used in commercial processing of foods.

These efforts have been rigidly and effectively controlled by law under the 1954 Pesticide, the 1958 Food Additive, and the 1960 Color Additive amendments to the Federal Food, Drug, and Cosmetic Act. When pesticides and food additives have been used in accordance with regulations and with what is accepted as good agricultural and manufacturing practice, they have caused no known harm to the human consumer. In spite of this fact the simmering controversy about the safety of these substances over more than a decade was brought to a boil recently by several restrictive actions against use of certain pesticides and food additives. The use of DDT as an insecticide, for example, has been drastically curtailed because it has progressively accumulated in our environment, apparently interferes with reproductive processes in certain forms of wildlife, and has been shown to produce liver tumors in laboratory animals fed high levels. The cyclamates, artificial sweetening agents, were officially banned as a result of some highly controversial evidence that they may be carcinogenic, mutagenic, and teratogenic. The use of monosodium glutamate, a naturally occurring amino acid widely employed as a flavor enhancer, was voluntarily discontinued by the food industry in its processing of baby foods when it was reported to cause cell damage in the hypothalamus in the brain when administered to infant mice. Though

there were certain elements of justification, aside from considerations of food safety, in such actions as these, there was still no evidence that the extensive use and presence of these agents in foods over many years had caused any adverse effects in the human consumer. Some years ago, use of coumarin and safrole, flavoring agents of natural origin, and agene, a bleaching agent for flour, was discontinued when it was shown that they produced toxic effects in experimental animals fed very large doses, again in the face of no evidence of adverse effect of these agents in humans after long use.

The toxicologic and regulatory philosophy behind these withdrawals of items longstanding in our diet is based on a mixture of ignorance and prudence. When a substance long present as an additive or residue in foods without apparent harm in humans is found to cause an effect of a serious nature in experimental animals, such as tumors, alteration in reproductive function, or unexplained cellular damage in a vital organ, even though fed throughout the animal's lifetime at dietary levels greatly in excess of those consumed under any circumstances in the human diet, then prudence may dictate cessation of use of that substance. It is frequently not possible to apply fully reasoned scientific judgment in the matter because of several unknown factors. It is not known if the effect observed in the animal would ever occur in man at any dietary level. Also assuming that man does respond with the same effect, it is not known how much more sensitive or resistant than the animal man might be. It is not known at what level in the diet there would be no effect in man, again assuming he is responsive. If the substance has a given observed harmful effect in the animal it is not known that it will produce the same type of injury in the human. Finally, since no group of human beings has been observed scientifically throughout lifetime exposure to any given substance in the diet, ultimate safety cannot be claimed with absolute assurance for any substance.

Thus long-continued and widespread dietary intake of a chemical substance without evidence of any adverse effects does not prove its safety. DDT, for example, has been in our diet for 20 years with no indication of injury to the public health, and much experimental evidence of its safety at existing dietary levels has accumulated. We cannot be certain, however, that it has not caused some injury to health, or that it will not in another 20 or 30 years. Similarly, we do not have scientific proof of the safety of saccharin, which has been in use for 80 years by millions of people with no sign of insidious injurious effects coming to light. Long-delayed harmful effects, especially when they are of infrequent occurrence or when they are mainfested as the common illnesses of mankind, are extremely difficult to attribute to their specific causes. Injury due to unrecognized causes may have been the result of substances that have long been thought safe for use in foods. We are forced, therefore, to be concerned about the possibility that some items lurk in our diet among the food additives and pesticide residues that may play a role in the production of cancer, birth defects, and genetic damage, and of various endocrine, cardiovascular, special sensory and mental disorders that plague mankind. It is this complex of unknowns that explains the conservatism displayed by those who have responsibility for protecting the public health from long-range injury through the food supply.

It was pointed out earlier in this chapter that the natural composition of common food products is much more complex and unknown chemically than is the additive and pesticide residue component, and that many known ingredients of natural products have toxicologic properties, the long-range hazards of which may be even more suspect than those imagined for additives and residues. An authority of the National Cancer Institute, for example, recently stated that he felt that naturally occurring environmental carcinogens are more responsible for cancer of the colon in man than are synthetic food additives. These comparisons of the suspected hazards of the natural and the man-added components of foods do not mean that we can relax our precautions in regard to the additives and pesticides that enter our diet. Indeed it means just the opposite. The presence of many unavoidable toxic chemicals placed in our diet by nature is a compelling reason for us to avoid adding any more, even though it may be only a small percentage increment.

Recommendations

Numerous occurrences in the last few years have brought to a focus what should be done in the next decade to assure the safety of our foods from the standpoint of food additives and residues of agricultural chemicals. The use of DDT has been widely restricted. The cyclamates were banned. The addition of monosodium glutamate to baby foods was discontinued. Broad and far-reaching recommendations were made in regard to the use and assessment of pesticides in the future.[10] The Panel on Food Safety of the White House Conference on Food, Nutrition and Health, in December, 1969, made numerous recommendations designed to improve the safety of foods. The Food and Drug Administration drew up more stringent protocols for the testing of food chemicals for their carcinogenicity, mutagenicity, teratogenicity, and other effects on reproductive physiology. The National Academy of Sciences published a report of its Food Protection Committee in 1970,[11] discussing the principles involved in the toxicological testing of chemicals proposed for use in the production and processing of foods. And finally, the federal budget for 1972 includes funding for a National Center for Toxicological Research at

Pine Bluffs, Arkansas, at which the Food and Drug Administration and other government agencies will participate in research to develop scientific guidelines and protocols for the testing and evaluation of the safety of environmental chemicals, with appropriate emphasis on those associated with foods.

The GRAS List In 1958 the Food and Drug Administration listed about 200 substances that had been used as food additives and were judged by qualified experts as "generally recognized as safe" (GRAS) for addition to foods without being subject to rigorous regulatory control and the requirement of extensive toxicologic testing. This list has since been expanded to include more than 600 items. Widespread distrust of the GRAS list developed when certain hazards of several of its members (such as the cyclamates, saccharin, monosodium glutamate, and the brominated vegetable oils) came under suspicion in 1969. As a result of recommendations from several quarters, the GRAS list is now under comprehensive review to determine the commercial output and the extent and manner of use in foods of each item, and to examine all the toxicologic data known about each. This undertaking will require several years. It is predicted that the GRAS list will survive without extensive changes because it is largely comprised of dietary supplements, such as vitamins and minerals, and of natural flavoring materials and spices that have been used down through the ages.

The Delaney Clause This clause of the 1958 Food Additive Amendment provides that no food additive may be used that is found to produce cancer when ingested by test animals even at excessively high levels in the diet. This concept applies also to pesticides that occur as residue in foods. Recommendations for the revision of this law came recently from two panels of the White House

Conference on Food, Nutrition and Health, from the HEW Commission on Pesticides, and from the Council of the Society of Toxicology.

The Delaney Clause restricts application of sound scientific judgment in determining the safety of chemicals for use in foods. It has never been strictly enforced because it is not possible to do so. Without the Delaney Clause, food-additive law provides adequate mechanisms for preventing addition of hazardous chemicals to foods. The clause does not accept the possibility that a substance that is carcinogenic at high levels in the diet is not carcinogenic at low levels, or that a substance that produces a tumor in one animal species may not produce it in other species or in man. Scientific evidence for both of these possibilities in relation to certain food chemicals is available.

No revision of the Delaney Clause would serve any useful purpose. It should be stricken from the law.

Research There are recognized gaps in our knowledge of the effects of chemicals in the body, of how to interpret subtle observed effects in animals or man in terms that apply to human health, and of how to devise tests that provide data that can be used with confidence in evaluating the safety of food chemicals.

The question of the comparability of man and other animals in response to chemicals has been much discussed. But only a little is known about what accounts for the differences or the similarities of men and other species in their responses to chemicals. Aspirin, for example, causes birth defects in rats but is safe in pregnant women, whereas thalidomide has no such effect in rats but is highly dangerous in pregnant women. Many have urged that the fate and metabolism of a chemical be studied in man as early as possible in its evaluation to ascertain man's similarity in these respects to an animal species that is to be used for complete toxicity tests. One cannot overemphasize the futility and waste of carrying out expensive, long-term, and complex programs of toxicity tests of a substance on a species in which its fate, metabolism, and biochemical effects are markedly different from those in man. This aspect of the safety evaluation of food chemicals should be developed vigorously.

The Dose-Response Relationship and the No-Effect Concept This is one of the most critical and elusive problems in the evaluation of the safety of chemicals. For a serious irreversible effect, such as carcinogenesis, some experts feel they cannot accept the possibility that a carcinogen can be fed at a no-effect level. They feel that we must assume, since the contrary cannot be demonstrated experimentally, that the carcinogenic effect will be seen at any level of the carcinogen in the diet if a large enough group of animals receives it. The mathematical trick of extrapolating the dose-response curve down to zero is of no avail because there is no knowledge of the behavior of the curve as the response approaches zero. Since no feasible way to solve this problem has been suggested, the toxicity evaluation of each individual food chemical has to be achieved on the basis of other accumulated information and judgments, including a consideration of the benefits expected from the use of the chemical in relation to the suspected risks involved in its use.

Perhaps in the near future the congregation of scientific experts at the new National Center for Toxicological Research can do some productive thinking on this problem of dose-response relationship and the no-effect concept. New ideas or philosophy in this area are, of course, as important in other aspects of environmental toxicology as they are in the consideration of food additives and pesticides.

Informing the Public The public should be provided a balance of perspective in mat-

ters pertaining to the safety of chemicals in our foods. The unfavorably biased view that has reached the public through numerous newspaper headlines has been eroding confidence in the safety of the food supply. The public should be assured that much has been and is being done to make its foods safe. It should be made aware of our outstanding record of safety, of how this has been accomplished, and of the reasons for expectations of the future safety of foods.

The number and variety of chemicals used in producing and processing foods are indeed impressive. The very number is the cause of much of the public alarm. But contrary to common opinion the great number of these agents is in itself a contribution to their safety. For example, the larger the number of different insecticides used to control pests on food crops, the more unlikely it is that any one of them will reach harmful levels in our foods. The Joint Food and Agriculture Organization-World Health Organization Expert Committee on Food Additives recently enunciated the same principle in regard to food additives as well as pesticides. This concept is based on the fact that although the body has a limited capacity to tolerate any single chemical substance it has an amazing capacity to tolerate combinations of small amounts of many different ones. The toxicities of each of many different toxic substances taken simultaneously are not additive. This is what enables us to survive a normal well-balanced diet comprised only of food products containing their natural ingredients.

Summary

The attempt has been made in this chapter to present a comprehensive picture, in breadth at the expense of depth, of potentially harmful agents associated with man's foods. Many of these substances have caused much injury to health, notably those present in foods as a result of bacterial infection or contamination by natural toxins, and those entering foods through accidental or unexpected means.

The many toxic chemicals that appear naturally and normally in foods eaten by man in his everyday diet rarely cause trouble under normal patterns of consumption except in cases of allergic sensitivities or individual intolerances. Some of them, however, may also be harmful under conditions of gross departure from a balanced diet or in persons made unusually sensitive by disease.

There is no evidence that food additives (whether they are intentionally added, as in food processing, or whether they enter food incidentally when used as packaging materials, as pesticides or as plant or animal growth regulators) are exerting any adverse effect on the public health. The existing laws and regulations controlling the use of these materials have been highly effective in insuring their safety when used properly. In the area of food additives and pesticide residues, however, the chronicity of their intake, and the fact that the general population is their captive consumer, necessitate rigid regulatory control and the continued development and practice of preventive toxicology. Since 1969 several episodes and numerous recommendations relating to considerations of food safety have set the stage for improved controls and pertinent research that promise greater assurance of the long-range safety of our food supply.

REFERENCES

1. Center for Disease Control, 1970. *Foodborne Outbreaks Annual Summary.* Department of Health, Education, and Welfare, U.S. Public Health Service, Washington, D.C.

2. Dack, G. M., 1956. The Role of Enterotoxin of Micrococcus Pyogenes var. Aureus in the Etiology of Pseudomembranous Enterocolitis. *American Journal of Surgery* 92:765–769.

3. Bergdoll, M. S., 1967. The Staphylococcal Enterotoxins. In Mateles, R. J., and Wogan, G. N., eds., *Biochemistry of Some Foodborne Microbial Toxins.* M.I.T. Press, Cambridge, Massachusetts.

4. Smith, N. R., Gordon, R. E., and Clark, F. E., 1952. *Aerobic Sporeforming Bacteria.* Agricultural Monograph 16, U.S. Department of Agriculture, Washington, D.C.

5. Molnar, D. M., 1962. Separation of the Toxin of Bacillus Cereus into Two Components and Non-identity of the Toxin with Phospholipase. *Journal of Bacteriology* 84: 147–153.

6. Thorne, C. B., Molnar, D. M., and Strange, R. E., 1960. Production of Toxin in Vitro by Bacillus Anthracis and its Separation into Two Components. *Journal of Bacteriology* 79: 450–455.

7. Johnson, C. E., and Bonventre, P. F., 1967. Lethal Toxin of Bacillus Cereus. 1. Relationship and Nature of Toxin, Hemolysin, and Phospholipase. *Journal of Bacteriology* 94: 306–316.

8. National Research Council, 1966. *Naturally Occurring Toxicants in Foods.* National Academy of Sciences Publication 1354. Washington, D.C.

9. Liener, I. E., ed., 1969. *Toxic Constitutents of Plant Food Stuffs.* Academic Press, Inc., Palisades, New York.

10. *Report of the Secretary's Commission on Pesticides and Their Relationship to Environmental Health,* 1969. Department of Health, Education, and Welfare, Washington, D.C.

11. Food Protection Committee, National Research Council, 1970. *Evaluating the Safety of Food Chemicals.* National Academy of Sciences, Washington, D.C.

Chapter 12

Distribution of Food

Gordon F. Bloom

The private-sector food-distribution system in the United States has been lauded and extolled as the finest in the world. No other nation spends such a small proportion of its total income for food as the United States and no other food system delivers such a variety of product at such low cost as that in America. It is no accident that when Khrushchev visited the United States some years ago, among the national institutions that he asked to see was a typical American supermarket.

It came as a shock, therefore, to the American food industry as well as to the public at large to learn that in this land of plenty there were millions of Americans who were undernourished and that this condition existed even among the more affluent members of our society. A study of approximately 7,500 housekeeping units conducted in 1965 revealed that 37 percent of the families in the lowest income groups (under $3,000) had diets rated "good" in contrast to 63 percent in the $10,000-and-over income group.[1] It is not surprising that the higher the income of a family, the better the diet nutritionally. What is surprising is that even in high-income groups almost two out of every five families had diets that evidenced some nutritonal deficiency.

The American food industry has demonstrated its ability to "deliver the goods." The question now being asked is whether the private-sector distribution system can deliver nutrition efficiently and at low cost to the American public.

In this chapter we shall direct our attention to the role that can and should be played by food retailers in providing better nutrition for American consumers. We shall be looking at the 208,000 food stores, chain and independent, supermarkets, superettes, and small stores, which in 1970, according to *Progressive Grocer* of April 1971, accounted for 88 billion dollars of food sales to American consumers.

The thousands of merchants who operate these stores are part of an elaborate and highly sophisticated system of distribution that has evolved over the years in response to the needs of consumers and the legal, institutional, and competitive conditions peculiar to food marketing. The primary objective of this system has been to deliver to customers at the lowest possible prices the products that they demonstrate they wish to consume by their purchases. Whether their buying behavior has been rational or not has not, until recently, been an issue. The system has responded to the dollar bill in the hands of the customer and has assumed that the customer can make an intelligent choice.

In a sense, the retail food industry in this country has served as the buying agent for the consumer. It buys and stocks what the customer wants. Frequently buyers for retail food organizations will purchase newly offered products that they believe customers will want, only to find that their judgment was wrong and that the new products will not sell. When this occurs, no amount of merchandising and promotion will make a "fast mover" out of a "dead item." The customer, not the store operator, makes the ultimate decision as to what will be stocked and displayed in our food stores.

Can this complex system be modified or adapted in such a way that customer decisions are influenced in the direction of more intelligent attention to nutrition? Can the supermarket function not only as a channel to the customer but also as a marketing counselor? It is to be hoped that the answer is in the affirmative and that these new functions can be assumed by the food-retailing system while still maintaining the essential principle of exercise of freedom of choice by the consumer. However, the manner of implementing such change is by no means clear. As will be seen from the following discussion, the private-sector food-distribution system operates under major limitations in the drive for improved nutrition and many of the major solutions to the problem of nutritional deficiencies are outside its purview.

One such key variable is income. Although, as has already been mentioned, nutritional deficiency can be found at all income levels, the single most important cause of malnutrition is lack of income. If we examine the makeup of the group of approximately 25 million Americans who constitute our poor, we can see very clearly how provision of adequate income is and must be the primary and essential step to better nutrition.

Twenty percent of the poor , or 5.1 million Americans, live in families whose yearly household income is less than the cost of the U.S. Department of Agriculture Economy Diet alone—less than the equivalent of $1,200 a year for a family of four.[2] Obviously the needs of this group must be met through food assistance by government or they are certain to suffer from chronic nutritional deficiencies.

Thirty-seven percent of the poor (9.3 million Americans) live in families whose incomes are less than twice the cost of the economy diet.[2] Unless they are receiving food assistance, they too are likely to be victims of poverty-related hunger and malnutrition. Like the first category, this group must look first to government for assistance.

Of the currently estimated 25 million poor 10.6 million have incomes between two and three times the cost of an economy diet or between $2,400 and $3,600.[2] While they are not certain to be suffering from malnutrition, they probably suffer from periods of nutritional deficiency.

The extent to which the existing private-enterprise food system can help bring better nutrition to these different groups varies, depending in part upon their income level and in part upon their location and buying habits. Unfortunately the very poor are often located in rural areas or in inner-city ghettos where the most advanced facilities and the most progressive operators in the food industry are least likely to be. The poor have little access to the food-distribution system in this country; this is one of the major limitations that we shall discuss at greater length in the following pages.

This brief catalog of the problems of the American poor serves to place the role of the private sector in clearer perspective. The major problem is not the functioning of the private-enterprise food-distribution system— it is the distribution of income. However, there are ways in which food retailing can assist in bringing better nutrition to all Americans. In the following discussion we shall examine a number of possible avenues that involve action by retailers in the following areas:

1. more efficient distribution with the objective of reducing the cost of food or preventing inflationary increases in food prices;
2. provision of adequate retail facilities, particularly in inner-city ghettos;

3. cooperative efforts to broaden the use of food stamps;
4. promotion and sale of enriched foods;
5. participation in a broad-based educational campaign to improve awareness of nutrition.

Before we turn to an examination of each of these possibilities, it may be useful to consider briefly some of the salient features of the retail food industry as it is conducted in the American economy.

The Economics of Food Retailing

At the White House Conference on Food, Nutrition and Health, suggestions were made that retail food stores carry special enriched products at low cost in plain packages for low-income buyers. Other participants recommended that the federal government purchase certain nutritious foods, package them inexpensively, and have them distributed through private food stores at a profit margin of 10 percent.

In order to appraise the practicability of these and other recommendations, it is important to understand how food stores operate. The retail food industry in the United States is a business that operates on large volumes at paper-thin profit margins. In 1970, retail food chains reporting to the Figure Exchange maintained by Cornell University in cooperation with the National Association of Food Chains recorded net earnings after taxes of only 0.92 percent on sales.[3] In other words, the retailer kept less than one cent as profit out of the dollar that the customer spent in shopping at the store.

Compared with other industries, the food industry shows meager profits. In 1970 there was only one retail food chain in the list of the 100 most profitable companies in the United States and that corporation—Safeway

Stores—was Number 100 on the list. In the same year only seven food chains made the list of the 500 most profitable corporations. The sales of these seven large chains totaled almost 20 billion dollars—more than twice the sales of Sears Roebuck Company—yet the profits of that great retail organization were almost twice as great as the combined profits of the seven large food chains, according to *Forbes*, pp. 115–127, May 15, 1971.

Not only is the margin of profits low in the retail food industry but the trend has been downward, whether measured as a percentage of sales or as return on net worth. As a percentage of sales, net earnings fell from 1.32 percent in 1961 to 0.92 percent in 1970.[3] As a percentage of net worth, earnings fell from 11.25 percent in 1961 to 9.34 percent in 1970.[3] The reduction in profit ratios reflects the combined effect of higher occupancy costs, increased wage rates, the spread of discounting, and other factors.

To most Americans the retail food industry is symbolized by the supermarket. In 1970, out of the total food industry sales of 88 billion dollars, slightly over three-quarters was accounted for by sales in supermarkets.* Although the bulk of retail food sales is conducted through supermarkets, the latter type of outlet represents only about 18 percent of total food stores. Of the total of 208,000 retail food stores in the United States, over 65 percent are small stores with annual sales of less than $150,000.* In considering the role of the retail food industry in bringing better nutrition to the poor, it is important to realize that a very high proportion of the poor in this nation, both in rural and urban locations, are served by such small stores.

The supermarket survives on its narrow margin of profit only through a delicate

Progressive Grocer, April 1971, p. 66. *Progressive Grocer* defines a supermarket as a retail food store, chain or independent, doing $500,000 in sales or more per year.

balance of its merchandise mix. Basic volume items such as coffee, butter, baby food, and shortening are typically sold at or near cost. In many areas the entire gross mark-up in the dry grocery department is 12 to 15 percent, yet the total operating costs of the store will approximate 20 percent. It is obvious that the supermarket must display and promote high-profit impulse items such as health and beauty aids, frozen foods, convenience foods, and similar products in order to meet its expenses.

The items it displays, therefore, must be carefully selected for movement and profit. Most products move very slowly—studies indicate that about 50 percent of the items in a market move only two to four packages per week. With close to 8,000 items in stock and a limited amount of display space, it is important for the store operator that every new item pay its way. The problem of shelf space is becoming more acute because of the continuing flood of new items. By 1980 many food-chain officials predict there will be 10,000 items on display in supermarkets.

In view of the foregoing circumstances, supermarkets could not take on a new line of enriched foods and sell them at, say a 10 percent mark-up without raising other prices to balance the marketing mix. On the other hand, enrichment of existing foods would not produce a similar problem. Recommendations with respect to the role of food retailing in providing better nutrition must take account of the peculiar operating problems of supermarkets if they are to be accepted and promoted by the food industry.

Nutrition and the Cost of Food

In May 1969, in his Message on Hunger, President Nixon stated, "Millions of Americans are simply too poor to feed their families properly. For them there must be first sufficient food income." The ability of poor families to purchase sufficient food for an adequate diet depends, on the one hand, upon the amount of their gross income or supplementary benefits (such as food stamps) and, on the other hand, upon the level of food prices. The private food-distribution system cannot do much about the former, but it must and can do something about the cost of the products it sells to consumers.

The cost of food has for many years been intimately related to the statistical concept of poverty in this country. For statistical purposes, the Social Security Administration—which sets the "poverty index"—designates a family as poor when its income does not exceed three times the cost of obtaining food. Thus any family (or unrelated person) that cannot buy the food it needs for 33 percent of its total income is assumed to have to go either without sufficient food or without other basic living necessities. It is therefore defined as a poor family.

In 1966, the poverty index was based on a yearly income of $3,335 or three times the assumed minimum food cost of $1,111.67. The latter figure was based on the Department of Agriculture's so-called "Economy Food Plan" which provided a minimum diet for a family of four. Figures in the *New York Times*, November 14, 1971, p. 41, show that as food and other costs have increased, the poverty threshold has risen and in 1970 stood at $3,968 for an urban family of four.

It is apparent therefore that if the private food-distribution system, through some superhuman effort, could reduce the price of food substantially, this would reduce the number of "poor" in our society. On the other hand, if food prices should commence rising rapidly, the consequence could be a rise in the number of persons statistically classified as "poor."

Wholly aside from the statistical effect of a rise in food prices, it is obvious that such a trend would impose a very heavy burden upon the poor. For the average American,

who spends only 17 percent of his income on food, a rise in food prices would be reason for resentment and complaint. But for the poor and the near poor, who must spend almost one-third of their incomes on food, such a contingency would be calamitous.

In a very real sense, therefore, the major contribution that the private-sector distribution system can make to the problem of hunger and malnutrition in this country is to improve its efficiency and productivity so that food can continue to be a bargain in our society. This will be no easy task in the years ahead, for a confluence of factors now threaten an unprecedented inflation of food costs.

These inflationary forces derive from the changing conditions discussed below.

Agriculture   Despite the rapid improvement of productivity in agriculture, farm prices may nevertheless advance sharply in the decade ahead. The fact is that the food on the table of the American consumer has been subsidized for many years by the substandard working conditions of agricultural—and particularly migratory—workers. These conditions are about to change. It seems likely that the next few years will see both an extension of the minimum wage on a uniform basis to agricultural workers and a major growth of union power on the farm. Farm operators are particularly vulnerable to strikes called at harvesting time—a fact that workers will hardly lose sight of in their bargaining strategy. The result will be strikes with a loss of crops and/or substantial increases in wages, fringe benefits, and improvement of working conditions. American housewives who participated in the grape boycott may be surprised to learn what the success of Cesar Chavez means when it is converted into the price they must pay for a head of lettuce.

Consumerism   The main thrust of the consumer-rights movement has been directed at the supermarket. The objectives of consumer advocates are legitimate, but they will unquestionably add to the cost of food in the years ahead. Programs such as unit-pricing add costs to the distributive process by requiring more administrative time, more labor at the store level, more computer operation, etc. One large food chain has calculated that the installation and maintenance of a unit-price system will cost about 0.1 percent of sales. This does not sound like much, but the reader will note that the whole profit of food chains after taxes was only 0.9 percent. Most studies have demonstrated that the poor have little interest in programs such as unit-pricing and that it is primarily the better-educated middle-income suburban shopper who makes use of these calculations in formulating buying decisions. (The question must be asked whether such programs are desirable if the net effect is to tax the poor for the benefit of the more affluent.)

Ecology   Legislation restricting emissions into the atmosphere will affect food-processing plants, warehouses, and stores along with all other establishments. Of particular concern to the supermarket industry, however, is the development of state and national policy that is directed toward banning the nonreturnable bottle. Such action, although possibly beneficial from the point of view of society at large, would impose major costs upon the food industry. For the retailer in particular, handling of the returnable bottle is time-consuming and requires considerable space for collection, sorting, and storing. One large food chain has estimated that total conversion to the returnable bottle would decrease productivity at the store level, as measured by sales per man-hour, approximately 4 percent and would increase store labor costs 0.26 percent. Again, these are small percentages, but the retail food industry is a business of decimal points, and these small amounts multiplied by the billions of dollars of sales mean millions of dollars of additional costs to American consumers.

The Wage Explosion   Of all the inflationary trends affecting the food industry, the most serious threat to cost stability is posed by the apparent acceleration of the rate of increase in wages. Food retailing uses labor intensively. About one-half of all store level costs are labor costs. For many years wages in the retail food industry advanced at an average annual rate of about 5 percent, while productivity increased at a rate of about 3 percent per annum. The net upward movement of food prices therefore was minimal.

Today, however, in many areas of the country, the rate of increase in wages in food retailing is in excess of that recorded in the construction industry. In Chicago, for example, recent settlements with the Retail Clerks Union amounted to 35 percent to 44 percent over two years. Male clerks won wage increases of $50 per week over the two-year period. In the same city the Meatcutters Union obtained wage increases of 31 percent to 39 percent over an 18-month period. Similar adjustments are now being recorded in other localities.

Obviously, cost increases of the magnitude described cannot be absorbed by an industry that already operates on such narrow profit margins. Nor is the present rate of productivity improvement likely to afford much relief. The U.S. Department of Labor, Bureau of Labor Statistics has estimated that the annual rate of increase in man-hour output in the retail food industry for the balance of the decade will approximate past performance and will average about 3 percent. With wage adjustments of the size indicated, and other costs added to this burden, it is quite possible that food prices could move up at an annual rate of 6 to 10 percent unless a major effort is made to improve productivity in the industry.

President Nixon appointed a National Commission on Productivity to study the problem of lagging productivity in this country and to determine what role, if any, government can play in stimulating the rate of annual improvement in man-hour output. The primary reason for establishment of this commission was apparently a hope that appropriate action might accelerate the rate of annual improvement in productivity and thereby dampen the inflationary forces in the economy. It probably was not recognized that, at least in the food industry, a national commitment to productivity is closely related to the national commitment for improved nutrition.

It is to be hoped that the commission will in the near future appoint a committee of industry leaders to investigate what practical steps can be taken to improve productivity in the food industry. Without affirmative industry action and appropriate support from government, there is a very real danger that food prices will begin rising faster than other elements in the cost of living index and will render even more difficult the complex task of delivering a minimum nutritious diet to the poor of this nation.

The food industry is basically a "pass-through" business. Because profits are already low, increases in cost tend to be passed on to consumers, although admittedly with some lag. While rising costs may force industries such as the shoe business and the textile business into bankruptcy and bring in a flood of imports, this is not likely to happen to the retail food business. Individual stores or companies may go out of business, but in the long run the increasing costs of operation will be paid for by the American public.

Adequate Food-Marketing Facilities for the Poor

As has already been observed, the benefits of the modern American food-distribution system are not uniformly distributed. By and large, the supermarket is a suburban development. The poor in both our rural and urban areas frequently have no choice but to shop at smaller, less efficient stores that charge higher prices than the large efficient markets found in our suburbs. However, the problems of urban and rural shopping are essentially different. Let us examine each of these problems in turn.

The Problem of Ghetto Food Marketing

Numerous studies that have been conducted by governmental agencies and other groups substantiate the fact that the inner-city poor pay more for food in our society.[4] Although some studies by private groups purport to show that higher prices are charged as a matter of policy by chain stores and that prices are manipulated so as to be higher when welfare checks are issued, investigations by governmental agencies such as the Bureau of Labor Statistics, the Federal Trade Commission, and by the U.S. Department of Agriculture[5] have generally refuted this thesis and have shown that the high cost of food for the poor is a consequence of two factors:

a. In the first place, persons with low incomes have different shopping patterns than persons with higher incomes. The poor resident of the ghetto shops many times a week, each time buying a few items. The shopper (usually a woman) does not have a car available and therefore cannot easily shop around for bargains. The typical pattern is a hand-to-mouth existence, buying on a daily basis what is needed. In poor neighborhoods, for example, small sizes are more popular than relatively cheaper larger sizes of packaged food.[4]

For ethnic and other reasons, the ghetto shopper often feels more comfortable in the small store where she may know the owner and where frequently she may require an extension of credit. For example, research findings indicate that Puerto Ricans prefer traditional small stores (perhaps because of the language problem) to large impersonal price-competitive outlets. The same is true of Negro migrants from the rural South.[6]

For these reasons, without a major change in income for families living in urban ghetto areas, it is not at all clear that if more supermarkets were available in such areas, residents would change their shopping patterns and leave the small corner store for the large impersonal market.

b. In the second place, it is a fact that there are few supermarkets in ghetto areas. The number of square feet of supermarket space per resident is much lower in all inner-city areas than in the suburbs. The primary reason is the lack of available land. The modern supermarket requires a large flat piece of land and such areas are difficult to find in cities. Sometimes the needed land area can be put together by tearing down old buildings, but then the land-acquisition costs and real-estate taxes may make the occupancy cost too high to permit operation of a profitable market.

There are other important deterrents to the construction of new markets in such areas. Experience has demonstrated that the operating cost of a market in a ghetto area can be 2 to 3 percent higher than that of a suburban market. High occupancy costs, low productivity of labor, high pilferage rates—all contribute to high operation costs. Even the small size of orders is a problem. Obviously it costs more to process ten orders of $2 each than one order of $20.

From the merchandising side, it has been found that poor people tend to pick up primarily the basic items such as coffee, bread, potatoes, milk, etc.—items that are generally sold at anywhere from cost to about 10 percent gross profit in the average market. Markets make their money by selling impulse items—the frozen foods, fancy produce,

health and beauty aids, etc. But poor people cannot include such items in their budgets. As a result, the operator of a market in the ghetto is faced by a squeeze between high operating costs on the one hand and low gross margin on the other.

Perhaps the greatest deterrent to construction of new markets in black ghetto areas is the fear of violence. Crimes of a violent nature are a frequent occurrence on ghetto streets, especially robbery, aggravated assault, forcible rape, burglary, and similar crimes. The National Advisory Commission on Civil Disorders found that low-income black areas have significantly higher crime rates than low-income white areas.[7] The ever-present threat of riots and bombing in such areas has made fire insurance extremely costly and in many cases impossible to obtain.

The most serious consequence of the violence that has become an integral part of black ghetto life is that it erects a barrier around such areas and effectively keeps good employees—both black and white—from working in such stores. Furthermore, supervisors are reluctant to visit the stores and employees are afraid to work late at night.

As a result of these and related problems, few if any new markets are being built in such areas. Many of those that are still operating are inadequate in size and do not contain modern equipment and satisfactory refrigeration facilities.

The situation is bad today, but it is likely to become even worse with each passing year. Trends in the retail food industry indicate clearly that within the next decade the middle-size supermarket will become obsolete. There will be only very large markets—averaging four to five million dollars per year—and small stores, which will provide convenience and speed in checkout time but will charge higher prices. Higher labor costs and the cost of new automated equipment are making the minimum size of a profitable market larger. Obviously this trend will further complicate the task of finding adequate land areas in the ghetto. With larger size will come greater automation, higher productivity, and lower prices. But these benefits will not be shared with the ghetto resident unless governmental assistance intervenes to make it attractive for private companies to operate in ghetto areas.

What needs to be done to assure adequate facilities to sell food at retail at low prices to the urban poor? A number of proposals have been made, but all have their shortcomings.

Black Capitalism. If white operators cannot run supermarkets successfully in black ghetto areas, why not sell such markets to blacks and let them operate them? The idea may seem sound, but it overlooks the fact that changing the color of the skin of the operator does not make the problems go away. As a matter of fact, most black operators of ghetto supermarkets have precisely the same difficulties as their white counterparts—and more.[8] Few black grocers are qualified to operate a store with such narrow profit margins, where success depends upon knowledge of fine operational details. Furthermore, instead of flocking to black-owned markets, most black customers have a deep skepticism as to the ability of a black to compete effectively with the big white food corporations. Therefore, most black operators have found it difficult to attract and hold their trade.

Despite the problems experienced by black owners of supermarkets, it seems likely that in the years ahead there will be more stores available for sale in ghetto areas than qualified black operators who can run them. It is essential therefore that the retail food industry, in cooperation with the federal government, inaugurate a large-scale intensive training program for black store managers so that out of this pool can come some people qualified to assume entrepreneurial roles in ghetto food marketing.

Community Cooperatives. A frequently suggested solution to business problems in ghetto neighborhoods is the utilization of cooperatives or so-called community development corporations. Advocates of such forms of business organization argue that cooperative community action assures wide community support, provides a broader capital base, and enables the new venture to prolong its staying power during the difficult first years of operation. Although any device that provides capital and strengthens the ability of a ghetto enterprise to survive deserves careful attention, actual experience with cooperatives in black supermarket operations has not been encouraging. The simple fact is that the cooperative idea—even when modified by the community development corporation form—is not an efficient mechanism for operating a business. In the ghetto, as elsewhere, cooperatives have typically been beset by internal conflicts and have failed to bring to management the expertise required to run a business profitably.

Government Subsidy. It seems likely that some form of government subsidy will ultimately be required to offset the cost differential of doing business in the ghetto. This is true not only of the retail food business, but also of other types of retail outlets. Some experts have suggested a tax credit as an incentive but this would be of little value to the one-store operator who was losing money in a ghetto operation, although it would be helpful to a food chain. Another kind of recommendation involves government guarantees against loss resulting from looting, burning, civil disorders, etc.[9] This would be helpful but would hardly bring an influx of new investors into the ghetto. The problems of ghetto retailing are too acute to respond to half-way measures. Perhaps we need to draw on the experience of Puerto Rico, which was able to attract new investment into its disadvantaged economy through a well-conceived and highly attractive package of tax benefits and subsidies. We need to look at our own ghetto areas as disadvantaged economies, and we ought to devise legislation that will not merely plug some of the holes but will actually make it more attractive and profitable for business to locate in such areas rather than elsewhere. This can be done, but it is doubtful that the American public at this juncture is ready to generate the tax dollars that would be needed to implement such a program.

Government Commissaries. In some large cities, if private enterprise fails to provide the needed retail food facilities, it may be necessary for government to take land by eminent domain, erect a large modern market, and then arrange to have an experienced private company operate the store on a fee basis, with the understanding that losses through inventory shortages over an agreed-upon figure would be absorbed by the government. Such an operation would bring lower prices for food to ghetto residents; however, it would also hasten the demise of the existing small stores and older markets in the area. Therefore, it is a step that ought not to be taken unless all other measures fail.

Other Possibilities. Not all ghetto areas are large. In many cities, there are modern retail food facilities in adjacent parts of the city that could be utilized by ghetto residents if more convenient low-cost transportation were available. Operation of special buses or perhaps issuance of transportation stamps to the poor that could be used on public transportation might enable more of the ghetto residents to shop at modern food facilities.

The Problem of Rural Food Marketing Almost one-half of all the poor in this country live in rural sections outside of the metropoliton areas of the nation.[10] Although numerous studies have been made of the marketing problems facing the urban poor, very little is

know about the problems of the rural poor. They have not been militant; many have scruples about taking government aid. Their voice has not been heard.

Do the rural poor pay more for their food than middle-class suburbanites? If so, how much? We do not have the answers to these questions. We know that only small food stores can exist in rural areas because of the lack of the sales volume necessary to support a large supermarket. How much higher are the prices of given items in such stores than in large markets in nearby cities? It is possible that low occupancy costs and low labor costs may enable operators of such small stores to operate with less of an upcharge than the typical small food store in the ghetto.

As has already been mentioned, the marketing problems of the poor in rural areas are essentially different than those in the ghetto. In the latter case, the density of population is available to support modern supermarketing; the roadblocks are lack of land and operational difficulties. In rural areas, by contrast, it simply would not be economical to build large modern markets in the backwoods of the nation. Furthermore, the pattern in most rural communities is to "go to town" for shopping. The trip to town is often an event, not just a shopping excursion.

Therefore in the case of the rural poor, governmental support of additional food shopping facilities would be impractical and unwise. Provision of adequate income coupled with convenient transportation are the major needs.

Retailers and the Food-Stamp Program

Until such time as the poor in our nation are provided an adequate cash income, the food-stamp program offers the best existing mechanism for supplementing inadequate incomes. The retail food industry welcomes the broader use of food stamps, since it brings the poor family into the mainstream of American life and gives them freedom of choice in the marketplace. However, there are a number of modifications that should be made in the food-stamp program to make it of maximum value to the recipient and more acceptable to the retailer.

1. Food stamps should be modified so as to make them as close to money as possible. This would facilitate their utilization in a busy market. Criticism has been directed against personnel in some markets because of their hostile attitude when stamps are offered at the checkout stand. Although such attitudes cannot be condoned, it is understandable why a busy checker may look askance at a food order that requires matching of food items with stamps. Considerable time could be saved if food stamps were issued in the same denominations as U.S. currency and if the stamps could be used for all items except for alcoholic beverages and tobacco.

2. Consideration should be given to the development of innovative programs whereby it would be profitable for food stores to seek out and attempt to attract persons with food stamps. The food-stamp program needs more publicity, and the holder of food stamps needs to feel welcome in the supermarket. One of the easiest ways to achieve such an objective would be for the government to offer food stores a premium of, say, 5 percent upon redemption of food stamps. Such a proposal would probably be criticized as enabling the food markets to make money on the poor, but anyone familiar with the competitive nature of the retail food industry would know that this premium would soon be eroded by various promotion devices designed to induce holders of stamps to shop at particular stores.

Thus some stores might offer free merchandise for the food-stamp holder, and others might offer special discounts at the checkout upon presentation of food stamps. The end result would be that the stamp holder would get more food for his stamps and the stamp program would achieve considerable publicity. Experience has demonstrated that promotional efforts of this type do attract food-stamp business. One large food chain has been offering extra bonus trading stamps for food-stamp customers and has been surprised by the increase generated in food-stamp business. The question that remains to be answered is whether such promotions merely shift food-stamp business from one market to another or actually attract more people to use food stamps.

3. There is a great need for more information and publicity about the food-stamp program. One recent survey found that in the average food-stamp county only 10 percent of the poor obtain food stamps.[2] A frequent reason is lack of funds to purchase the stamps. Yet in another study,[11] four out of five of the nonparticipating households were found to be spending more on food than they would have spent to purchase stamps. It is apparent that lack of adequate information about the food-stamp program is one of the major causes of its limited use. Retail food stores should be encouraged to display leaflets explaining the food-stamp program and to include in their ads reference to the fact that they welcome food-stamp holders as customers.

Enrichment of Foods

Although some retailers have manufacturing facilities, by and large the enrichment of foods must start with food manufacturers. Both manufacturers and retailers agree that it would be a mistake to attempt to bring out a new line of specially enriched foods for the poor. The poor may be hungry, but they have their pride; they want to be able to buy the same products as everyone else. As has already been mentioned, retailers would resist adding such new items for a limited number of customers; experience demonstrates that such items would have very little sales appeal. If a low-cost nonadvertised vehicle is sought for enrichment, private-label foods can serve this purpose. Since nutritional deficiency is a problem that affects all income groups, enriched foods should be attractively packaged and generally available to all shoppers. It therefore makes more economic sense to fortify conventional foods than to attempt to change eating and shopping habits by introducing special enriched foods to meet nutritional needs.

Although enrichment of foods is a reasonable goal, it also raises many questions that need to be carefully considered. Will consumers begin to compare the nutritive value of Brand A versus Brand B so that companies soon will be involved in a nutrition race? Can consumers get too much enrichment if particular vitamins are added to too many products? Will stores be required to carry nonenriched products for the benefit of the relatively few people in the population who may be allergic or unable to tolerate the enrichment factor?

A case in point is iodized salt. Only about half of the salt sold in retail stores is iodized. Many stores carry both iodized and noniodized salt on their shelves. This means that double the amount of shelf space is required for a relatively slow moving product. If the same condition is multiplied for hundreds of products, the impact upon costs could be substantial. As more products are enriched, it is important that the enriched product become the item that is generally available and that the nonenriched item should be available only on specialty counters or in "health

food" stores. There is no reason why all salt should not be sold in iodized form through conventional food stores, as long as sources for the noniodized product are available to the few persons in the population who cannot tolerate the iodized version.

Retailers can use various devices such as shelf-talkers, eye-level displays, end displays, and other merchandising methods to stimulate the sale of fortified products. However, their ability to do so depends upon modification of current regulations that would require many enriched foods to be labeled "imitation." It would be a difficult task for a market to promote the sale of peas to which vitamin D had been added if the peas had to be labeled "imitation."

Nutrition Education

Recent surveys have revealed a surprising lack of knowledge concerning the essential elements of good nutrition among persons in all income groups. The retail food industry talks to consumers every day—either in stores or through advertising. It would seem that a real contribution could be made in this area by the private sector. The basic question is whether the food industry can succeed in getting the nutritional message across in a believable fashion; other efforts to do so have quite obviously failed.

The first move in this direction was undertaken in September and October, 1970, when the first Nutritional Awareness campaign was launched by the food industry. This campaign was one of the first actions to come out of the many hundreds of recommendations at the White House Conference on Food, Nutrition and Health. At that conference, the Food Retailing and Distribution Panel had recommended that the Food Council of America be reestablished to conduct nutrition education campaigns.

The Food Council is an intra-industry group composed of the chief staff officer of all the national food industry associations who choose to join. Its membership includes associations representing food chains, grocery manufacturers, convenience stores, wholesale grocers, canners, and numerous specific food institutes. Overall, it constitutes an excellent cross-section of the leadership of the American food industry.

For the first campaign, the Food Council decided to adopt a simple theme and to give it wide publicity. The theme selected was: "Eat the Basic Four Foods Every Day". The council's thinking in selecting this slogan was that although nutrition is a vastly complex subject from the scientific point of view with many basic issues still subject to controversy, from the average consumer's point of view it is really quite simple. People who consciously choose a balanced diet from among the four basic food groups will probably meet necessary nutritional needs, although it is possible that specific nutrients could still be lacking from the diet.

Each of the members of the Food Council pledged to volunteer its efforts and support for the 1970 campaign and to continue the program on an annual basis for at least five years. During the 1970 campaign supermarkets all over the country displayed the "Basic 4" symbol. Stores were decorated with attractive in-store display material spelling out the message of good nutrition. Newspaper and magazine ads also picked up this theme. Moreover, many stores continued promoting the theme of nutrition after the major fall campaign had ended.

This program was repeated with more emphasis and expanded coverage in the fall of 1971. Obviously, such efforts are not going to change America's eating habits overnight. As *The Nation*, of October 19, 1970 critically remarked, "Good nutrition cannot be promoted like a National Donut Week." Nevertheless, the program and others that will follow represent a long overdue recognition on the part of the retail food industry of its obligation to educate its customers as well as to sell to them.

In addition to participating in the program outlined above, food retailers have also offered to assist the U.S. Department of Agriculture and other agencies, including public schools, in the development of community teaching programs aimed at reaching all Americans, with special attention being paid to the problems of the poor. The food industry is also assisting in the training of homemaker aides and other volunteer groups who are reaching low-income families through existing programs. Many large food chains have home economists on their staffs and have volunteered the services of such trained specialists in developing programs and educational material to spread the message of better nutrition.

The task of changing eating habits is a staggering one. It will take years of coordinated effort by our educational institutions, advertising media, government, and the food industry. It will be easier to deliver the message to middle-class Americans, whose need is less than that of poor Americans, whose need is great. The poor resident of the slum or of the rural village may never shop in a supermarket and may not read the newspaper; if he is exposed to nutrition education in either of these ways, he may have no interest in the subject. Actually, it is possible that the greatest impact would be registered on the poor in our economy by broad participation of small and outlying stores in such a program, yet, as a practical matter, it will be very difficult to insure such participation.

The diet problems of the poor and the affluent in our society are both highly complex, rooted in both physiological and psychological factors. For example, if milk cannot be tolerated by disadvantaged minority groups—a condition that is quite common—it is difficult to provide a readily available source of calcium. According to one nutritionist, a family living on the USDA

Economy Food Plan would have to eat liver at least once each week in order to get sufficient folic acid in its diet.[12] But many people—both rich and poor—do not like the taste of liver. The Basic Four is a simple rule, but it remains to be seen whether or not it is really meaningful for poor people.

For the affluent with nutritionally poor diets, the problems are also complex. How can the retail food industry convince the busy executive that breakfast should consist of more than a hurried cup of coffee? How does the supermarket convince the teenager—who has already been preached to about the dangers of cigarette smoking, speed, and marijuana—that a coke and potato chips is not a nutritious lunch?

Nutrition must be taught and repeated every day and every week, not once a year. From this point of view, the retail food industry is not in a position to do a very good job in getting the message across. The advertising budgets of most retail food stores are limited and their ads are a hodgepodge of bold prices and banal copy. Food stores have not been particularly effective in getting other institutional messages across to their customers. People do not like to be preached at. (For example, the retail food industry's effort to convince customers that "Food is a Bargain" had little lasting effect. Also, despite continued advertising of private-label merchandise, customers still pick up national brands that are identical in composition and pay more for them than the private label of equal quality.) Retail food advertising is generally considered to be unimaginative and monotonous in content. If "nutrition" is incorporated in such ads on a regular basis, it may become an overworked word and lose its meaning and impact.

It has been urged that supermarkets should advertise particularly nutritious foods. They do this now. Look at a supermarket ad. There will almost always be several produce items, meat items, cereals or bread, and dairy products included within the features. Since most people build their meals around these basics, it is simply good business to include them in the ads. Will more people make the proper selection simply because the market labels certain items as especially nutritious? It is probable that the appelation will simply get lost in the multitude of messages in the typical food ad.

In the long run, television almost certainly is the best medium for conveying the nutrition message in an interesting and informative way. The clever ads debunking cigarette smoking probably had as much to do with the decline in the consumption of cigarettes per person in this country as all the scare headlines about cancer. The retail food industry is not a large user of advertising on television, but the food manufacturers are, and perhaps it is the manufacturing sector of the food industry that can contribute the most on a continuing basis to keep the public aware of nutrition.

The ability of retailers to promote good nutrition depends upon the adoption of a coherent national nutrition policy. If, for example, cholesterol is a problem in American diets, food retailers ought to promote the sale of lean meat. This is difficult to do when the prime and choice grades are reserved for the fattiest meats. Similarly the system of pegging milk prices (and, in consumer thinking, milk quality) to butterfat content ought to be revised. The food industry can promote good nutrition, but first government must set the goals and policy on a coherent basis and adopt standards and grading that will facilitate the implementation of such objectives through the commercial marketing system.

Conclusion

The retail food industry in the United States has pledged its cooperation to assist in the campaign to improve the nutritional content of the diets of American consumers. This is a giant step forward.

Yet, as the first flush of enthusiasm wanes and the problem is subjected to closer scrutiny, the limitations imposed upon effective action by the distribution sector of the food industry become apparent. Most of the needed solutions are outside its purview. Efforts to improve productivity are impeded by restrictive labor practices, retarded by antitrust laws, and made costly by the lack of tax incentives. The need for development of modern retail food facilities in ghetto areas becomes more critical with each passing day, but companies cannot afford to apply their expertise without subsidies or special tax incentives. Retailers can help to publicize food stamps, but the real need is not publicity but a liberalization and extension of the program so that all persons below the poverty level can participate in the program wherever they may dwell. Markets are ready to sell and promote enriched foods, but the actual process of enrichment awaits the action of manufacturers and government regulatory agencies.

Most of all, the chronic malnutrition of the poor is an income problem, and this is not going to be solved by building more and better supermarkets in the ghetto or by conducting annual nutrition-awareness campaigns. Poor people are relatively undernourished because they have too little money with which to buy proper food. If government will provide the poor with the necessary purchasing power, the private-sector food-distribution system will perform its function of delivering food as cheaply as possible with a maximum opportunity for freedom of choice by the consumer. Furthermore, with respect to all those Americans who do have sufficient funds to buy proper food, the private-sector system has an obligation to use its marketing expertise and its promotional ingenuity to make good nutrition a byword (and a "buy-word") among all consumers.

REFERENCES

1. Consumer and Food Economics Research Division, Agricultural Research Service, 1965–1966. *Food Consumption of Households in the United States*, Spring, 1965. Household Food Consumption Survey 1965–1966. Report No. 1. U.S. Department of Agriculture, Washington, D.C.

2. *The Food Gap: Poverty and Malnutrition in the United States*, 1969. Interim report of the Select Committee on Nutrition and Human Needs, United States Senate, 91st Congress, 1st Session, August.

3. *Operating Results of Food Chains 69–70*, 1971. New York State College of Agriculture, State University of Cornell University, Ithaca, New York.

4. **Croom, P.,** 1966. Prices in Poor Neighborhoods. *Monthly Labor Review*, October: 1085.

5. **Taylor, E. F.,** 1970. Food Prices Before and After Distribution of Welfare Checks. *Marketing and Transportation Situation*. Economic Research Service, U.S.D.A., November:34.

6. **Richards, L. G.,** 1969. Consumer Practices of the Poor, in Sturdivant, F. D., ed., *The Ghetto Marketplace*. The Free Press, New York.

7. *Report of the National Advisory Commission on Civil Disorders*, 1968. Bantam Books, Inc., New York.

8. **Bloom, G. F.,** 1970. Black Capitalism in Ghetto Supermarkets. *Industrial Management Review*, Spring: 37–48.

9. **Sturdivant, F. D.,** 1968. Better Deal for Ghetto Shoppers. *Harvard Business Review*, March–April:136.

10. **Downs, A.,** 1970. *Who Are the Urban Poor?* Committee for Economic Development, Supplementary Paper No. 26.

11. Subcommittee on Employment, Manpower, and Poverty of the Committee on Labor and Public Welfare, 1968. *Hunger in America*. U.S. Senate, 90th Congress, 2nd Session, October.

12. **Calloway, D. H.,**   1969. *Working Paper on the Food Budget for the Poor*. Submitted to Panel VI, White House Conference on Food, Nutrition and Health, October.

Chapter 13

Grading of Foods

Emil M. Mrak and Vera G. Mrak

The quality of foods is a subject that has received a great deal of consideration during the past few years, and yet it is something that can hardly be defined and that very few people understand.

For example, a recent book concerned with quality of food states that the farmer produces for his market, and unless his market will pay a premium for high consumer quality (acceptability), he has no choice but to produce as much as he can or, in other words, the highest yield. This, therefore, supports the view that quality is simply a function of what the consumer is willing to pay. On the other hand, over the years, our government has acted on different assumptions and has increasingly engaged in the establishment of standards of quality.

History

The first use of regulatory powers by government to control the safety and purity of foods is really lost in antiquity. Mosaic and Egyptian laws indicated how cattle were to be selected, slaughtered, and the meat handled. There were also ancient regulations prohibiting the adulteration of a number of products, including fats, oils, grains, and spices.

We can trace our own regulations pertaining to quality back through history. For example, England established standards for bread, spices, wines, and other products in the twelfth century, and some of these standards survived into our own colonial era.

A hundred years ago, the food industry of the United States and the standards of quality were relatively primitive. Livestock were driven to the cities for slaughter, and the meat was sold as soon thereafter as possible; there were no formal standards of quality pertaining to toughness, fat content, or taste. Fruits and vegetables were, to a large extent, grown in home gardens or at least near the cities. Acceptance standards for home-grown items were, in general, set at the family dining table. Little was known about the safety of foods, and for this reason, it was of little concern.

Conditions, however, have changed, especially with the great movements of people to the cities. Americans have come to depend on the food-processing industries for their food. Accordingly, it has been necessary to establish laws to protect the consumer and to initiate the development of standards of quality and grades. Our manner of living is still changing, and without doubt, there is a need to continue to modify our foods to comply with our changing needs.

Our first pure food law was passed in 1906, and the Meat Inspection Act followed shortly. Accordingly, the Meat Inspection Division was established in the USDA and was made responsible for quality, grades, wholesomeness, and the safety of all red meats and the many products in which red meats are used for human and pet food purposes. Standards for butter were defined by Congress in 1923, and enforcement was assigned to USDA. This agency also has the responsibility for nonfat dry milk, the only other food receiving such special congressional consideration. In 1957, Congress enacted the Poultry Products Inspection Act, which is also administered by the U.S. Department of Agriculture. In 1946, Congress passed an Agricultural Marketing Act as an aid and stimulus to orderly and good practices. All other federal standards and definitions of foods are officially established, promulgated, and revised periodically by other administrative agencies of the government.

Since the establishment of these acts to enforce regulations pertaining to quality standards and grades of foods, there has also been an expansion of activities relating to food quality in other governmental agencies.

In spite of all these acts, however, it is often extremely difficult to attain a clear indication of what the standards are in practice, or the basis for establishing them. It would be well, therefore, to discuss some of the confusing considerations that lead one to wonder if we really do have satisfactory and up-to-date standards of quality.

Quality is defined in Webster's Unabridged as "a standard of excellence." Accordingly, our standards should change as our perception of excellence changes. "Standard" is defined as "that which is established by authority as a rule for the measure of quantity, weight, extent, value, or quality." "Grade" is defined as "a step or degree in any series, rank, quality, order; relative position or standing; as grades of flour."

It is apparent that the interpretations of standards and grades as well as of quality can vary greatly depending with specific situations, and this is just what occurs in practice. Variations are great indeed.

Frank L. Gunderson, in his very useful book entitled "Food Standards and Definitions in the United States—A Guidebook,"[1] pointed out that, generally speaking, standards, grade standards, definitions, and specifications are of very essential and far-reaching importance to farmers, processors, distributors, and, above all, to consumers.

Gunderson also stressed the fact that standards help to assure and safeguard an ample supply of wholesome food, to require that each product is what its label claims to be, and to minimize deception or misunderstanding. Nevertheless, authorities vary in their views of what grades are and should be. This becomes quite clear if one reviews the presentations of several authorities at an American Association for the Advancement of Science symposium of food quality held in 1965 and published in a book entitled "Food Quality—Effects of Production Practices and Processing."[2] It is interesting to summarize the views of several of these authors on quality and grades.

With respect to fruits and vegetables, Amihud Kramer defined quality as "the composite of those characteristics that differentiate individual units of a product, and has significance in determining the degree of acceptability of that unit to a user." Kramer indicated, too, that hidden characteristics that may affect the degree of acceptability of a food item, such as the nutritive value or wholesomeness, are not considered, since they are not usually of direct importance in market quality evaluation. (On the other hand, many who attended the White House Conference in 1969 were greatly concerned with the failure to consider nutritive value as a factor in quality.)

Karl F. Finney defined the quality of cereals as "suitability for a given product." Presumably this refers to the performance characteristics of a product.

For dairy products, V. H. Nielson gave a detailed definition of quality as that which reflects the long-time effort of industry to improve sanitary conditions and furnish the consumer with safe and wholesome products that can be consumed without further cooking. He stressed the importance of freedom from microorganisms that cause spoilage of the product or pathogenic infection of the consumer. He also indicated the importance

of flavor, aroma, color, texture, appearance, and ability to maintain desirable quality characteristics for a required period. This is certainly a deviation from the butterfat philosophy of quality.

With respect to poultry products, Owen J. Cotterill called attention to the long-standing concept of freshness as an indicator of quality. More recent concepts of quality, however, are based on performance when used in considering food preparation. H. D. Naumann, on the other hand, used the definition, "that which the public likes best." W. J. Stadelman expressed the view that it is "any attribute that has or might have an economic value." Furthermore, with respect to the nutritive value of poultry and eggs, Stadelman indicated that quality attributes used in procedures for the evaluation of nutritional qualities deserve reevaluation in the light of newer knowledge, and that practically no application is made of nutritional values in the direct measurement of quality in poultry, meat, and eggs in market channels. Furthermore, he indicated that gross composition (for example, protein, fat, fiber, moisture, vitamin and mineral content) included on the label would be of great help to the consumer in evaluating the quality of these products.

With respect to meat, T. C. Byerly indicated "quality can be improved to better suit our taste, or nourishment, through selective breeding, nutritional or physiological control, or a combination of these." This statement leads one to wonder if quality in meat is not a thing that may vary from place to place and from year to year.

In a book entitled "Introduction to Livestock Production Including Dairy and Poultry"[3] edited by Dr. H. H. Cole, it was pointed out that meat quality refers to its expected palatability—tenderness, juiciness, and flavor, and that the most important factors considered in evaluating the quality of a carcass are: (1) firmness of the lean and its degree of marbling or intramuscular fat, and (2) indications of the maturity of the animal from which it was produced. Futhermore, the excellent quality in meat, as evidenced in cuts, usually implies a full, well-developed, firm muscle of fine texture and bright color, containing a liberal amount of marbling and a minimum of connective tissue.

In addition, there is discussion in the book of yield grades and of the need to change standards. Finally, a footnote gives another point of view. It states "the term quality is also used, at times, to refer to the general excellence or acceptability of meat for a specified purpose. When used in this less restricted sense, quality may also include such factors as proportion of fat to lean, color of fat, and so forth."

It is apparent that the general concept of food quality evolves from the best that is produced and the development of strains or products better than those on the market. The question then is: What should these really be and what will they be?

In any event, it must be remembered that the concept of quality for any given product will change from time to time, since it depends upon what the public likes or dislikes, acceptability, and changing needs. To meet these changing requirements poses a serious problem, especially so in view of established standards of grading and identity, which are rigid and not easily updated or upgraded.

Why Have Grades and Standards of Quality?

It is interesting to note that the development of food standards and grades parallels the increase in scientific information relating to foods. In 1890 there were practically no food standards, and even 50 years later there were relatively few. Food research was indeed meager in the early nineteen-hundreds and only started to gain momentum during the thirties and forties, with the greatest amount being done during the past 30 years. Likewise, the greatest number of food standards have come into being during the past 30 years. Scientific contributions have provided a sounder base for the establishment of standards and grades as food habits and needs have changed during the past several years. These developments have made it essential that standards and grades be established and that our philosophy with respect to standards and grades change with our changing needs and habits.

The Situation at Present

The number of federal, state, and local standards is almost astronomical, and the number of agencies administering these standards is large indeed. It is, therefore, almost impossible for anyone to keep track of all that have been and are being established.

Accordingly, in 1963, Gunderson et al. wrote their book in an effort to bring together the information concerning grades, where they might be found, sources of information, and so on. There was then no simple method or place where one might get information pertaining to all federal food standards, and, in fact, this was the case until quite recently. There were few people who could locate and organize in a logical manner the far-flung parts of this sprawling though important subject. Yet, ostensibly, these grades, standards, and specifications are made for the protection of the consumer. Consumers, as a rule, however, have little knowledge of what grades are all about, or where to get information on them. Without doubt, it was for this reason that on October 26, 1970, the President issued a directive relating to consumer product information.[4] In issuing this directive, the President pointed out that numerous agencies of the federal government purchase from private industry a wide variety of consumer products for government use. This requires the keeping of detailed documents, reports, and other information for evaluating the products purchased. The President realized, therefore, that the federal government had an opportunity to help the consuming public by sharing the knowledge accumulated in the process of purchasing items for the government with tax dollars. A Consumer Product Information Coordination Center, therefore, was established and the General Services Administration assigned to implement this center and to promote and develop public dissemination of these government documents and information.

This is a great step forward in bringing order out of chaos; unfortunately, there are several types of standards and grades not related to purchasing, which are not disseminated by the new center. It would be helpful if these, too, were included in the order so the consumer would have one central place to obtain all such information.

The Food and Drug Administration, of course, is well known for its interest in safety, spoilage, aesthetics, wholesomeness, and proper labeling. At present the Food and Drug Administration is giving more consideration to nutritive values and certain acceptance factors of foods. It also has the responsibility of establishing and administering standards of identity.

As already stated, the U.S. Department of Agriculture has established grades on meats and poultry and certain other animal products. Some of these are at present undergoing change but not to the extent or at the rate necessary to meet the needs and desires of consumers. The USDA also administers the Marketing Act, established in 1946, which has enabled the establishment of many grades for fruits, vegetables, and other plant products. These are based to a large extent on visual measurements such as uniformity,

size, color, workmanship, and texture. Now and then consideration may be given to flavor but not very often. Nutritional value is rarely if ever considered.

Other grades are established by the Public Health Service; the Bureau of Commercial Fisheries; the Treasury Department, which is concerned with alcoholic beverages; the Bureau of Standards; the Federal Trade Commission, the Department of Defense, the Department of State, and even local governments.

The Need for Revision and Changes

There are definite weaknesses in our present system of establishing grades and standards of quality. As already indicated, many agencies are involved. For this reason, the approaches and points of view, of course, are bound to vary—and they do.[5,6,7]

The greatest weakness in our present systems is that they have not changed to maintain pace with the needs of our changing habits.

Strange as it may seem, there is practically no mention of nutritive value in the literature relating to grades, and it appears that there has been a tendency to underrate the food buyer's interest in this quality.

Generally speaking, our standards of quality are based on appearance, texture, uniformity, marbling, and so on. We do not need as much fat today as perhaps we did some years ago, we should not have it, and above all we should not be forced to throw this costly meat constituent away if we don't want it. Much of the fat occurring on meat is actually discarded, for it is neither needed nor wanted. Yet the grades tend to ignore this fact. In milk, too, butterfat stands as the basis of quality, and we do not need this fat either.

Jams may be given as another example of outdated standards of identity. The standards require such high concentrations of solids that they are not nearly as palatable as they would be if the product were more dilute and the moisture content higher. Without doubt when the standards were originally defined, the philosophy was to guarantee the purchaser a full share of richness and calories. But we do not need such calorie-rich foods today, and we have reached a point where taste and flavor are indeed important, yet we retain outdated standards that are no longer useful or appropriate.

The process employed in the establishment of standards of identity is so tedious and time-consuming that it has become almost impossible to update and upgrade them. Unfortunately, as presently developed, they encourage uniformity and discourage ingenuity and improvement that might well make it easier to meet modern day needs from the standpoint of nutrition, acceptability, and even costs. It might be said, therefore, that inflexibility, insofar as updating and upgrading are concerned, has inhibited the application of many of the advances in food research and has inadvertently denied improved products to customers, products more suitable to their present wants, needs, and way of life.

In a judgment of quality, there are factors other than nutritional value that should be considered today. Some of these are acceptability, stability, and convenience, as well as safety.

Acceptability includes such food characteristics as flavor, color, texture, tackiness (as in peanut butter), pain (as in Mexican foods), and even the noise one experiences when eating potato chips or celery. These and other characteristics make up the important but complicated composite called food acceptability, which, unfortunately, is rarely considered in formulating grades or standards of quality.[8]

Another factor of great importance is stability. Foods when packed may abound in nutritional value, flavor, and acceptability, but as time goes on (and particularly if storage is unfavorable), they may very well change adversely in flavor, appearance, color, odor, nutritional value, and even in texture. Stability is generally ignored when establishing grades, which, of course, become meaningless if a product is not handled and stored properly. Even though a housewife may purchase a product packed recently, upon storage in the home under adverse conditions it may very well be poorer in quality when consumed than a product stored for several years under favorable conditions. Thus attempts to require the dating of all products miss the mark somewhat, although dating may be worthy of consideration for certain products (such as milk, which deteriorates in a relatively short period of time) and for certain cheeses that improve with age for a period of time.[9]

Convenience built into new foods is another factor that is ignored in establishing grades and this needs consideration, for by introducing the convenience factor, the nutritive values may very well be influenced adversely.

Safety, of course, is something that is of prime importance and given high priority by the Food and Drug Administration.

Recommendations

At the White House Conference there were many comments relating to grades and standards of quality. It was clear that there is a strong feeling that the factors on which grades and standards are based must be reevaluated and in many cases extended. Nutritional value and acceptability in particular were emphasized. It is of interest that the need for these changes was related to changes in our living habits. Our diminished need for calories and increased need for a well-balanced diet were apparent and especially so in view of the large body of scientific information that has accumulated concerning food nutrients, flavor, and other factors of acceptability. Improper diets of the affluent were discussed at length and attributed to a lack of understanding, standards of quality, and labeling.

A great deal was also said about people suffering from hypertension and the need to produce special foods for these people. Reference was made to the rigid standards of identity as related to low salt foods and the importance of taking into consideration special needs for foods with low salt content. For foods not covered by such standards, it was indicated that food processors should be encouraged to minimize salt, especially in special packs for special situations.

Recently the Food and Nutrition Board of the National Research Council pointed out that there is a growing deficiency in certain essential nutrients in our diet. Specifically, iron is now considered as a deficient but important element. The conference recommended that the Food and Drug Administration together with other federal and non-federal agencies, including the food industry, review current policies and practices with the objective of increasing the amount of available iron and certain other nutrients in typical American diets, through appropriate enrichment of food products, and that these foods be defined and labeled accordingly.

There is a need to change some of our existing foods. The conference referred, for example, to the need to produce milk lower in fat but higher in protein content and recommended that this should be encouraged by (*a*) amending Milk Marketing Orders so that milk prices can be based on protein content rather than fat content; and (*b*) supporting research that aims to increase the production of milk protein.

There was also a strong recommendation that

> Lesigglation that governs the utilization of dairy products should be reviewed to mitigate restrictions on:
>
> a. the composition of dairy products in ways which discourage further product improvement and development, and
> b. the pricing, distribution and marketing of milk in ways which unnecessarily increase the cost to the consumer.

Here again, however, we are enslaved to antiquated rules, regulations, and policies.

A great deal was also said about the need for the use of generic names, which would accurately describe (in as simple and direct terms as possible) the basic nature of the food or its characterizing properties or ingredients. The generic name, it was indicated, should describe the food affirmatively to show what it is—not negatively to show what it is not. Oversimplified and inaccurate terms such as "imitation," it was pointed out, should be abandoned as uninformative to the public. Yet, the present law requires the use of the word "imitation" when foods do not meet our present standards of identity.

The Panel on Food Quality indicated that for a food product to have acceptable nutritional quality, it must be capable of providing those nutrients normally associated with its food group when consumed by a human population of known dietary habits. For example, nutritional quality of a specific food may be sufficient for one consuming group and not for another, depending upon the defined population, or the manner in which the food is consumed in its normal diet.

Furthermore, the panel's acknowledgement of the importance of acceptability was well indicated when it pointed out that acceptability encompasses all of those attributes, both tangible and intangible (including enjoyment during consumption) that lead an individual to choose a particular food.

With respect to standards for nutrition, it was pointed out that the mounting importance of factory-formulated foods and others differing from traditional patterns causes the previous experience and education of many, or even most, people to be unreliable in the selection of a properly nutritious diet. We are moving away rapidly from the use of the basic commodities for the preparation of food in the home to the use of convenience foods and especially newly developed products, and we tend to know little about them.

It was indicated that a processor who wishes to design nutritionally sound new products not only has no guide in present national policy; he is often actually prevented from doing so by existing rules and regulations.

The panel recommended that the government take action to change this situation as soon as possible. It was also recommended that standards of nutritional quality for specific foods or classes of foods be established to indicate a minimum and maximum value for nutritional properties of significance in accordance with the use of the product in the daily diet. Such nutritional values should include vitamins, minerals (including sodium), proteins, fats (including total saturated and polyunsaturated fatty acids), and calories. Consideration should also be given to establishing maximum fat levels

for foods high in invisible fat and to permitting optional replacement of saturated fats with polyunsaturated fats in certain foods.

Accordingly, it was recommended that the grade standards for beef and lamb be designed to encourage the breeding and feeding of animals that produce high-quality meat with a low ratio of fat to lean meat, and that consideration be given to the possibility of setting meaningful grades for pork. Furthermore, it would be highly desirable to develop a single code of regulatory requirements pertaining to the grading standards that can prevail in all jurisdictions: federal, state, and municipal.

Labeling

It is difficult to discuss grades and standards of quality without making some reference to labeling. A great deal was said about labeling at the White House Conference. Some of the recommendations for changes are clearly desirable, but others would create problems because of variations in raw materials used in processed products. It has been pointed out that many persons are attempting to modify their diets, either on their own volition or because they have been medically screened and found to be high risks. In addition, many physicians are prescribing special diets for patients who have had a heart problem, or who, for other reasons are thought by the physician to merit such management.

Following such modified diets is made difficult by lack of good information on fat content and the fatty-acid composition of foods found on the grocery shelf. Current regulations prevent manufacturers from providing such information.

There was a strong feeling at the White House Conference that the regulatory agencies should permit and encourage the food industry, on a voluntary basis, to label as to their content of fat and fatty acids those foods that constitute major sources of fats in typical diets. In line with this, consideration is being given to the possibility of stating on the label the percentage of fat by calories as well as by percent of weight. Furthermore, if the fat content is over 10 percent and over 3 grams per serving, it has been suggested that the processor be permitted to declare the percentage of polyunsaturated fatty acids and of saturated fatty acids in the fat. Since the occurrence of excessive fat in certain products, and especially meat and meat products, was of such great concern, these suggestions are signs of progress.

It should be pointed out, however, that changes in this direction, though desirable, should be done with care so they may be feasible as well as worth while. Raw materials do vary greatly, and of course, the conditions of handling and storage are important factors that could cause labeling to be more misleading than informative.

Some believe that a complete statement of ingredients should be required on every label regardless of whether or not there is a government standard for the product.

It has been suggested that labels contain information about any food additive that has health implications and that information about the major nutritional contents of processed foods be provided to the consumer at the discretion of the producer.

The latter part of this suggestion is probably in order, but the first part would place an almost impossible burden on the processor and the regulatory agency too, for judging whether or not a food additive has nutritional implications is difficult indeed.

It has even been suggested that the labels provide statements regarding the types and quantities of fatty acids present. This is almost impossible because of variations in raw materials.

The Food and Drug Administration is taking the recommendations with respect to labeling seriously and is considering (a) the use of figures to indicate quantities supplied for the daily need of children and adults, supplied by an eight-ounce serving or (b) a system whereby a rating for nutrient elements will be "good" or "very good."

Summary

The situation with respect to food grades and standards of quality in the seventies can be summarized very briefly by stating that our pattern of living has changed and is continuing to change dramatically. Furthermore, the body of scientific information has increased greatly and is continuing to increase.

We are eating more prepared foods, newer foods, different types of foods, our activities are changing, interest in the preparation of food in the home is declining, and we are, as a whole, a population of uninformed consumers of food. A great deal of this can be attributed to the fact that we do not exert any effort in our junior high schools, high schools or even medical schools to instruct students in foods and nutrition. On the other hand, there is a clear indication of the need to change our present philosophy with respect to regulations, grades, standards of identity and quality, and labeling. At present, however, it is difficult to make constructive changes in our foods because of legal restrictions that make it so often difficult to update and upgrade standards of identity.

The need, therefore, is not only for education, but for a revision of the whole governmental approach to regulations, grades, standards of quality, and labeling. Changes need to be made, but they should be made in collaboration with the various interested groups. There should be a constructive interest on the part of government, the processor, and the buyer in working together to make desirable changes. Unless this interest exists, we will continue to live with the present unsatisfactory, uninformative, and antiquated system of grades, standards, and labeling.

REFERENCES

1. **Gunderson, F. L., Gunderson, H. W., and Ferguson, E. R., Jr., eds.,** 1963. *Food Standards and Definitions in the U.S.—A Guidebook.* Academic Press, New York, N.Y.

2. **Irving, G. W., Jr., and Hoover, S. R., eds.,** 1965. *Food Quality: Effects of Production Practices and Processing.* American Association for the Advancement of Science, publication number 77. Washington, D.C.

3. **Cole, H. H., ed.,** 1966. *Introduction to Livestock Production, Including Dairy and Poultry,* Second Edition. W. H. Freeman and Company, San Francisco, California.

4. *Consumer Product Information,* October 26, 1970. White House Executive Order.

5. Food and Food Products, Part 10 (Sub-chapter B), Definitions and Standards for Food, pages 181–397, January 1, 1970. *Code of Federal Regulations,* Washington, D.C.

6. *Protecting Our Food,* 1966. Yearbook of Agriculture. U.S. Department of Agriculture, Washington, D.C.

7. *Food for Us All—Yearbook of 1969.* Yearbook of Agriculture, U.S. Department of Agriculture. Washington, D.C.

8. *Flavor Research and Food Acceptance,* 1958. A survey of the scope of flavor and associated research compiled from papers presented in a series of symposia given in 1956–1957, sponsored by Arthur D. Little, Inc. Reinhold Publishing Corporation, New York.

9. **Slavetz, L. W., Chichester, C. O., Gaufin, A. R., and Ordal, Z. J., eds.,** 1963. *Microbiological Quality of Foods.* Proceedings of a conference held at Franconia, N.H., 1963. Academic Press, Inc., New York, N.Y.

Chapter 14

Labeling

Jean Mayer

Nutritional labeling—the quantitative description on labels of all processed foods and the posting in the store of the caloric and nutrient content of meats, vegetables, fruits, and other produce—is the key to effective nutrition education, improvement of our food supply, and food law enforcement. The availability of information regarding ingredient content is also important—particularly to any attempt to keep the cost of food down. This is already apparent to practical nutritionists who have wrestled with the problem of maintaining the integrity of our nutritional health in a period of rapid change. Extensive acceptance of—and popular clamor for—nutritional labeling are necessary for this important measure to become a daily reality in the face of resistance by parts of the food industry and the inevitable governmental inertia.

The Need

Our food supply has changed drastically since World War II. In the thirties, the bulk of our diet was made of unprocessed foods—meat, milk, fish, potatoes, beans, corn, other vegetables, fruit, with bread and noodles the main processed foods. Canned foods were available, but by and large the cans contained unmodified fruits and vegetables (or sardines). At present, our food supply has become highly processed (over 55 percent of our foods are canned, frozen, milled and combined, or "convenience" foods). Not only are the old "food groups" obsolete (what "food group" does a pizza belong to? or a spinach soufflé?) but the information as to their composition is not available to the public. The "Food Tables" established by the U.S. Department of Agriculture, reprinted in many manuals and dietetic books, give the composition of "common foods"—essentially those of the old food groups; the composition of the new foods cannot be found except by writing to the manufacturer—and hoping that he will consent to answer.

Under these conditions, nutrition-education programs acquire an unreal character. Because the composition of most of our food supply is no longer known by the public, nutrition educators limit themselves to discussion of the "old foods," members of food groups, ignoring the fact that their listeners are perforce making use of canned soups, convenience foods and other products of our modern industry without any guide as to what these contain in terms of calories and nutrients: Is mushroom soup high or low in calories? Is spinach soufflé a high-fat or a low-fat dish? Is fruit in heavy syrup to be avoided by a dieter or does it make little difference? And what of television dinners? The fact is that, if we want to preserve the nutritional integrity of our food supply in the face of transformation of the architecture of our meals and the change in the nature of our foods themselves, we shall have either to legislate enrichment of all foods with all nutrients—or give the consumer the information he or she needs to consume a modern balanced diet. Most nutritionists feel that the second method, which respects the idea that variety is essential, is the preferable solution. For one thing, we don't know with certainty

all the requirements of the human species. For another, not all foods can be used satisfactorily as carriers for all nutrients. The need for doing something, however, is increasing; recent surveys are showing that the nutrient intake of Americans, after improving for decades, has started sagging in some respects since 1960. And introduction of new food products is constantly accelerating. Taking all these factors into account, the 1969 White House Conference on Food, Nutrition and Health strongly recommended new labeling methods, covering both nutritional labeling and ingredient labeling.

Labeling Schemes

A number of different schemes have been proposed for nutritional labeling. The most comprehensive was devised by a committee that included consumer representatives (such as James Turner, author of the Nader report "The Chemical Feast," Helen Nelson of the Center for Consumer Affairs of the University of Wisconsin Extension Service, and Sidney Margolius, the well-known consumer reporter); representatives of industry (National Canners, the American Meat Institute, retailers); representatives of government (the Food and Drug Administration and the Federal Trade Commission). This scheme was put into effect by the Giant Food Stores in the Washington, D.C. area, a progressive organization which had already pioneered the now near-universal "unit pricing" practice. In this system, the label indicates the calories per household portion (specified per ounce, cup, glass, or whatever the common measure is). It also gives grams of carbohydrates, protein, and fats per portion and a rating based on the percentage of recommended daily allowance of other nutrients contributed by a common portion of the food: vitamins A, C, B_1, B_2, and niacin, iron, and calcium. (Vitamin D is given when added to milk or to cereals as specified by law). Ratings are 0, $\frac{1}{2}$, 1, 2, 3, and so on to 10. A rating of 10 means that 100 percent of the daily recommended allowance is contributed by a portion (as for vitamin C by a glass of orange juice), 4 no less than 40 percent, 1 no less than 10 percent, ½ no less than 5 percent, 0 below that. Jewel Stores has adopted a similar system. Other stores such as First National, Kroger, etc., are experimenting with simpler, less comprehensive descriptions, which omit mention of any nutrient not in appreciable amounts and describe the food as "an excellent·source of . . . ." or "a good source of . . . .". The model labeling scheme proposed by the Food and Drug Administration is similar to the Giant Food type, except that it gives ratings based directly on rounded percentages of the Recommended Dietary Allowances rather than on a 1-to-10 scale.

The more comprehensive, Giant Food Stores-type labeling is preferable on a number of grounds: (1) It is not promotional, and looks least like one more advertisement. Its honesty—it shows what is in the food and what is not in the food—makes it much more effective to a public saturated with and tired of promotional material. (2) By reminding the customer that no single food contributes all nutrients in optimal amounts, it testifies to the need for a varied diet, the best recipe for good nutrition. (3) Its rating system gives a simple guide to reaching the daily allowance for all main nutrients: the sum of the ratings on the portions consumed during the day should add to 10 for each nutrient.

Reactions to Labeling Proposals

Although the supermarket chains—which consider themselves the buying agents for the public—appear relaxed in their search for the labeling that will be most informative and, even more important, most educational, there is little doubt that some manufacturers are very nervous about the effect of a comprehensive nutritional labeling system on the sales of at least some of their products. Some manufacturers oppose the concept altogether, others are pushing hard for the "promotional" scheme (". . . is an excellent (good) source of . . .," with no mention of the missing nutrients). Pressure for the "promotional" scheme is reminiscent of the old song (to be sung, one presumes by the absent vitamin), "If you can't say anything real nice, honey, please don't talk about me when I'm gone." Opposition to the comprehensive schemes is usually based on male commiseration for the poor women who, faced with a dozen numbers on the label, are supposed to completely fall apart. Almost every middle-class American male reads the thousands of figures daily printed in the newspapers on the stock exchange pages. Many ten-year-old boys know the batting averages of their favorite baseball teams to three decimal places. But the mother of the family, who, instead of playing games, is working to preserve the nutritional health of her family, is presumed to be unable to comprehend a system based on a few numbers ranging up to 10 or rounded percentages like 5, 10, 20, and so on percent. Quite the contrary is the case. Women are glad to see the task of composing a balanced meal placed on a more interesting, less empirical basis than it has been until now. And customers are clamoring for the extension of the labeling system (and the posting of the same indications on meats, vegetables and fruits, cereal products, etc.) to as many foods as possible as fast as possible. More important, buying habits are changing rapidly for the better—even in poor "inner city" areas, where the housewives are presumed by the opponents of nutritional labeling to be baffled. Liver consumption has risen. Apparently, it is one thing to hear nutritionists praise liver but quite another (and more effective) thing to see for yourself how favorably it compares to much more expensive meat in terms of the ratio of protein to fat to calories (liver has as much protein but well under one-fifth the fat and one-half the calories as steak), iron (twice as much per calorie), vitamin A (about 10,000 times as much per portion), and the B vitamins (about ten times as much). Poor black women rediscover with great pleasure that the traditional chicken and greens is an excellent dish; mothers in general find that while donuts are as empty a mass of calories as they thought, pizza is, in fact, an excellent food, high in protein and calcium, and that they can, therefore, direct the choice of their children's snacks in a positive rather than killjoy role. Generally speaking, comprehensive nutritional labeling makes marketing more interesting and less confusing—and increases the assurance with which the housewife operates.

The objection is raised that comprehensive nutritional labeling still does not cover all nutrients—namely, vitamin E, some of the B vitamins (such as vitamin B_{12}, pyridoxine, and biotin), and about 20 trace minerals. This objection was taken into account in devising the scheme. It was judged very unlikely that a diet adequate in all the labeled nutrients would be inadequate in the unlabeled ones. Should this turn out not to be so, additional nutrients will have to be added to the label list. Such a situation could arise if more and more "synthetic" foods and drinks, rich in purified protein and a few vitamins and nutrients, invaded our food supply in important proportions. The Food and Drug Administration is mindful of this risk and, at this time, is trying to determine vitamin and mineral enrichment policy for all-vegetable protein meat substitutes; vitamin B_{12}, possibly other B vitamins, and a number of trace minerals may be included. The FDA is also studying the limitations to be placed on enrichment of cereals, snacks and other products so that we don't jump from the extreme of unfortified foods (e.g., unenriched white flour) to overfortification (when every mouthful promises to cover your requirements for the whole day, at least for a few nutrients). Obviously, nutritional labeling, useful though it is, is not a substitute for a number of needed regulatory measures.

Benefits of Labeling

Calorie Control   Nutritional labeling is essential to calorie control. Calories do count, and only the knowledge of the number of calories per portion will dispel some of the old chestnuts (or canards) that have spelled the doom of many a dieter's efforts. One is the belief that meat is all protein, that protein is calorie free, that only "carbohydrate" foods are fattening. Many misguided dieters will pass up bread (60 calories per slice) and eat instead a three ounce beef hamburger pattie (320 calories), thinking that he or she has struck a mighty blow for weight control. Nutritional labeling will inform the consumer in this instance that bread, in weight and calories, is 13 percent protein and that the calories of hamburger may be over 70 percent fat. More generally, the lesson that there are no "thinning" foods as opposed to "fattening" foods—that all foods contain calories and that portion size is important—is an essential basis for weight control, which is quickly learned from perusal of nutritional labels and which may not really be learned without them.

A label giving the caloric content of household portions is the only way in which the dieter will be able to use processed and "convenience" foods. Even if one were willing to keep a table of calories handy to the dining table, such compilations do not give the caloric content of the "new" foods—nor would they ever be inclusive enough to keep up with the seemingly endless variety of modifications brought out on the market by competing firms. There are now thousands of such foods, and only "tables" as thick as telephone books, with monthly supplements, could cope with the numbers involved. How is the meal planner to know whether a spinach souffle is primarily spinach, a low-calorie vegetable, or a high-fat, high-calorie dish, in which spinach is only one of the ingredients, unless he is told by the label?

In this regard as well as others, nutritional labeling will probably be an important factor in improving the quality of our food supply. The informed dieter already knows that by buying pineapple canned in its own juice instead of in "heavy syrup," all one passes up is sugar—and a great many empty calories. Nothing will decrease faster our ridiculously high national sugar consumption (100 pounds per year per American—equivalent in calories to 52 pounds of body fat) than the desire of manufacturers to offer a combination of high nutritional value and relatively low calories. When you add the preoccupation of Americans with weight control to their growing wariness of additives, nutritional labeling insures that, in the post-cyclamate era, instead of going back to sweetening additives, we will make full use of the natural sweetness of fruit—perhaps bolstered by the synergistic effect of such natural potentiators as passion fruit.

Fat Control The current attention to cardiovascular diseases—our number-one health problem, with half of the men over 40 falling victims to diseases of the heart and vessels—makes it imperative that we know the amount of fat in our diet. A high-fat diet, particularly a diet high in saturated fats, promotes high blood-cholesterol levels. As cholesterol goes from 150 milligrams per 100 milliliters of serum to 250 milligrams per 100 milliliters of serum, the risk of coronaries triples and increases even faster

above that level. The FDA Commissioner is considering special legislation applicable to shortenings and oils that would make it mandatory for any manufacturer who wants to use the word "polyunsaturated" to provide a quantitative statement of the amounts of saturated and polyunsaturated fatty acids. Quantitative description of the components of fat, including the cholesterol content, ought to be available on the label of any food which makes a substantial contribution to the fat intake of Americans.

Salt Content Similarly, because there are over 20 million hypertensives in this country, mention of the salt content of processed foods would be useful to an enormous number of consumers. Such labeling might also induce manufacturers to lower the salt content. Many soups and convenience foods, otherwise excellent, are too high in salt (even though it is easy enough for those not at risk who want to do so to salt them after tasting them).

Ingredient Labeling

Ingredient labeling, oddly enough, is somewhat more difficult technically than nutritional labeling—though, of course, by no means impossible. Consider some of the problems: one problem is that if you make a stew containing chunks of meat and dehydrated carrots, you end up with apparently less meat (because some of it gets dissolved or dispersed in the liquid phase) and more carrots (because they absorb water during rehydration) than you started with. Obviously, an answer to that problem is a "recipe" rather than a "final-content" type of quantitative listing. Another problem is that often economic considerations change the proportions within a given category of certain ingredients without much effect on taste or nutritional value: mutual replacement of peanut oil by soy-bean oil or corn oil is a frequent example. And yet to some people—patients with allergies associated with the protein present in traces in this or that oil—the indication is important. This dilemma can be solved by adding to the "nutritional label" a "percentage main ingredient label" which also gives a quantitative indication of the main, characteristic ingredients—no less than (so much) turkey in "turkey pie" or beef in "beef pie" or beans and pork in "pork and beans"—and continues to simply list the nutritive (and potentially allergenic) ingredients. The detailed, chemical description of additives has been opposed on the reasonable basis that such terms are not only unintelligible to the enormous majority of the public, they are very long and their inclusion in the label would mean the necessary use of such fine print as to be self-defeating. An answer seems to be the continuation of description by class names (preservatives, vegetable coloring matter) coupled with recognition of the right of any consumer to write to the manufacturer and obtain a prompt, detailed answer. After all, the old Roman maxim of "Caveat emptor"—let the buyer beware—is no longer a reasonable one if it presupposes that the buyer has at his or her disposal an analytical laboratory with almost unlimited means. To continue to accept this principle in the nineteen-seventies may spark a rejection of all processed foods containing additives and a headlong rush for the illusory aims of an all-"natural" or "health" food supply.

The veterans of "consumer campaigns" base their advocacy of at least limited ingredient labeling—over and beyond nutritional labeling—first on the type of Gresham's law that operates in the food field. Gresham's law—often summarized as "bad money drives out good"—was the name suggested in 1857 by H. D. Macleod to describe the fact first observed by Copernicus and by Sir Thomas Gresham in the sixteenth century that the worst form of currency (underweight or debased coins, for example) regulates the value of the whole currency and drives all other forms of currency out of circulation. In the food field, consider, for example, the case of turkey pie. Conscientious manufacturers A and B have recipes that call for a lot of chunks of turkey meat in their frozen turkey pies. Manufacturer C enters the market with a frozen turkey pie, lavishly advertised, encased in a box adorned with the picture of a steaming turkey pie as succulent as those on the covers of existing pies, and appreciably cheaper. Recent history has been that, in the absence of obligatory labeling conspicuously describing the quantity of turkey in the turkey pies, manufacturers A and B have been forced to lower the turkey content of their pies. In some areas, this process has taken place in several documented downward steps. Proper labeling is thus a guarantee to the quality manufacturer that he will get, at the point-of-sale, the advantage that will justify the premium that his product entitles him to. Proponents of adding some ingredient labeling to nutritional labeling recognize that, in the situation just described, nutritional labeling would give the necessary advantage to our friends A and B. But they fear that C would then add in his gravy enough suspended soy or wheat protein to equal the protein content of his competitors A and B. While he would have to upgrade his product—to his customers' nutritional benefit—they are still entitled to know that C's products are more inexpensively made and although as high in protein, are not as high in turkey protein. The difference may not have nutritional significance; it would still have economic significance.

Generally speaking, the "right to know," particularly when applied to commodities as basic as foods, should become a fundamental tenet of our economic life. When applied to a particular food, it should entail (*a*) a quantitative description of the nutritional value of the food; (*b*) an indication of the percentage content of the named, characteristic (and expensive) ingredient; and (*c*) a complete list of all ingredients, whether the food is subjected to a "standard of identity" or not. Standards of identity, which, in effect, are recipes defined by regulatory agencies that dictate the nature and amount of the main ingredients, do nothing for the information of the public and are, in particular, of little assistance in helping allergic individuals to avoid ingredients to which they are sensitized.

Chapter 15

The Family: Nutrition and Consumer Problems*

Effie O. Ellis

The family is the basic unit of our society and a most important institution. It is the family that molds the early years of a child's life and establishes the life pattern of the individual. It is the family that determines the physical, mental, and spiritual growth and development of its members, and establishes patterns of discipline, communication, and personal relationships.

Food and feeding have served from time immemorial to establish man's family relationships, to transmit tradition and cultural patterns from one generation to another, to fulfill family roles and to provide basic satisfactions in so doing.

Many experts in child growth and development have commented on the vital role of food and the act of feeding in establishing warm human relationships, first within the family, and later with others. After all, man's first experience with love and security is intimately related to food and the feeding process. The family meal can help to nurture and cement family life and enhance individual and group growth. It affords an occasion for parents and children to talk with each other and provides an opportunity for sharing and developing understanding. It can reinforce the role of parents as providers and givers of love and security.

*The author wishes to acknowledge the valuable assistance of Mary C. Egan of the U.S. Department of Health, Education, and Welfare in the preparation of this chapter.

Today, many traditional functions of the family are increasingly being assumed by other institutions—schools, restaurants, community agencies, and so forth. In all social strata fewer meals are being eaten at home. This development could weaken the stability of the family and threaten the uniquely important role it plays in shaping its members' destinies.

For these reasons, the recommendations of the White House Conference on Food, Nutrition and Health (1969) include suggested solutions to major nutrition and consumer problems at the family level. Full recognition was given by the conferees to the need for national policies that will enable the family to continue to function as a major food-delivery system.

Three Problem Areas

The policies that affect the family regarding food, nutrition, and consumer problems can be placed in three main categories: (1) problems associated with an inadequate income or inadequate assistance from federal, state, and local programs; (2) problems associated with budgeting, marketing, and food pricing; and (3) problems associated with a lack of education (in foods, nutrition, child care, home management, and consumerism).

The problems associated with budgeting are dependent upon an adequate income, since no person can obtain a nutritious diet unless he has the financial means to do so. The problems of marketing and food pricing, however, often stem from a consumer's lack of basic knowledge of food labeling, quality, and selection. Therefore, one must consider the total interplay of these three problem areas before one can determine the fate of the family and therefore of society itself.

Adequate Income Adequate income is of major concern to millions of families in our country at the present time. (This is true,

particularly, of the nonwhite minorities and the residents of Appalachia.) There is considerable variation in the amount of a family's income that can be allotted for food, even among higher income groups; other essentials that the family needs—housing, clothing, transportation and health care—compete for the dollar.

The high and constantly rising cost of food is considered to be the primary reason for the high cost of living. At least it seems safe to say that the food dollar buys very little. In order to make ends meet, it is common practice for families to cut the food budget, which provides some elasticity, to meet unexpected emergencies.

Although the existence of poverty and malnutrition is widely deplored, efforts to ameliorate these social conditions clash with the commonly held belief that a person's need for help is evidence that the person is not willing to work. There is an amazing amount of mixed feelings about the root causes of poverty and the remedial measures and methods that are needed for the prevention of poverty. This widespread ambivalence in public opinion is reflected in the provisions of the 1962 and 1967 Amendments to the Social Security Act.

In general, welfare policies and practices present the needy family with many complex problems. Consider, for example, the almost unbelievable restrictions encountered in the provision of aid to dependent children of unemployed parents: the full-time earnings of an employed father may not be supplemented even if they fail to meet the family's needs. Also, assistance may not be given with federal matching funds until the father has been unemployed for 30 days—and then only if he has been previously employed for certain periods of time.

There are earned-income exemptions for adults and older children—the first 30 dollars they earn per month plus one-third of the balance of their earnings are not counted as family income. But this applies only to families who are already receiving assistance. Families who apply for assistance are not allowed such exemptions and for this reason may be unable to get help.

Supporting social services are limited only to welfare clients in many states. As a consequence, potential and former welfare clients are denied preventive and maintenance social services. Thus, families who are near-poor or in need of special services are penalized for not being on welfare; because they are not on welfare, they cannot receive family-planning services, day-care services or family-counseling services.

Such policies yield a house divided, largely because the socioeconomic realities of the life of the poor are not generally understood by those in power. In part, they are not understood because the problems of communications across socioeconomic lines are mammoth. Program-planning input from the families in need has been small, at best, since so many of the poor are unable to speak for themselves. Through a lack of understanding and ill-advised restrictions, the stated intent of the law does not prevail.

The ADC (Aid to Dependent Children) law, which was designed to keep families together, has failed to enhance the capability of the family to function and indeed leads to family decay. The law was based on the premise that the father in the home would be capable of working and supporting his wife and children. All too frequently this premise has proven to be false.

When a hard and honest look is taken of the situation, we recognize immediately that willingness to work is only a part of the picture. It is the actual earning power of the workers that is of highest importance. It is a well-established fact that opportunities for employment are limited by race, ethnic background, place of residence, age, training, education, union regulations, state of the economy, etc.

For whatever reasons, when a father fails to earn enough money to support his family,

he is in trouble. He is in danger of being alienated from society. In order to obtain aid for his family under the ADC law, he must abandon them. Should he seek help under the General Assistance Program, which is set up to cover family needs not provided for by ADC, he must be prepared to be treated as an unworthy person and willing to go through miles of red tape. As a rule, the funds for this program are insufficient, and the eligibility requirements and administrative policies exclude many needy families.

As a further handicap, recipients of these services, particularly those of very low incomes, are often subjected to much criticism by the general public. There is widespread belief that even when the poor are given sufficient resources, they are unable to improve their well-being. Examples of this belief are evident in statements as: "Those people are too lazy to learn.", "Look at what they buy—the food carts are full of potato chips and soft drinks.", "All these people want is money for alcohol and cigarettes.", "They don't know how to buy.", "How can these people be hungry when there are television sets and radios in every household?" In reality, most poor people would like to work, but are physically unable to work or cannot find a job. The reason their food baskets at the checkout counters emphasize quantity rather than quality is because the first object of eating is to avoid physical hunger. As for tobacco and alcohol consumption, they are far from being the monopoly of the poor.

An impoverished family that cannot provide all basic essentials, including nutritious food for its members, is without a doubt at high risk of falling apart. And, without a doubt, widespread disruption of family structure will weaken the nation.

The highest priority should be given to the development of policies that will enable every family to have an income that will allow for the purchase of a nutritionally adequate diet. Attainment of this goal would reduce the need for current government programs such as food stamps, food (commodity) distribution, and others. It would reduce the stigma and red tape associated with these programs as well. In addition, the responsibility for budgeting for the family food would be shifted from the government to the family.

A guaranteed adequate family income of necessity must be a long-range goal. Until such time as this goal can be accomplished, strong effort must be directed toward improvement of current food programs.

Food-Stamp Program. Since the White House Conference, the food-stamp program has been strengthened substantially as a money-equivalent resource. However, there is still much room for expansion and extension of the program. The purpose of the program administered by the Department of Agriculture is to improve the diet of low-income consumers by supplementing their food-purchasing power. Presently, the maximum purchase price of stamps cannot exceed 33.5 percent of a family's total income. A family of four with a monthly income of $100 would spend $25 for food stamps in order to receive $106 worth of food. Although this amount may seem to be adequate at first glance, the consensus is that this allowance falls slightly below the standardized USDA low-cost food plan. (This is a menu plan that meets the minimal nutrient needs of a family without any provision for the family's cultural food likes and dislikes.) In addition, no provision is made for nonfood items necessary for personal hygiene, cleanliness, and home sanitation.

Eligibility for stamps varies within and between states because of the differences in the standard of living. Problems of welfare impose an additional hardship in providing for the needs of the family. For example, a father or mother who gets a job loses food-stamp allowances. Usually the decrease is not compensated for by the increase in family income, because the latter is taxable.

A method of self-certification would help to alleviate the humiliation of applying for stamps, which today strips away a person's right of privacy. Since no one knows his needs better than himself, criteria for eligibility should be established by the government only after consultation with the poor person. Presently the food allowance is determined by USDA, which defines an average meal cost at 35 cents per person. The free-food-stamp plan, for which the poorest of the poor are eligible, is still in an experimental stage and is not available nationwide. Under this plan, a family of four with an income less than $100 per month will be able to receive $125 worth of groceries. Presently that family pays a maximum of $22 per month.

Eligibility requirements arbitrarily define the meaning of the word "household" to include family members under 60 years of age. As a result, a large percentage of elderly people who are living alone or with families are deprived of food-stamp benefits. The elderly are perhaps the most neglected group in the United States nutritionally, socially, and culturally. That more efforts are not made to meet their needs is a fault of all programs.

Food-stamp procedures should be flexible enough to benefit recipients with special needs. This would include a provision for increased benefits for those with a special nutritional requirement for additional foods or special dietary foods. In times of emergency, such as a loss of a home due to fire, stamps should be provided free or at a greatly reduced price. In addition, ways should be developed to strengthen the use of stamps for people in nursing homes, communal groups, or other similar groups. Special consideration should be given to those families who have no cooking facilities and depend on higher priced prepared foods.

The present method of distributing stamps from a central office directly to the recipient is humiliating for those who pride themselves on their independence. This could be remedied by establishing the policy of issuing stamps by mail. Such a plan would be most beneficial to people who are unable to pay the round-trip bus fare and to those who are disabled.

For people who receive a daily or weekly paycheck instead of pay on a monthly basis, the policies should be flexible enough to permit weekly stamp distribution. Likewise, clients should be allowed to determine the amount of stamps they need to buy at a given time; minimum purchase requirements should be eliminated.

School Lunch. For many children the school lunch is the primary source of nutritious food. Many others who need additional food are prevented from participating in the school-lunch program because of restrictive administrative policies. New policies should be designed to utilize food stamps as payment for the school lunch.

In the light of the poor food habits of large numbers of children and youths, efforts should be directed toward providing a free school lunch for all regardless of income.

Problems Associated with Budgeting, Marketing, and Food Pricing   There are many interrelated factors involved in the development of a meaningful, workable budget. Often problems of budgeting are easily traced to lack of consumer education and unfamiliarity with public services available to consumers in the community. The nutritional needs of the family must be viewed within the family context in relation to other basic family needs—housing, clothing, health care, etc.

Services should not be limited to a specific family member or age group. Witness the feelings of frustration and inferiority which are generated when a pregnant mother is given supplemental food for her personal use and her young children are hungry. Imagine what happens in terms of sibling relationships when the young children in a poor family are given food at school and the older

children are hungry during the school day. Careful coordination of community education, public health, social service and other agency programs can go a long way in reducing problems for many families.

In this connection, people with small sums of money sometimes cannot spend money for adequate food because of health problems that need immediate attention. On the other hand, a mother may decide to forego needed prenatal care because she cannot afford the high cost of baby sitting or day-care services. A working father may postpone needed medical attention because he cannot take time from his job without losing pay. Nutritious foods, which are furnished by the Commodity Distribution Program, may not be utilized because they fail to meet the family's ethnic needs. It is difficult to overstress the fact that food must be consumed in order to nourish. To make food available is not sufficient. It is of little value to suggest that the family can obtain sufficient calcium to meet nutritional needs from nonfat dry milk if families refuse to drink this milk.

Knowledge of food labeling is helpful, if not essential, in planning budget-wise meals. The consumer relies upon labels attached to packaged foods as a prime source of information about the contents, nutritional value, and safety of those foods. Policies that will improve food labeling are essential.

Three actions that would provide needed consumer information are:

1. Improvement in labeling all packaged and processed food products by listing the name and amount of each ingredient, including the nutritive value of each major ingredient per serving. Food ingredients should be declared in terms of these sources, such as: "wheat-protein hydrolysate" rather than "protein hydrolysate"; "potato starch" rather than just "starch"; and "peanut oil" rather than "vegetable oil."

2. Strict enforcement of existing standards of actual nutritive values to which food manufacturers must conform if they promote, advertise, or label a given product as nutritive.

3. Informative labels on all foods and food products including those that have an established standard. These standards of identity are not defined for laymen. Certain food items are exempt from listing ingredients because the contents follow a recipe that is consistent for all brand names. United States standards have been set for a large number of foods such as ice cream, peanut butter, catsup, hamburger, etc. Consumers cannot be expected to remember all of these standards when making purchases.

Every shopper knows the burden of comparing food items, particularly canned goods, when the content varies between brand names. Weights should be standardized in order that "unit pricing" can be a facilitating factor in budgeting for family needs.

There are many problems of budgeting and food purchasing simply because food-distribution facilities are not conveniently located. In small, inner-city neighborhoods, the conveniently located, privately owned store is known for higher priced items. Often the produce is of lower quality, and display cases are not maintained in accordance with public-health regulations.

It follows that the larger chain economy stores are located away from ghetto areas and also from rural residents. Three actions that would improve distribution of foods to these areas include: development of new facilities in needed areas or improvement of existing facilities; provision of mobile food stores, particularly in rural areas; transportation of residents to nearest food distribution centers.

Nutrition Education   Nutrition education is a necessary component of any program. The head of the family can set an example for its members that will give them a foundation in good nutrition. For the basic concepts of good nutritional habits and health to be learned at an early age, it is essential that the parents have sound information in these areas. Some people have emphasized that attempts at parent education have been directed to the middle class and that the parents who need it the most don't get it. However, recent programs conducted by various voluntary and service organizations have shown that parent education for low-income people is succeeding. This is evidenced by the fact that low-income mothers are eager to take advantage of the opportunity to learn and to have their children increase their living skills. Evaluation of the success of these programs cannot be made objectively, but many mothers have expressed their appreciation for this type of assistance.

While it has been more common for women to be involved in nutrition education, it is equally important for the father to be involved. A mother who has accepted a new idea and prepares a new recipe for a meal will be depressed to find that the father won't accept the new dish.

Nutrition education is particularly important for adolescent girls. Current statistics indicate that one out of every four babies is born to an adolescent and that many are born prematurely following a lack of total prenatal care. Childbearing is an example of a situation in which appropriate care can prevent untimely death or lifelong disability, and may simultaneously serve to move an entire family forward to new levels of healthier living. However, in producing normal, healthy infants, nutrition begins at (or before) the moment of conception and depends on the health of the mother. Of prime concern is the fact that many adolescents are malnourished and suffer from anemia. Often, the adolescent's only nutrition advice is provided by sources that may not be reliable, and the adolescent's dietary habits are conditioned by peer group approval. For this reason, a great effort should be made in schools, clinics, community health centers, privately owned centers, and more importantly, at home, to see that accurate information is relayed. It is of extreme importance that adolescents are motivated enough to seek these services when in need. The same is also true for non-adolescent housewives. If nutrition education programs are to succeed, they must give much attention to the women that produce the next generation.

There are various considerations to be made for any nutrition education program. Persons living in poverty are those who have the least—and yet are expected to know the most. They lack such basic necessities as stoves and refrigerators, yet they need ways to prepare nutritious meals. Because of these drawbacks, the woman resigns herself to preparing the same monotonous meals. Many do not have the confidence to try something new. Acceptance of new ideas must begin with demonstrations using familiar recipies, showing ways in which the recipe can gradually be improved.

Eating fulfills a psychological need. In order for education to be effective, the family's food preferences in meeting this psychological need should be known. In this way, the family culture is maintained. The satisfaction derived from a family eating together or a mother nursing her baby can hardly be overemphasized.

The important contributions of the family members in determining the quality of family life also need to be recognized. Business, industry, and communications media can do much to emphasize the importance of the homemaker's role. Even in financial terms, the services provided by a mother for her family—and society—are hard to overestimate. Too often, we disparage the homemaker's role, as in the phrase "only a housewife."

Efforts to provide family-life education should be supported. The subjects studied should include the importance of good nutrition in relation to family relationships; home management; cognitive and intellectual development of the children; the stages of life and their relation to nutrition. Materials can be developed to illustrate "The Family Life Cycle" and explained by trained para-professionals. This education can be made a part of the elementary and high school curriculum.

Much can be done to illustrate the role of the father or father-substitute as family provider. It is estimated that it costs between $15,000 and $19,000 for a family to raise one child to age 18 if they live on the low-cost food plan. If one multiplies this factor by the number of children and includes additional family expenses, it is not hard to see the importance of the father as family provider. Anything that denies this family member's right to provide for his family is threatening to fragment the family unit. In our strongly work-oriented, money-based society, profitable productivity is vastly more popular than idleness in poverty.

Recognizing the need for education in the areas of foods, nutrition, child care, consumer education, and home management, there are various ways in which this need can be implemented. A comprehensive program should be provided to the public by a trained home-service corps of para-professionals. Community-sponsored programs can be carried out in neighborhood centers, supermarkets, by public instruction in schools for children and adults, as well as in churches and other community meeting places. Nutrition associations are planning on sponsoring consumer-education programs in large chain supermarkets nationwide. One is currently in progress in Chicago in which free nutritional advice is given on topics of current interest such as weight control.

Nutrition education based on past experience, current knowledge, and research can make a difference in the quality of life for many Americans. Nutrition alone can play an important role in the growth and development of all people, and be a major influence on the way a person performs on the job, at home, and in society as a whole. What we need is the best way to educate the public with the resources at hand in order for families to attain a new status in life. Factual information presented in an understandable way at the time of decision is needed in solving some of the nutrition and consumer problems at the family level.

READINGS

Working with Low-income Families, 1965. American Home Economics Association. pp. 103–117.

Chilmore, C. S., and Kraft, I., 1963. Helping Low-income Parents Through Parent Education Groups. *Children,* July-August: 127–136.

Chapter 16

Consumer Problems in Relation to the Food Industries

Robert J. McEwen

Food Prices

The most important consumer problem in regard to food is the extremely high and rising cost of food in retail stores. Volumes have been written in a bitter dispute attempting to explain away the problem of food prices or to fix the blame on one party or the other in the production and distribution chain. The food buyer of the seventies is not interested in such explanations or debates about relative blame. He is convinced that the food industries have allowed their prices to run wild and he wants action to reverse that trend.

Of the priorities suggested by the Consumer Task Force of the White House Conference, the very first one singled out for emphasis was the lowering of food prices. The report of the Consumer Task Force said:

> Recent inflation has caused great injury to both low- and moderate-income families. In many inner-city areas, the proportion of family income spent for food exceeds the proportions spent in underdeveloped countries. The high cost of food, and resulting malnutrition, is a burden on both the low-income family and the tax-

payer. High costs and poor quality of foods have been an important factor in the riots and discontent of the past decade.

The goal of consumer action in this connection was stated by the Consumer Task Force as follows: "to lower food prices by reducing forms of promotion that have little to do with nutrition or other food values supplied to consumers." The report had singled out the reduction of expenditures for promotion as "one of the most significant ways by which food industry costs and retail food prices must be lowered."

No significant progress on the achievement of this goal is apparent. One action that should be considered is a complete ban on the use of chances, games, and prizes in connection with the sale of food. The usual gimmicks, games, and gadgets offered by supermarkets as prizes have an incongruity that is somewhat revolting.

While on this subject of chances, games, and trading stamps, it is interesting to note the emergence of challenges to supermarkets who advertise "we have eliminated trading stamps and therefore our prices are lower." The present challenge to such advertising is taking the form of a demand for proof that the saving of money formerly put into trading stamps has truly been passed on to customers and not diverted either to other forms of promotion or to the profit of the store.

Another form of consumer action that will come into increasing prominence in the next few years is the selective boycott of certain foods. Consumer groups and their leaders will have to organize effective boycotting of food products whose supply-and-demand situation permits a steady inflation of prices. Beef is a case in point. Sooner or later, U.S. consumers will have to switch to other meats, fish, or poultry if the price of beef is to be kept within reason. At the same time, more attention will have to be given to the farm policies and import restrictions that affect the supply of beef.

Food Advertising

As a result of the conference's recommendations, we have seen some improvement during the past year in food advertising. A great deal more attention is now paid to nutrition, the nutrient value of food, and nutrition education in some of the advertising by food sellers.

It will now be necessary to police such advertising very carefully to be sure that the nutrition information given to the public is accurate and the best available from the current state of the science.

Problems associated with the advertising of food specials have received much public and private attention recently. Two main problems were noted in the long series of surveys and studies that led to the Federal Trade Commission's recent rule on the matter. Unavailability of advertised specials and failure to sell at the advertised price were the two chief customer complaints. Both have now been declared an unfair trade practice by the FTC rule effective July 12, 1971. Consumers will now be urged to watch for violations of this rule and report them promptly to the FTC local offices.

There is some evidence that stores tend to feature too many of the same items in their advertised "specials." If further examination bears out this initial impression, serious doubt will have been cast on the usual advice to shoppers—that it is wise to travel from one store to another just buying the specials. Maybe all the housewife is doing by this process is wasting time, gas, and energy.

The Federal Trade Commission has exhibited increasing concern for misleading and fraudulent advertising, both in relation to claims concerning product value and to pricing methods. Charges have been brought against major producers for exaggerated and false claims as to the nutritional quality and content of food products.

Diet-aids and "children's" foods are areas where the customer may be easily influenced by persuasive advertising. Often it is not only misleading (for example, the potential value of "Wonder Bread" in contributing to normal growth as opposed to regular bread), but it is presented in a manner that implies that the mother who really cares for her family would buy only the advertised product.

In regard to pricing, methods are often employed whereby the consumer is unable to determine whether or not the advertised price actually represents a bargain, unless the normal retail price is known. Both the FTC and the FDA have proposed legislation pertaining to "cents-off" sales. Included in the proposals are the requirements that the sale represent a reduction of at least 8 percent in the normal price and that the old as well as the new price appear on the package.

The degree to which heavy advertising expenditures enable the food industry to influence the media poses a threat to fair news coverage of consumer issues, which may be presented with a bias or completely ignored because profitable accounts are involved.

Also relevant for consideration is the effect that advertising may have on certain classes of people. Much of advertising is annoying and irritating in general. Beyond this however, is the possibility that advertising may unduly "exploit desires, fears and anxieties." Children and lower-income group members are especially susceptible to advertising claims, and as a result of them often formulate unrealistic expectations concerning product fulfillment. Because they are so influenced by what they see advertised, children are often able to successfully pressure their mothers into buying foods that they would rather their children didn't eat.

The Function of Government in Relation to Food

Another pressing problem is the improvement of governmental structures and operation in the food field. Organized consumers are seeking the following goals:

1. Greatly strengthened and expanded representation of the consumer in all structures and levels of government dealing with food inspection or regulation. Not enough progress has been made on this matter, and the willingness and eagerness of some agencies to listen to consumer opinion leaves much to be desired. Many federal departments and agencies, for instance, have not yet established a special consumer-advisory group for their operation, and there seems to be quite a bit of hesitancy on the part of timid bureaucrats to move in this direction. However, if the government and its bureaus are ever to convince the public that they really pay attention to consumer needs and consumer desires, a greatly expanded consumer participation in policy making is going to be required.

2. Adequate budgets for federal agencies in the fields of food inspection, labeling, and standards. There is no indication that such budgets will be available. On the contrary, the demands of the general budget and the costs of the war and the military establishment have usually imposed at least a standstill in budgets for these consumer programs, and, at times, we see actual reductions in the amount of budgeted funds for efforts at food protection.

3. Evaluation of the work of federal agencies by an independent outside group with strong consumer orientation. We see very little evidence that this is being done with much aid or encouragement from the government itself. Some of Ralph Nader's groups are attempting to fill this vacuum but they are doing it entirely on their own or with some help from private foundations. The foundations are derelict in their duty in not supporting consumer activities on a much wider scale than they have in the past.

4. A program of federal grants and technical aids to state and local authorities to implement nutrition policy, to improve food and health inspection, and to strengthen weights and measures enforcement on state and local levels. This highly recommended and necessary suggestion is still waiting for effective implementation.

The Wholesome Meat Act is testing the good intentions of both federal and state officials. The federal government has to decide whether state programs have been improved sufficiently for federal certification or whether the federal government itself will have to take over all the meat inspection activity for delinquent states. The theoretical desirability of a joint federal-state program, which was a cornerstone of the Nixon Administration's "federalist" approach to the problem of meat inspection and which was adopted by Congress as a premise of the Wholesome Meat Act as passed, may not be successfully vindicated by the course of events. One wonders whether the U.S. Department of Agriculture is going to be as insistent with the states on the upgrading of their meat-inspection systems as it should be or whether the federalist concept will turn out to have been a snare and a delusion by which all segments of government share joint irresponsibility in the field of food inspection.

Consumer Expectations, the Press, and the Broadcasting Media

One also has distressing doubts about the way the press and the media in general operate to keep the public informed about the realities of governmental functioning in the area of food inspection and regulation. One problem is that the news media tend to act like bees instead of tigers. Instead of attacking an issue (such as the adequacy of the state's food-inspection system) and worrying it to death until the public has enough information to understand both the problem and the possible solutions, the news media flit from one sensational flower to another, presenting a few charges, facts, or allegations with very little effort to put them in any meaningful context.

Obviously, the reader or viewer's judgment is no better than the information he receives. The "flitting bee" approach does not provide the public with enough information about problems and possible solutions; instead, it serves to confuse the public, and generally draws the lesson that efforts to bring change are largely a waste of time. Clearly, the news media must learn to meet their responsibilities as organs of public information in these matters.

In fairness, it should be noted that at least some newspapers recently have assigned teams of reporters to do "in-depth" studies and surveys of certain problems. These teams do attempt to put the whole immediate situation into some kind of focus. This practice should be more widespread. Commercial television should put its best talent and resources to work in this manner in an effort to show the public what the situation actually is with respect to governmental activity in protection of its food supply.

The worst of all possible worlds exists when the consumer mistakenly assumes that government is performing certain protective activities for him. He therefore relaxes his own guard and his own investigations because he relies on the supervision of the government. If the government is not doing this, the consumer ends up with no protection at all.

Labeling and Consumer Information

Special emphasis should be placed on informative labeling and an expanded consumer-information program. These two topics are linked quite closely. Ideally, the label of a food can or package should, within the limits of its size, be as informative to the purchaser as possible. In the whole area of labeling and consumer information and education, there are two somewhat contradictory schools of thought. One approach suggests that the label should contain precise and rather technical descriptions and identifications of contents and nutritive value. The other approach says this would be unintelligible to the average consumer and, therefore, confusing. This second approach recommends some effort at popular labeling in nonscientific terms with whatever sacrifice of accuracy is required to achieve this goal. This debate is not peculiar to the food field, but is one that arises whenever consumer information is at issue.

It is true that the average consumer will have neither the educational background nor maybe even the inclination to use full and detailed, precisely technical information about food or any other product. (A long program of education of the consuming public would have to be undertaken to make them a little more able to profit from information furnished by sellers in pursuance of these campaigns for full disclosure of pertinent facts about products. But this is a long-range goal.)

There are three key objectives of labeling and a consumer-information program:

1. *Complete information.* Packages and labels should show, to the extent possible, all of the precisely technical information about the product that would be useful in judging its suitability for customer needs and its required conditions of care, storage, preparation, and use. In regard to food, we need also whatever information is necessary to relate this particular food to the total diet and the total nutritional needs of a person. In other words, the producer should publish as much pertinent information about his product as a customer would ever need or use, even though a complete interpretation of the information might require expert assistance from the consumer groups.

2. *Clear information.* Recognizing the fact that the average customer will not be immediately able or disposed to understand or to use all this technical information, an effort should be made to develop popular symbols, numbers, letters or other signs that can be used to identify for the purchaser those qualities of a product that are most critical for him to understand.

3. *Increased competition.* The third objective of a consumer-information program is to increase competition among manufacturers. Publication of pertinent facts about products will reveal a manufacturer's weakness relative to competitors—and the bright light of full disclosure will reveal deficiencies in many products that enjoy highly advertised but unearned reputations. Given the economic pressures of a free market, producers of inferior goods will be forced to improve their products. (Although it may be initially marginal, the influence of a group of informed buyers constitutes a risk that no manufacturer will want to endure voluntarily for long if his product is inadequate or much inferior to his competitor's.) It is almost impossible to overemphasize the potential of this approach.

Because the use of the free-market mechanism does not depend on widespread and immediate understanding of consumer information for its effectiveness, all the recent surveys of what consumers in general now understand or want or will use are irrelevant to the question of full disclosure. This point must be stressed because opponents of consumer-information programs are constantly making the unfair, illogical, and impossible demand that those who advocate consumer information must be able to show that the average consumer will *immediately* be able to make use of the information that manufacturers are asked to provide. This tactic is an attempt to delay or prevent imposition of the legal requirement that producers have to tell buyers the whole truth about their products.

Some of the information in question is indeed technical, but this is no reason to withhold it. It simply means that consumer groups and agencies will have to rely on knowledgeable specialists who can acquaint themselves with all the technicalities of at least certain groups of products. These specialists can then help organized consumers form judgments about products, and through them, can influence even wider circles of the general public.

In this connection also should be mentioned the valuable and praiseworthy efforts of newspapers, radio stations, and television stations to handle programs of consumer problems and consumer information. This can be a good method of spreading public awareness of the interpretation and meaning of the data furnished about products by their labels and packages.

Food Dating

One of the most important aspects of informative labeling now coming to the fore is the problem of open dating of packaged food. As the system of distribution of food becomes more and more remote and complicated from the point of view of producer and consumer alike, it becomes almost impossible for the average customer to judge for himself questions involved in the freshness of foods.

In this connection, there are at least three problems associated solely with age and dating of food. A consumer needs to know (1) when a thing was canned or packaged and (2) when it should no longer be used or eaten. Of course, sellers must have information about (3) how long they should leave a product on their shelves. This, of course, implies some judgment of how soon after purchase a consumer is assumed to eat or use the product.

The present shameful confusion in the marketplace on the subject of codes and dates and dating is a real blot on the reputation of the food industry and should be ended immediately. As a matter of fact, the situation, instead of getting better, may be getting worse. Some companies that previously practiced open and intelligible dating of their products have suddenly abandoned that in favor of secret codes.

This problem of dating and coding of food can lead consumer groups to utter frustration. No sooner do they learn how to read and interpret a certain code than they find, after a few weeks, that it has been changed. The situation almost has the appearance of a deliberate conspiracy on the part of sellers to keep the consumer off-balance and to prevent him from ever penetrating the secret of how old the food product is when he buys it. Therefore, the Consumer Task Force's recommendation 3B asked for the (1) labeling of packages with the date of packing, (2) storage recommendations, and (3) the expiration date.

We should also ask supermarkets and other sellers to upgrade the information in the possession of their employees. Students, investigating this subject for some months, have gotten answers from store personnel to their questions about age, dating, and storage of food that betray abysmal ignorance. Frequently the employee either denies there is any age code or in answer to a question about how long a consumer can keep a product, they'll tell them "forever."

Considerable progress in the matter of open dating of food has come from voluntary action by certain chains. The most common date stamped on the product by these chains is the so-called "pull" date (the date on which it is supposed to be removed from retail stores).

One chain of stores has taken full page ads in Washington newspapers to boast that it has made available in its stores "Code books (which) cover more than 2,000 perishable and semi-perishable foods." Sadly enough, it had to admit in print that

> Because there is no uniform system of dating and coding in the food industry, it took us months to compile, research and interpret the codes so that you can interpret them. Here's what we found: Some manufacturers code by number. Others, by color. Some use a combination of both. Some manufacturers use a "package" date. Others, a 'pull date'. Some have no freshness date whatsoever.

It seems obvious that what the consumer ultimately needs is the *expiration* date—beyond which a food should not be consumed. The seller can presume or even include in the instructions adequate storage conditions for his product. But too many products are discarded because of fear that they are too old, or, on the other hand, some foods are consumed after they have been kept too long or under improper conditions of storage. These situations result in unnecessary consumer waste and risk.

Unit Pricing

For many years consumer spokesmen have been demanding that the price-per-unit be supplied by sellers in order to facilitate price comparisons between competing goods. Now several chains have taken the lead in experiments with unit pricing and at least

one state, the Commonwealth of Massachusetts, has passed legislation requiring it after hearings and regulations issued by the Consumers Council, an official body of the Commonwealth. One supermarket executive has said that his chain "broke its back" to meet the deadline established by the Massachusetts regulation. In the process, according to this same source, they discovered and overcame every conceivable problem and difficulty with unit pricing. It has proven feasible, and it will not be very costly—as its critics and opponents maintained.

This should go a long way toward eliminating the baffling array of prices and sizes that made a rational choice almost impossible except for a mathematical genius among the shoppers. It remains now for customers to show that they use and value the unit-pricing information.

New Industry Moves

Many supermarket and food firms have established posts with titles like "director of consumer relations" or "director of consumer affairs" and in some cases have put knowledgeable consumer people into those jobs.

It remains to be seen how effective the consumer's voice will be through these spokesmen, because it really depends on how sincerely business management desires reform. Management may not really want a "vice-president in charge of revolution," which is what a consumer spokesman should be; on the contrary, it may really want no more than "window dressing"—the respectability acquired from the use of a famous name. If businessmen and industrial groups see such corporate consumer advocates as a means of heading off consumer complaint before it has chance to crystallize, then these moves will turn out to be nothing more than public relations, with very little profit to the public.

PART 3

Improving Education Concerning Nutrition

Chapter 17

The General Public

Helen D. Ullrich and George M. Briggs

Nutrition education is a complex field that is, in many ways, supportive of the other areas of nutrition discussed in this book. (For example, a program to improve the nutrition status of young children would include providing nutritious food for the children, but it must also educate the young children to eat, enjoy, and ask for foods and that meet their needs.) For this reason, almost every panel at the White House Conference on Food, Nutrition and Health mentioned nutrition education in their recommendations.

Nutrition education in an individual life is part of the continuous learning process that begins at birth and ends only with the end of life. Nutrition is affected by the culture, behavior, and attitudes of each individual; good nutrition must meet the special needs of each person within his own environment. To attain good nutrition, each individual must be motivated to utilize his knowledge of nutrition for his own physical benefit. (For example, nutrition education is not effective for the overweight person until he is motivated to apply his knowledge of nutrition to the loss of weight.) There are, of course, many factors that influence the use of nutrition knowledge. These will be described later in this chapter. The objective of nutrition education is to promote optimum growth and health through the consumption of appropriate foods, thus contributing to an individual's potential for achieving his goals in life.

If each individual in our society is going to effectively implement his right to and need for proper food, then he must be given the opportunity to know enough about food and nutrition to choose for himself those foods that will supply his nutritional needs throughout life.

Nutrition education must be carried out at all levels of education, government, industry, mass media, and family. The approaches may vary with income, age, education, and environmental conditions, but there is always a need for knowledge of nutrition.

Nutrition Education and Malnutrition

Nutritionists, agriculturalists, and politicians alike were considerably shaken when the USDA Food Consumption Survey of 1965,[1] Hunger USA,[2] and reviews of previous nutrition status studies in the United States,[3,4] all documented that there was considerable malnutrition in the United States. This condition existed in spite of the fact that American agriculture was providing adequate food for the population, legislators were providing protection of the food supplies, and people were being informed about what to eat.

There are many factors affecting people's diets that can bring about the conditions of hunger and malnutrition. For example, people must have enough money to buy food or have a resource such as food stamps with which to buy it. They also need the education and motivation necessary to make a good choice. Some people live in areas and under conditions where an adequate supply of nutritious foods is not available; educational programs can show them ways to obtain these foods; for instance, they can learn that food stamps are available and how to put them to best use. Even when food and income are available, there are other influences such as religious beliefs, food habits, family traditions, and food fads and taboos that will affect the choice of food. Any educational program that motivates people to improve their eating habits must take these factors into consideration. Enrichment, supplementation, or development of nutrient rich foods will improve nutritionally the foods available to people, but educational programs are needed to inform the public about the nutritive value of these foods and to encourage their use. Mass feeding programs can provide millions of people, young and old, with nutritious meals, but these meals have to be eaten to nourish the individual. Here again, nutrition education is needed.

Malnutrition must be eradicated. Any programs, therefore, that are provided through legislation to improve conditions must include provisions for nutrition education in order to be effective.

Who Are Nutrition Educators?

In one respect, almost everyone is a nutrition educator. The ideas that influence what we eat come from many sources. In the home, all family members influence one another. In the school, teachers and children influence each other. In the community, the market place, the church, the health facilities, and social organizations have an influence. The total environment, including all kinds of mass media, has its influence. However, there are certain people who are especially fitted to act as nutrition educators.

These people might be grouped as follows:

a. *Nutrition research scientists.* These are the people with the greatest degree of specialized knowledge. They are the educators of other professionals in the field of nutrition and related fields.

b. *Those who have advanced training in nutrition and biochemistry.* This group includes dietitians, nutritionists, public-health nutritionists, extension nutrition specialists, most college food and nutrition teachers, some home economists, and some physicians and dentists.

c. *Professionals whose work involves some aspects of nutrition.* This group includes home economists, nurses, school-lunch supervisors, health educators, some elementary physical education, biology, and science teachers, most physicians and dentists, food technologists, and welfare workers. These people require some specialized training in nutrition. There is a great need for more effective programs for this group.

d. *Para-professionals.* The comparatively new para-professional workers in community nutrition, health education, and welfare consultation who work as nutrition aides require specific training in nutrition at a level that will be effective in their work.

Then there is constant informal education for which very specialized training is needed, particularly in the area of mass media. Because the means of nutrition education are so wide and varied, the kinds of nutrition education are also varied. It has been shown in more recent years that nutrition education must employ the insights provided by behavioral science. While the nutrient needs are the same for individuals of the same age, sex, size, and physical activity, the environments in which their needs are obtained can be extremely different. For example, the homemaker with limited cooking skills, almost no storage facilities, and very limited reading ability must take very different steps to provide an adequate diet than does the middle-class homemaker who has an electric kitchen, a college education, and adequate money to buy what she chooses from her market places.

Sources of Nutrition Education

In addition to formal teaching of nutrition at colleges and universities, there are several other areas of nutrition education. This chapter will concentrate on the roles of elementary and secondary schools, the community, the public-communications media, and the food industry.

The Schools   There is a great need for more effective nutrition education in elementary and secondary schools. The time has come to recognize that the food served in the schools as breakfast and/or lunch is an excellent teaching resource. Unless the student is taught to eat and enjoy nutritious meals, part of the educational obligation of the school has been overlooked. Food habits are formed early in life. Nutrition education must be incorporated into the elementary school curriculum. Elementary teachers must be provided with training in nutrition. Coordination of nutrition-education programs on local, state, and national levels is needed. Some method of evaluation of these programs needs to be built in so that we have a means of evaluating the effectiveness of such education through the school systems. These areas are discussed in greater detail later in the chapter.

The Community   One of the developing resources of nutrition education is the community or neighborhood program. The people of a given community or neighborhood must be drawn into participation in such a program. Care must be taken to coordinate all phases of nutrition programs that may be taught by community aides and workers. One of the outstanding things about community nutrition education is that people who live within the community and have empathy with its cultural and social conditions can be trained to teach others nutrition and family health. The Extended Nutrition Education Program of the Cooperative Extension Service of USDA has been particularly successful in this approach. The Congress recognized these results and for the years 1970–1971 increased the funds available to this program as a result of its initiation in 1969–1970. There are many others who are carrying on effective programs such as Head Start, maternal and child-health centers. This will be discussed in greater detail later.

Public Communication One of the purveyors of nutrition education that reaches the largest numbers of people is the mass media—radio, TV, newspapers, and magazines. This is also probably one of the areas where the least effective job is being done. Part of the reason may be that the effective utilization of the mass media requires a special kind of expertise, which most nutrition educators do not possess. A step forward has been made since the White House Conference in trying to reach the mass media. The Advertising Council of America[5] at the request of the President, has agreed to coordinate a nutrition-education campaign with government agencies and industry. The purpose of the campaign will be to promote better eating habits. The food industry has proven that advertising can change food habits. It is time nutritionists make use of advertising to sell one of the best products in existence—good nutrition.

The Food Industry The food industry, of course, provides most of the food people eat. Whether this food is nutritious is, in part, the responsibility of the food industry. In the past, the food industry has placed such things as storage life, color, texture, and flavor before nutritional quality. One of the responsibilities of the nutritionist is to educate the

food industry to recognize first of all that food provided for people must meet their nutritional needs. The industry should offer information in its advertising or promotions about the nutritive content of food, as well as its desirability. It would be wrong to say that the food industry has had no concern about nutrition; however, the food industry has not always provided the best available information to its customers. There must be a closer cooperation between industry and nutrition educators. For over 30 years, the food industry has provided some nutrition education through the Nutrition Foundation. However, the industry's major contributions have been given to research projects in colleges and universities for research in the nutritional sciences rather than for education of the public. The emphasis is now being changed, and the foundation can provide leadership to the food industry. More detailed suggestions are given later in the chapter.

Government Several departments of the executive branch of the federal government have some responsibility for nutrition education, but most responsibility lies in the Department of Agriculture and the Department of Health, Education, and Welfare.

During World War II, the Inter-Agency Committee on Nutrition Education of the Federal Government was formed.[6] This group has functioned through the years and provides leadership at the national level. At five-year intervals, it has sponsored national meetings to bring key nutrition educators up to date. There are also interagency state and local committees of nutritionists who function cooperatively. Some are more active than others.

The Inter-Agency Committee on Nutrition Education has been active in setting up guidelines for concepts in nutrition education. It was also instrumental in providing information leading to the Four Food Groups as a teaching tool. Within the government, there is need for further leadership to coordinate all areas of nutrition education. The tools for nutrition education need to be revised. Some specific recommendations are given in the resource section of this chapter.

Nutrition Education in Schools

Curriculum An effective program that begins when the child enters elementary school and continues through the secondary school will enable children to acquire positive attitudes toward foods and make wise food choices as a part of their maturity. As was stated in the introduction to the recommendations of Panel IV-I of the White House Conference: "As future citizens in a democracy, children must develop acceptable nutritional practices and a sense of social consciousness to enable them to participate intelligently in the adoption of public policy affecting the nutrition of people."

There are many curricula into which nutrition can be coordinated, or it can be taught separately. Nutrition can be a part of learning arithmetic, social science, geography, history, science, health, physical education, and home economics. It has been traditional that nutrition be included as a part of the home-economics curriculum of our secondary schools. However, this kind of a program reaches only a very small part of the school population. Only a segment of girls in junior and senior high school receive this training. Also, by this time, attitudes and habits toward food are quite firmly established.

Children should start to learn about the foods they need as soon as they are in school. While the elementary school is the usual time to start, preschool children also can benefit. Juhas[7] describes the interest and accomplishment of the preschool child in learning about food in relation to the world around him. This is the time when one's food habits are forming. Acceptance of simple food patterns can be established. Unfortun-

ately, there are very few nursery school teachers who have received any training in concepts of nutrition.

There are many good nutrition-education programs being carried on throughout the country. There are examples of interest: elementary school teachers weaving food choices into their mathematics and reading sessions; volunteer mothers with professional training who carry on a rat experiment for fifth and sixth grades; science teachers who use nutrition as a basis of their experiments; school nurses who carry out lessons about food and teeth. In many schools, it is the rare teacher or nurse who is able to present this sort of lesson.

Training and materials must be provided to enable teachers to carry out such programs.

Food Service as a Part of Education The passage of the 1970 Child Nutrition Act,[8] which liberalized the school-lunch program, was a major step toward providing adequate nutrition as a part of the school child's development. It should be a national goal to provide free or reduced cost lunches to all school children. Along with food, the act provided for nutrition education, which received 1 percent of the appropriation. These funds are available for in-service training of food service personnel as well as education programs for the children. The adults who serve the food must understand the needs of the children in order to feed them effectively. With this financial support for a nutrition-education program, there should be more cooperation between the lunchroom and the classroom.

In order to effectively carry out these new school-lunch programs at all levels—federal, state, and local—the direction, supervision, and monitoring of food services must be provided by personnel trained in nutrition and food management. Continuous in-service and workshop training must be given employees at all levels.

Coordination of Effort To coordinate nutrition in the curriculum of elementary and high schools at the national level, a nutrition-education specialist has recently been appointed to the Office of Nutrition and Health, which was charged with the responsibility for coordination of resources for nutrition education within the U.S. Office of Education. For example, one of the first efforts was to form a working committee that contributed ideas for the preparation of a booklet directed toward administrators, teachers, and school-lunch personnel. The booklet focuses on attitudes as well as "how to" ideas for coordinating feeding with instructional periods.

The White House Conference panel on nutrition teaching in elementary and high schools recommended that such a position should be established in HEW. It was further recommended that state and local personnel should be appointed to coordinate nutrition-education activities and nutrition services at state and local levels within each state. In addition to providing personnel at national, state, and local levels, the administrative leadership personnel—from the state commissioner of education to principal of the smallest elementary school—must understand, accept, and actively support a nutrition-education program if it is to be implemented and carried out with any appreciable degree of harmony and effectiveness.

The participation and coordination of various professional groups concerned with school programs is essential to the strengthening of the nutrition education and nutrition service in the schools.

Training for Effective Teaching The various professionals who would be carrying on nutrition education must have appropriate training as well as teaching materials that are accurate, attractive, and educationally sound. This means that undergraduate programs must incorporate nutrition as a part of the requirements for the teaching credential for all professionals, such as elementary, science, physical education, and health-education teachers.

Continuing education courses must be developed, as well as workshops and conferences that include nutrition and sound innovative teaching methods for application to the curricula. Parents and other adults who influence children must also be provided with nutrition education. Children must have adults' interest and support before they will change their food habits.

Since 1968, several states including Louisiana, Georgia, Delaware, and Pennsylvania have prepared teaching guides for elementary teachers and others. These booklets outline concepts and learning experiences that can be developed at each grade level. Usually these are prepared by an authoritative group that represents areas such as the department of education, school food service, public health, cooperative extension services, and home-economics departments at the state universities.

There is need for an interdisciplinary study group at the national level to assess the current status of nutrition education in the schools and to prepare guidelines and resource materials.

Nutrition Education in the Community

When considering the large segment of the population that is not in school, we realize that there are vast numbers of people who do not know how to cope with nutrition problems. This may be due to lack of interest or lack or resources (both money and information). There are people who are suffering from malnutrition and even hunger as well as persons who suffer from serious health handicaps because of nutritional deficiencies who must be reached by nutrition-education programs.

A program of nutrition education has been

available to the rural population of the United States since 1918 through the Agricultural Extension Service of USDA. This program is extended to the rural communities through cooperation with the land grant colleges in each state. Its success can be attributed to the participation of the community and to training of local leadership.

The same type of local participation and leadership is being used by several different agencies to reach "hard-to-reach" groups in the inner-city poverty areas. Community aides are trained in the areas of health, welfare, and education. Nutrition education is an integral part of the program of work with the poor. Nutrition education is a component of public service agencies such as public health, visiting-nurse associations, and welfare.

Continuing education classes at high schools and colleges should be developed to train people to be community aides. Informational classes in nutrition for adults—men and women—could serve to supplement what they learned as children in school. It would equip consumers with knowledge to cope with all of the forces affecting their food choices.

A nutrition committee of all persons concerned with nutrition conditions in the community could serve as a coordinating group for dissemination of nutrition information.

Some methods for reaching people have been effectively developed within the last couple of years. The following examples of methods of taking nutrition education to the people were cited in the recommendations of Panel IV-3, Community Nutrition Teaching, of the White House Conference.

Some Methods of Taking Nutrition Education to the People:

1. Training para-professional workers, aides, and volunteers how to adjust to the people they will be teaching basic nutrition concepts.

2. Family-life education programs based on group work methods and focused on food and nutrition.

3. Mobile nutrition units equipped and staffed to provide nutrition education to people of various levels and backgrounds. Such units also would serve as a central base for teams of food aides and other community volunteers.

4. Food fairs including cooking demonstrations, movies, and question-and-answer sessions. These would provide an opportunity to reach the public with nutrition education in an entertaining way.

5. Educational television programs on nutrition in an entertaining and dramatic way, with follow-up discussion of application and information with homemaker groups conducted by a para-professional worker. This would assure reaching a fairly large group at one time with sound nutrition information.

6. Use of games for developing skills in selecting foods which provide the greatest returns in nutrition and family satisfaction for the money spent.

7. The nutrition-education component of portable-meals programs and group-feeding programs for the elderly should be expanded.

Local involvement is essential to the community programs. New methods must be found to effectively reach all segments of the community. It has often been pointed out that grassroots organizations should participate in the development, implementation, and evaluation of programs that affect them.

Nutrition Education in Mass Communication

Because television, radio, newspapers, and magazines are popular sources of information, the White House Conference Panel on Popular Education recommended that the President should appoint a task force of leading communications professionals to undertake an immediate (and continuing) program of mass communication in behalf of existing nutrition-education programs. Such an effort should be supported by public and private funds.

That panel also recommended that the task force should be guided in its work by the following guidelines:

1. The task force should maintain a continuous, close contact with all activities in nutrition information and education—particularly in problem areas—linked to a program of action where action is needed.

2. The task force should offer expert advice to independent groups and governmental agencies in connection with programs they operate.

3. The task force should have available the advice of nutrition scientists, social scientists, students of motivation, educators, specialists in communications, marketing, and advertising. It is of paramount importance that it should consult with and be guided by representatives of the racial and cultural groups to be reached.

4. The task force should enlist the support and cooperation of food companies and food-industry groups, foundations, and other private donors.

5. The problems of good nutrition being of national concern, the group should function on a national scale. However, it should certainly have close contact with local and particular situations and should devise special programs to deal with special problems.

6. Since educational materials and resources already developed are widely scattered throughout the country, with no central repository, the task force should establish a national information service to see to it that the most effective educational materials are used. Periodical listings should be published.

7. The task force should enlist the interest of influential popular personalities to help

where they can in spreading good nutrition information in the media in which they appear: sports figures, actors and entertainers, and disc jockeys—particularly those who are popular with the nutritionally vulnerable groups.

8. The program can have an identity in the form of a graphic symbol and a slogan to aid in its popularization. The idea of good nutrition must be easy to identify wherever it is written about or wherever it is talked about or exhibited.

9. The task force should address itself to the need for the reconciliation of some basic concepts and techniques in nutrition education. There is need for an evaluation of the general applicability of the simplified (Four Basic Food Groups) daily food guide. Variations of food groupings may be required to suit different audiences.

The Panel on Popular Education at the White House Conference was mainly concerned with the establishment of a national task force. However, task forces on regional and local levels could also be effective in carrying out programs of mass communication concerned with regional and local nutrition-education programs. Many fine programs exist that reach only a small portion of the audiences for which they are intended because the people don't know about them.

Food Industry Role in Nutrition Education

Malnutrition can result from overeating as well as from being underfed. The choice between enriched, fortified, or unrefined food against highly refined, sugar-filled foods can make the difference between an adequate and an inadequate diet. Adequate knowledge of nutrition to make a wise choice must be made accessible.

Nutrition education, in a broad sense, is the dissemination of information about food and nutrition. The 100-billion-dollar food industry of this country has a strong influence on the attitudes of the public towards certain foods. The food industry disseminates information through advertising, labeling, and "educational" materials. Some promotional material contains accurate information and some contains inaccurate information. Legislation should be passed to require that labeling and advertising contain information of help to consumers.

Advertising as Nutrition Education   The purpose of advertising is to sell products, so most food advertising speaks to the emotions rather than to the biological need for food. Those trained in advertising techniques have a good deal to teach nutrition educators about influencing their audience. The reverse is also true. Persons trained in nutrition are qualified to evaluate the accuracy of the advertisers' message, and to place that message in the right perspective in relation to total daily food needs.

Labeling as Nutrition Education   Although the Federal Trade Commission and the Food and Drug Administration have authority for surveillance of labeling and advertising, this is restricted to the statement being correct and not to the value of the statement. Within recent years, some legislation has been passed to provide better information on the label. This includes such information as number of servings in a package of convenience (premixed or partially mixed) foods.

The consumer is still not satisfied with the information available on packages. As an example, in October, 1970, a group of consumers, professional nutritionists, and representatives of the vegetable-fat industry concerned with the labeling of the kinds of fats in foods met and proposed a change in the labeling of certain foods to describe the kind of fat they contained.[9] As consumers become more knowledgeable about nutri-

tion, they wish to know more about the food they purchase. The FDA has shown an interest in learning about these concerns of consumers and industry.

Knowledgeable groups of interested persons should be encouraged to make recommendations to the Food and Drug Administration concerning what they expect to be included on food labels.

Studies are currently being started by the Food and Drug Administration and Grocery Manufacturers of America to test new nutrient labeling and to determine what the consumer wants on the label. Consumers have to be educated on what to look for before they can intelligently decide what is needed.

Nutrition Awareness   The food industry organized a "Nutrition Awareness" campaign in the latter part of 1970. This came about as a result of the industry's concern for its reputation after the 1969 White House Conference as well as a serious review of the recommendations of the conference. A symbol representing the Four Basic Food Groups was prepared and appeared in the advertising of food companies participating in the campaign. The impact of the symbol as a teaching tool for improving food habits is hard to measure. More needs to be done to carry the campaign beyond the advertising gimmick stage.

Unfortunately, very little money was allocated for the campaign; although the response and interest generated by the campaign were great, the whole project became bogged down. It would be hoped in the years to come that the food industry would support this cooperative effort with enough money to adequately promote a true awareness of nutrition by the public.

Educational Materials   There are some industry-prepared materials being used in and out of the classroom that are truly educational. All too often, however, these materials are prepared as promotional rather than nutrition-education material.

Materials such as some of those prepared by the National Dairy Council and the National Livestock and Meat Board have gained wide acceptance by nutrition educators. These have been carefully worked out by consultants who are well recognized in their fields. Even though these are excellent materials, it is difficult to overcome the fact that they are prepared by certain commodity groups.

The Nutrition Foundation (99 Park Avenue, New York, N.Y. 10016) is an organization to which a cross-section of the food industry belongs. The foundation is charged with distribution of funds for the support of nutrition education and research in this country. It has been in existence for 30 years. Unfortunately, funds for nutrition education are limited. If this group is to provide leadership for the food industry in developing innovative nutrition-education programs and materials, adequate funds must be made available.

The food industry has budgets totaling about four billion dollars for advertising. In 1969, General Mills' total TV budget for advertising was $29,425,100. Kellogg's budget was $22,505,900.[11] An allocation of only one per cent of each of those budgets would provide $519,310 for nutrition education programs. That amount would be about five times the total budget now available to the Nutrition Foundation for nutrition-education purposes.

Needed Resources

Nutrition Education Media Center   Nutrition education must be directed to people on every level of experience, age, income, and education so that everyone can benefit from scientific knowledge of nutrient needs. It is increasingly apparent that there is a need for a national learning, research, and infor-

mation center. The need for such a center has been described in the recommendations of all the White House Conference panels on nutrition teaching and education. This center should be established at a university. It should serve as a training laboratory, as a research and development resource, and as a clearing house for educational material with facilities for information retrieval and delivery to all persons involved with nutrition education.

Teaching Tools   On a national level, there have been two classic tools developed (a) a food guide and (b) a conceptual approach to teaching nutrition. It is time for both of these to be revised.

Food for Fitness—A Daily Food Guide (USDA Leaflet 424) places daily nutrient needs in four food groupings: (1) milk and dairy products group; (2) meat, fish, poultry and eggs groups; (3) fruits and vegetable group; (4) breads and cereal group.

The Four Basic Food Groups, a teaching tool that has been used extensively for the past ten years, should be reevaluated for its effectiveness.

A simple teaching tool must be meaningful to be effective. Grouping of foods has seemed to be the most easily understood concept of nutrient need. However, in explaining why foods are grouped in this way, some knowledge of nutrients must be taught. There are protein-rich foods, certain vitamin- and mineral-rich foods, and foods for energy. Advertising almost never mentions a food group; food is usually promoted on the basis that it builds muscles, gives energy, or contains vitamins and minerals. It seems that it is time to change the basic teaching tool.

A conceptual approach to nutrition education was developed by the Inter-Agency Committee on Nutrition Education in 1963.[12] At the present time, it is being reviewed by this same group. With the establishment of basic concepts, more effective teaching at all levels can be developed. Suggestions for revision of the basic concepts were incorporated in recommendations of the White House panels on nutrition teaching and education. The following framework was suggested by the panel that discussed elementary and secondary schools. However, it could be adapted for a wide range of nutrition education.

Conceptual Framework for Nutrition Education

1. Nutrition is the process by which food and other substances eaten become you. The food we eat enables us to live, to grow, to keep healthy and well, and to get energy for work and play.
2. Food is made up of certain chemical substances that work together and interact with body chemicals to serve the needs of the body.
   a. Each nutrient has specific uses in the body.
   b. For the healthful individual the nutrients needed by the body are usually available through food.
   c. Many kinds and combinations of food can lead to a well-balanced diet.
   d. No natural food, by itself, has all the nutrients needed for full growth and health.
3. The way a food is handled influences the amount of nutrients in the food, its safety, appearance, taste, and cost; handling means everything that happens to food while it is being grown, processed, stored, and prepared for eating.
4. All persons, throughout life, have need for about the same nutrients, but in varying amounts.
   a. The amounts needed are influenced by age, sex, size, activity, specific conditions of growth, and state of health—the amounts are altered somewhat by environmental stress.
   b. Suggestions for kinds and needed amounts of nutrients are made by scientists who continuously revise the suggestions in the light of the findings of new research.
   c. A daily food guide is helpful in translating the technical information into terms of everyday foods suitable for individuals and families.
5. Food use relates to the cultural, social, economic, and psychological aspects of living as well as to the physiological.
   a. Food is culturally defined.
   b. Food selection is an individual act but is usually influenced by social and cultural sanctions.
   c. Food can be chosen to fulfill physiological needs and at the same time satisfy social, cultural, and psychological wants.
   d. Attitudes toward food are a culmination of many experiences, past and present.
6. The nutrients, singly and in combinations of chemical substances, simulating natural foods, are available in the market; these may vary widely in usefulness, safety of use, and economy.
7. Food plays an important role in the physical and psychological health of a society or a nation just as it does for the individual and the family.
   a. The maintenance of good nutrition for the larger units of society involves many matters of public concern.
   b. Nutrition knowledge and social consciousness enable citizens to participate intelligently in the adoption of public policy affecting the nutrition of people around the world.

Research   There has been very little research in the field of nutrition education over the years. Methods of evaluation of the effectiveness of programs need to be developed. There is a need for nutrition education to be determined in a sociocultural framework. Very little is known about the behavioral motivations that bring about changes in food habits. Studies should be carried out on the motivation and effectiveness of nutrition education at all levels. A study supported by the Dairy Council of California points up the need for teaching by behavioral objectives at the elementary school level.[13] There has been no similar research at any other age or education level.

A New Resource

Society for Nutrition Education   It is interesting to note that better communication among professional nutrition educators exists now than ever before. The Society for Nutrition Education, an organization formed in 1968, has members all over the United States and the world who have expressed common needs. The Society has a publication, the *Journal of Nutrition Education*, which reviews materials for all phases of nutrition education and acts as a focal point for information about nutrition programs. Its planned activities follow along the expressed needs of the White House Conference.

The overall goal of the Society for Nutrition Education is to promote good nutrition for all by making nutrition education more effective. Nutrition education will be promoted at all levels: international, national, state, and local. The Society states that its activities, in addition to publishing the *Journal of Nutrition Education*, are threefold: education, communications, and research. (More information is available from the Society for

Nutrition Education, P.O. Box 931, Berkeley, California 94701.)

Summary

Nutrition education must be an integral part of all efforts to alleviate hunger and malnutrition. Money or its equivalent in food or food stamps must be made available for all individuals and families at low-income levels to guarantee that they will have enough food to eat. An adequate diet is a basic right of babies, children, and the indigent.

Enrichment and fortification can serve to improve certain foods in the diet. However, *motivation* to choose the right foods goes hand-in-hand with knowledge of what to eat. People's eating habits are influenced by family traditions as well as social, cultural, and religious traditions.

Nutrition education must begin with the very small child before he enters school and continue throughout his lifetime because new knowledge of food technology and nutrition will affect his choice of food. People learn about food and nutrition from a variety of sources including television, newspapers, advertisements, teachers, friends, and family. The food industry must realize its responsibility for nutrition education. Through education, people can make wise food choices. Research on nutrition education is badly needed. Nutrition education must be taught effectively. Ways must be found to reach the national population. The national policy should provide for further expansion of training of teachers in knowledge of nutrition to make them cognizant of the importance of nutrition in the lives of people.

REFERENCES

1. *Food Consumption of Households in the U.S., Spring 1965*, 1967. USDA Preliminary Report, Agricultural Research Service ARS 62–16.

2. Citizen Board of Inquiry into Hunger and Malnutrition in the United States, 1968. *Hunger U.S.A.* Citizens' Crusade Against Poverty, Washington, D.C.

3. **Davies, T. R. A., Gershoff, S. N., and Gamble, D. F.,** 1969. Review of Studies of Vitamin and Mineral Nutrition in the United States (1950–1968). *Journal of Nutrition Education* 1(2) Supplement 1: 37–58.

4. **Kelsay, J. L.,** 1969. A Compendium of Nutritional Status Studies Conducted in the United States, 1957–1967. *Journal of Nutrition* 99, Supplement I, Part II:123–142.

5. The Advertising Council, 1970. *Food and Nutrition Newsletter,* USDA, No. 7, October 26.

6. **Hill, M. M.,** 1969. Nutrition Committees and Nutrition Education. *Journal of Nutrition Education* 1(1):14–16.

7. **Juhas, L.,** 1970. Special Food Service Program for Children: San Francisco, California. *Programs for Infants and Young Children Part II, Nutrition.* Appalachian Regional Commission, Washington, D.C., October, p. 16.

8. Children's Food Service Programs, 1970. *Journal of Nutrition Education* 2:8, Summer.

9. FDA Weighing Special Dietary Rule for Fatty Acids, 1970. *Food Chemical News* 12(33):18, November 9.

10. FDA Negotiates with GMA Institute for Consumer Survey, 1970. *Food Chemical News* 12(38):12, December 14.

11. **Choate, R. B.,** 1970. The Seduction of the Innocent. Testimony to Subcommittee of Consumer Committee on Commerce, U.S. Senate, July 23. (Quoting: National Advertising Investment Report, 1969, Leading National Advertisers, Inc.)

12. Interagency Committee on Nutrition Education, 1964. Basic Concept for Nutrition Education. *Nutrition Program News*, USDA, September-October.

13. **Lovett, R., Barker, E., and Marcus, B.,** 1970. The Effect of a Nutrition Education Program at the Second Grade Level. *Journal of Nutrition Education* 2(2), Supplement I:79–95.

Chapter 18

Special Problems of the Very Poor

Robert Choate

Ideas held of American eating habits include the misconception that the poor have unbalanced diets because of ignorance. Actually, the vast majority of the poor are heavily influenced in their food selection by the limitations of their pocketbook. In many instances, their diet is amazingly balanced, considering the expenditures available. If a study of market prices indicates that a family of four should spend $1,570 a year for a modest but varied nutritious diet (according to USDA), many adjustments have to be made when the reality of poverty limits one to $600 to feed four hungry stomachs over a 12-month period. The adjustments include:

1. eliminating fresh milk, fresh fruits, and spoilables such as eggs and frozen foods;
2. increasing the mush-and-gravy routine, the mush to be from some cheap grain or tuber and the gravy to be high in meat-derived fats such as lard and pork drippings;
3. eating two meals a day or making one from a water base—such as coffee, colas, or other sugared syrups.

When the dollar crunch is this severe, the kitchen may be nothing more than a burner on top of a room heater. The sink may be outdoors. Storage space may be orange crates or abandoned iceboxes. Spoilage, infestation, and contamination under these conditions may further deplete the already marginal food supply. The poverty cook prepares food in spurts, generally when the money comes in. The meal served on Saturday may not taste the same on the following Wednesday after it has been stretched, added to, diluted and seasoned—but more often than not Wednesday's meal is a product of Saturday's origins. The nutritional depletion from cooking and recooking and drying and evaporation should not be underestimated.

To teach good nutrition to families under such economic stress is like teaching a little girl to swim and then pushing her overboard in mid-Atlantic. Such education can't hurt, but it has little chance of changing the eventual outcome. History has taught the impoverished family to rely on collards and grits, fatback and tomatoes, or tortillas and beans with chile for warmth. Such diets are not based on ignorance but on practical economics. They may be too high in calories for the nutrients gained, but at least they sustain life, though full vitality may be reduced and vigorous activity eliminated; the end result is flabby flesh—flesh unprepared for sustained physical effort. Since hunger hurts but onsetting malnutrition is experienced at worst as malaise, an unbalanced diet high in low-cost starches and fats is often chosen as the lesser of two evils. Thus, the poor first need dollars before any nutrition education reasonably can be expected to stick.

It may be true that the proper blend of peanut butter, yams, tomatoes, and rice can sustain one in healthy condition for a small sum per day, but the monotony will undermine morale just as malnutrition does, and make Jack in the classroom a dull boy.

Nutritional Illiteracy

Beyond improving the diet of the poor by providing them with greater funds, what can be done to contend with the nutritional illiteracy that pervades all economic groups in the United States?

If a $600-a-year family is given access to $1,200 for food, some of the additional funds probably will be squandered on imprudent purchases—the convenience foods, which are often high in calories and certainly are high in cost per nutrient. Enriched bread, milk, fruit, and the leaner meats might be the first things reinserted in the low-income family's diet, but endless advertising on television might also instigate purchases of sweet rolls, snack foods, ice cream, dry cereals, and canned fruit drinks. These are the foods that jingles sell so well, which have made television today's unmatched food educator.

Grandma's Kitchen versus Mother's TV The kitchen was once the learning place for food habits as one helped shell peas or bake cookies. From grandmother to mother to child, inherited food wisdom was passed down daily. Today the ever-present television set beckons the young as mother, rich or poor, seeks to reduce her work load by buying the more expensive preprepared foods. (Those who work eight hours a day and then commute home to a house full of kids appreciate work-savers and time-savers even more than the suburban housewife.)

Nutrition Teaching in the Schools With inherited food wisdom rapidly disappearing, the classroom teacher or nurse or coach has tried to fill the gap; these educators have been provided with teaching materials by segments of the food industry, following the lead of the powerful lobbies that created the "Four Basic Food Groups." The schoolroom nutrition educator now often is but one more salesman at the end of a tremendous line of public persuasion.

Inadequacy of the Four Basic Food Groups. The Four Basic Food Groups might have made sense decades ago, if one overlooks milk; placing milk in a special category even in those years still seems peculiar. Was it the protein? Was it the riboflavin? Was it the calcium? Was it the vitamin A that begot for the dairy industry a special food category? Today's complex foods, sometimes synthesized and often blended, transgress freely across the Four Foods boundaries. The foods of 1975 and beyond will be even more complicated. Teaching children of today by the Four-Basic-Food-Groups method is to invite ignorance a decade ahead. Perhaps unaware of the datedness of their teaching materials—in any case unable to develop exciting nutritional messages—today's classroom salesmen are defending a failure-proven system. We are still a nation of nutritional illiterates.

Television Commercials Almost by default, the tube has taken over. For the poor as well as the rich, the food information distributed by television and radio needs radical upgrading. Instead of promoting good nutrition, many advertisements of edibles on mass media today actually promote malnutrition. Instead of selling nutrients or the role nutrients play in the body's health, they sell calories. As we know, a calorie is a measure of heat, of energy, perhaps of mass of food; nutrients are the individual characteristics, each of which contributes to the well-being of the body. To confuse the public with the sloppy interpretation that calories are nutrients is similar to informing an automobile driver that it matters not what he puts in his gas tank, as long as the gallons are there. Advertisements also need a little tiger in their tank.

Sesame Street demonstrated the power

of commercials to teach and emerged with an exciting instructional message that now penetrates the ghetto. Madison Avenue's advertisers can learn from Sesame Street. Commercials *can* educate as they sell. It will require an intellectual effort by those who write the slogans and jingles. This effort must be made, for no amount of eleemosynary education put forth on public-service time will be able to win a child away from the salesman's hard-sell pitch, even if it promotes ignorance of food values. This brings us to ethics; ethics too must change. The sloganeer who wrote that one cereal "improves your wind" was simply not telling the truth. "Go power all day long" cannot reasonably be attained from any dry cereal; nor will any make you a tiger. "Hi-C" is not a term to describe a fruit drink that is really low in vitamin C. Although Sesame Street-type short announcements can sell nutrition to this nation of nutritional illiterates, the message won't stick if the commercial liars are left unchallenged. For that reason, currently pending lawsuits, petitions, and challenges to the ethics of the advertising industry bode well for consumers.

For years the food industry has claimed "you can't sell nutrition." Reviewing their past efforts, one wonders if they ever really tried. Certainly leaving nutrition education to nutritionists invited a fiasco. The food industry, seeking communication advice from this group of experts, could not have been envisioning a very vigorous campaign. Until recently, the vitality of nutritionist, dietitian, and food-technologist conferences resembled that of a wake. Even today many nutritionists who have consulted for industry think it beneath them (or malicious of them) to comment on the accuracy of their sponsors' media message. As one well-known nutritionist said not long ago about Saturday-morning TV commercials to kids, "I don't give a damn." One must search widely today for a professionally accredited independent critic of the advertising of edibles. Industry does not deal kindly with those who point out its foibles.

The default of nutritionists has shown that they should not be involved in future popular nutrition-education campaigns except as technical advisers on the validity of the presentation.

Nutritional Literacy

It is the box designer, the cartoonist, and the jingle writer who, made cognizant of Sesame Street's values and educated into new nutritional wisdom, can apply the proper talent to teach over 200 million Americans improved food habits.

Games Rich and poor would gain from modern versions of Jack Spratt or "one-potato-two-potato" and the like. If counting fingertips and knuckles can identify the length of calendar months or if jingles such as "Thirty days hath September" can remain popular and useful over generations, someone should be able to advocate nutrients by verse. Professionals may say that poor children cannot remember words like "riboflavin," but they have forgotten that the Mets' baseball roster is remembered by Harlem's ghetto child. Why not the nine players on the "good nutrition team"?

Vocabulary It might be wise to go back one step further and reconsider nutrition's vocabulary. Why should we have to remember words like "riboflavin?" Now that we realize that nutrients should become familiar in the everyday vocabulary, perhaps it would be wise to separate the vitamins and to better describe protein building blocks by a new simplified vocabulary.

Comic Books Comic books advocating nutrients offer opportunities. Members of the Supermarket Institute might be willing to distribute them en masse in both full-color and coloring-book form. Were the message to be duplicated over television, perhaps in a Romper Room setting, the coloring of certain nutrients might help children remember their advantages.

Nutrition History for the Pre-Teens One of the more intriguing ideas for reaching the preteen group comes from Cornell's Dr. Michael Latham. Nutrients have played an overlooked but important part in history. For example, Arctic explorers died from overdoses of vitamin A, consumed in the liver of polar bears common to the Arctic region. The vitamin-A level of such livers is far above mankind's toxic range. Marco Polo used protein from dried yak milk to sustain long expeditions. Geophagia, as evidenced by clay-eating in nonmilk consuming African countries, gets bone-building calcium into the diet.

A talented group of radio artists could easily produce one-minute historical vignettes designed to pique children's curiosity. One can imagine a scene verbalized over radio: an Arctic explorer crouches in an igloo seeking shelter from the driving blizzard outside; he learns to avoid the liver of the polar bear from his Eskimo host. What child could resist finding out more about vitamin-A and polar-bear diets if the sound track set the mood?

Teen-Agers For the 16-year-old crowd, nutrition education might gain from a set of wheels. That's the age when the paint job, the chassis, and the fuel supply often become an obsession. Why not compare one's skin condition to the paint job of the car, or one's skeleton to the chassis and nutrients to the octane rating?

Nutrition Education in the School These types of approaches, done in printed form, graphics, tapes, films, games, and skits can be bolstered on the school's own grounds. It's only a matter of time before some recreation-equipment company brings Cuisinier rods to the outdoor playground. Why not bring out a version of nutritional hopscotch; why not design play building blocks with the nutrient on one side and the sources of that nutrient pictured on the other sides? There are nutritional "Monopoly's" already on the drafting board.

More conventional but still effective would be a nutritional scorecard for the classroom wall. Showing desirable nutrient levels in at least nine categories, a changeable scorecard could reflect the nutritional worth of the upcoming school-lunch menu. At the steam-table line itself or on the paper milk carton accompanying the meal, the nutrient worth of the parts of the meal could be shown.

Another part of the new nutrition education effort must consider the best means for identifying nutrient *bargains* in the marketplace—those foods that fill yet provide nutrient balance at minimum cost. It should become part of elementary education for males and females alike to learn how to gain the most nutrients in all needed categories for the fewest dollars. One can envision a classroom whose walls show in perspective various foods in cans, packages, and wrappers. The labels would clearly state the size, weight, and unit cost. Geometry, addition, multiplication, algebra as well as nutrition could be taught in such a setting.

A Multi-Disciplinary Success

Alone, each of these approaches would fail. Together, backstopped by food commercials that popularize the nutrition message, the public will respond. The synergistic impact of a nutrition message from comic book, television ad, radio spot, drive-in theater screen and school-lunch scorecard could eliminate the nutritional illiteracy that pervades our country. That the population is interested in nutrients was shown in the cereal controversy in the summer of 1970 and in the wide sale of Linus Pauling's book on vitamin C. It is now time for the nutrient message to fill today's vacuum. Communicators have been very successful in selling "foodless" foods—the calorie-and-little-else group. Their powers of persuasion can be turned to a much more worthy task. It should help sales of quality foods at the same time.

As the grits-and-fatback, poverty-stricken family finds dollar relief from welfare or the food-stamp reform, as such families receive the new food direction of food advertising, as they learn from their children's experiences at the school-lunch table—their food buying habits will take a more healthful direction. Soda pop and candy bars will remain an attraction, but all Americans, rich and poor, will have learned the toll they take.

Chapter 19

Professionals and Para-professionals

Grace A. Goldsmith

A nutrition program is a fundamental aspect of a national policy of public health and preventive medicine. A comprehensive program in this area should be considered a cornerstone in developing and maintaining a healthy population capable of its most creative productivity. Good nutrition is a prerequisite for the normal growth and development of children and for the maintenance of health in adult life. Nutrition not only affects physical growth, but also influences learning and behavior and, as a result, has major social consequences. The dietary intake of all essential nutrients in proper amounts, and their effective utilization by the human body, can provide a basis for maximum fulfillment of the potential of every individual. The primary focus of a national nutrition program should be on the individual person and on making available to him the necessary information and resources to enable him to obtain good nutrition.

Many different professions provide health care for citizens, and each of these professions has need for accurate and up-to-date information about nutrition. Such information is essential also in functions and activities of many institutions, e.g., schools, private and commercial establishments, social agencies, hospitals, nursing homes and health departments, as well as in individual families, where most food is consumed and where most eating habits are learned.

A National Policy for Advanced Academic Training in Nutrition

Provision of a national policy for advanced academic training in nutrition in this country implies some assumptions about future health-care delivery systems and the manpower policy necessary to provide the personnel that will be required. A national nutrition and health policy should be focused on the community level to ensure that adequate food, and knowledge of how to use it, is available to provide health benefits in the daily lives of people. Community nutrition services should be expanded as part of the comprehensive health and welfare program of every state in order to utilize more effectively the available food supply and to facilitate both maintenance of health and recovery from illness. These services can be carried out in facilities that are currently available, such as universities, medical centers, health clinics, neighborhood centers, community hospitals, and other independent community-based operations, or in new facilities that can be developed.

Community nutrition centers should be responsible for promotion of the following services: (1) public-education programs to provide nutrition information for every citizen, (2) consultation services to health professionals relative to the nutritional needs of their patients, (3) consultation with individuals and families concerned with nutritional problems, (4) provision of nutrition-training programs for community-health aides and technicians, (5) provision of opportunities for field training for students working toward degrees as specialists in nutrition and for other health professionals. Such centers also could afford support for school programs in nutrition education.

A national nutrition program will require a major increase in manpower with competence and commitment in the field of nutrition—including physicians, dentists, basic scientists (biological and social), dietitians, public-health nutritionists, nurses, health educators, food scientists, and technologists. The manpower policy recommended by the Panel on Advanced Academic Teaching of Nutrition of the White House Conference on Food, Nutrition and Health[1] included provision for four primary areas of training.

1. Training of nutrition leaders (physicians, dietitians, nutritionists, basic scientists, and others) for teaching and research in universities and colleges and for administrative positions in health agencies. This training requires advanced study and specialization in nutrition leading to degrees at the master and doctorate levels. These graduate training programs in nutrition should have the highest priority.

2. Training of nutritionists and dietitians at the baccalaureate degree level who will be responsible for the direct delivery of services in the community and who can be assisted by health aides and technicians who have received training in nutrition.

3. Training of personnel in the health professions whose primary commitment is not in nutrition but who can play a supporting role in a national nutrition program. This group includes physicians, dentists and dental hygienists, nurses, health educators, home economists, social workers, physical education directors, and persons in other allied health specialties.

4. Training of health aides and technicians in nutrition. This training can be correlated with the utilization of baccalaureate personnel trained in nutrition and dietetics who, in turn, can train and supervise these aides. Opportunity and incentive should be provided for health aides to continue their education toward baccalaureate degrees. People who are recruited primarily from communities that have the greatest nutrition problems can be particularly effective as nutrition aides in their own communities.

The Panel on Advanced Academic Teaching of Nutrition of the White House Conference recommended that the Department of Health, Education, and Welfare be assigned responsibility for the national nutrition program and that an Office of Nutrition be established in this department to formulate policy and coordinate all food and nutrition activities. It was suggested that one of the responsibilities of this office should be to work with public and private agencies at national, state, and local levels to revise civil service and other job descriptions to permit employment of nutrition personnel with educational preparation below the graduate level, as well as at the graduate level, and to provide a "career ladder" opportunity for the employment of such nutrition personnel.

At present, programs in food and nutrition are scattered throughout many government agencies. It is essential that these programs be administered as a total system rather than being dealt with piecemeal. The National Nutrition Survey, which was conducted recently, showed that there are serious problems of undernutrition and malnutrition in the United States, particularly among the poor but also in other segments of the population. A nutrition program must be implemented now to alleviate existing problems. Effective nutritional surveillance must be instituted in the future to periodically determine the nutritional health of the people and to evaluate the effect of education and service programs in alleviating malnutrition and in teaching the basic tenets of proper nutrition to consumers.

Advanced Academic Training and Research in Nutrition

A national program in nutrition can be effective only with major increases in the numbers of competent personnel, namely, teachers, investigators, and practitioners, who have received nutrition training as part of the curriculum in the various professional health disciplines. The overall objective is to train leaders who can plan, administer, and evaluate nutrition programs; provide nutrition information; and deliver nutrition services to the people.

Current programs of advanced training and research in basic and applied nutrition should be strengthened and new programs should be established in colleges and universities. Nutrition leaders of the future should receive preparation for their careers in centers devoted to training in one or more of the several disciplines that can involve nutrition, that is, as:

a. Basic scientists in either the biological or social sciences. This group includes biochemists, physiologists, anthropologists, psychologists, and behavioral scientists. Much of the basic research in nutrition has been carried out by biological scientists. More recently, social and behavioral scientists have contributed to nutrition research, particularly in epidemiological and clinical studies.

b. Dietitians, public-health nutritionists, and community nutritionists. These are the only health professionals concerned solely with translating the findings of the science of nutrition into action and nutritional care of people. Expansion of training in this area should have high priority and should include both baccalaureate programs to provide personnel to work at the community level and graduate programs, at both master and doctorate levels, to provide future scientists and leaders.

c. Nutrition teachers for colleges and schools of home economics, teachers in health education and physical education, specialists in food science and technology, and others. In addition, all teachers in both elementary and secondary schools should receive some training in nutrition, since they have an opportunity to integrate nutrition teaching throughout the school experience.

d. Physicians, dentists, nurses, and allied health workers. Some health professionals in this group will specialize in nutrition, whereas others will use nutrition as only a part of their professional practice. The latter should learn the basic principles of nutrition and its application to human health; the specialist will require much more extensive nutrition knowledge.

The strength of future programs in nutrition will be dependent in large part on the scholarly productivity and investigative efforts of the leaders of nutrition in academic institutions. More financial support for research in many aspects of nutrition science is urgently needed in these institutions. The search for new information and for elucidation of unsolved problems must be continued and expanded. The important discoveries of the future can change the whole course of society. It should be emphasized that the caliber of research being carried out in institutions is closely correlated with the strength of the overall academic program.

Financial Support for Expansion of Nutrition Manpower

In order to train nutrition leaders (i.e., administrators, teachers, research scientists, and practitioners) it will be essential that the federal government provide substantial increases in funds for both institutional support and for traineeship for prospective students. Universities and colleges will not be able to develop these new programs without financial assistance. Support must be provided for teachers and institutions to carry out the training, as well as for students during the period of training.

One approach to the preparation of the necessary manpower for a national nutrition program is the development of centers in at least one university in each state that can provide high-quality educational programs for baccalaureate and graduate-level personnel and can develop important research programs in nutrition. These centers can, serve, also, as a regional resource for assisting in the establishment of community nutrition centers and for aiding other institutions in the development of training programs in nutrition at the baccalaureate or technician (aide) level.

General Recommendations for Curricula for Training Nutrition Scientists

The meaning and value of nutrition in the whole life span should be the principal emphasis. In the past, many curricula have stressed the nutritional-deficiency diseases rather than the role of nutrition in growth, development, and the maintenance of health. Relationships of nutrition to illness should receive due consideration, of course. It has been suggested that the nutritionist's laboratory should be the home and the community in which the person lives, as well as the traditional basic research laboratory. Nutrition training must include experiences in both basic and applied research.

New systems of delivery of nutrition services must be developed in conjunction with programs of total health care that include prevention as well as treatment of illness. There is a marked increase in interest in community medicine and ambulatory care at the present time. These are good areas for nutrition teaching in which basic information can be applied at a practical level.

More time for electives should be provided as part of the curriculum for all students. This time can be devoted to special nutrition projects or courses, or to nutrition services in the community. More emphasis should be given to applied nutrition, not only in the classroom, but through field experience in hospitals, clinics, and community centers. More interdisciplinary teaching in health services should be incorporated early in the course of study. The team approach is of great value in understanding and solving nutrition problems, which are many faceted.

In recent years, numerous advances have been made in food science and technology, resulting in marked changes in the food supply of the American public. The scientific principles of modern food processing that are involved in the preparation of well-known standard foods, new convenience foods and special dietary foods should be included in the nutrition curriculum.

Attention should be directed to continuing education of all persons engaged in the teaching and practice of nutrition, from the elementary teacher and community worker through the university professor and high-level administrator. Authoritative, attractive and readily understandable information derived from nutrition science should be prepared for the use of these various kinds of personnel. All types of communications media should be employed in this endeavor.

Recruitment of Nutrition Personnel

A massive program of recruitment to the nutrition professions should be undertaken to fulfill the needs expressed at the White House Conference. Teachers and students in schools and colleges, and the general public as well, should be made aware of the value of good nutrition and its contributions to health, growth, learning, alertness, and ability to work. The fascinating opportunities for service to mankind for persons educated in nutrition should be delineated. The positive values of nutrition in the lives of people

should be stressed. The social, psychological, and cultural implications of nutritional care, as well as its scientific application, should interest many young people who are seeking to be involved in helping individuals to a better life. The personal rewards and satisfactions in this profession are great and should be used to recruit personnel to this field. Expansion and improvement of existing nutrition training and research programs and the development of new programs (such as interdisciplinary projects where future professionals are exposed to important problems in nutrition under new systems of health care) should attract more students.

Adequate financial support for trainees is an essential part of the recruitment process. Increased numbers of scholarships and training stipends must be made available, and the levels of the stipends must be increased.

Recruitment should draw from all parts of American society, with emphasis upon those who have not had an opportunity to participate previously in responsible positions in health and nutrition. Recruits drawn from a community should be especially well-equipped to return to that same community as competent leaders. The many career opportunities in nutrition include teaching and research in an academic environment; public-health nutrition, dietetics; interpreting nutrition in health-care agencies and institutions; the educational and technical fields of food and nutrition in industry; and the broad area of nutrition education, including the communications media.

Special Recommendations for Training of Public Health and Community Nutritionists and Dietitians

As mentioned previously, this group of health professionals is the only one whose professional training is grounded solely and specifically in the knowledge, skills, and art required in translating the findings of nutritional science into action and the nutritional care of people. The nutritionist and dietitian must know nutritional needs in health and disease throughout the life cycle; the role of nutrients in metabolic processes; the nutrient content of foods, food habits and practices; planning and evaluation of diets; food ecnomics and budgeting; and the psychological and social significance of food and eating. Educational methods and knowledge of ways of meeting the nutritional needs of individuals, groups, and communities are important.

Educational requirements for dietitians and public-health nutritionists are essentially the same at the undergraduate level and may be similar at the graduate level. Dietitians usually work in hospitals or clinics while public-health or community nutritionists usually work in agencies in the community. Both dietitians and nutritionists may function as administrators, teachers, research workers, and consultants or be involved in direct-service activities with individuals or groups.

The American Dietetic Association[2] has developed requirements for association membership that include minimum academic requirements and requirements for four areas of specialization: general dietetics, management, therapeutic and clinical dietetics, and community nutrition.

A committee of the Faculties for Graduate Training in Public Health Nutrition and the Association of State and Territorial Public Health Nutrition Directors[3] has prepared a detailed report on nutrition personnel in public health that describes the responsibilities and qualifications of various categories of public-health nutritionists, including guidelines for undergraduate and graduate training. The public-health nutritionist may work in general or specialized areas of public health, such as maternal and child health, the mentally retarded or multi-handicapped, chronic diseases, geriatrics and rehabilitation, clinical or therapeutic nutrition (dietetics) or group feeding. A discussion of the role of medical, research, and administrative public-health nutritionists and community-health aides is included in this report.

Dietitians usually have an internship, which means that they spend a year in a hospital under supervision after completing their academic studies. Public-health nutritionists may or may not have an internship but do have training in public-health areas. In the future, it would seem desirable to provide a wide variety of internships, field experiences or opportunities for on the job training after, or as a part of, academic requirements. This could be done through various agencies and centers that deliver nutritional services to the public. Some dietitians and public-health nutritionists will need more training in psychology and the social sciences than they have received in the past. Others may need more training in business management and administration.

The Panel on Advanced Academic Teaching of Nutrition of the White House Conference estimated that the number of dietitians and public-health nutritionists needed to provide even moderately adequate service to the American people should be at least doubled within the next five years. It was pointed out that there is an urgent need for these services in antipoverty programs; school-health programs; consultation for patients of private physicians; programs of local and state health departments; and of various community agencies, clinics, hospitals, nursing homes, and other medical-care facilities.

In the future, the responsibilities and services of the dietitian and public-health nutritionist will probably change. Some of their current activities will be delegated to nutrition aides and technicians. Dietitians and public-health nutritionists will be engaged to a greater extent in planning, evaluating, consulting, and supervising.

The funding of educational programs in this whole area of training must be expanded. New programs for the development of nutrition technicians, aides, and assistants should be developed in community colleges. More baccalaureate and graduate professional training should be instituted. New programs in dietetics and public-health nutrition at the doctoral level should be provided. Graduate-level trainees are needed for the training of teachers and practitioners in schools of public health, medicine, dentistry, nursing, home economics, and other areas.

Research funds should be made available for development of new methods and techniques in nutrition education for both the professional worker and the general public. For example, the most effective ways in which information can be brought to the ordinary citizen to improve the quality of individual and family nutrition should be the subject of extensive investigation.

Nutrition Training of Physicians, Dentists, Nurses, and Allied Health Professionals

In view of the fundamental importance of nutrition in normal growth and development and in the maintenance of health, it is essential that all physicians, dentists, nurses, and allied health personnel receive some training in basic nutrition and its application in preventive and therapeutic health care. Some of these health professionals will be interested in studying nutrition as a speciality and will require advanced training in both basic and applied nutrition science.

The teaching of nutrition in schools of medicine, dentistry, and nursing is most inadequate at the present time and is almost nonexistent in some schools. The number of specialists in nutrition among physicians, dentists, and nurses is very limited; a few hundred persons would be an optimistic estimate. It has been suggested that an individual or a committee be assigned responsibility for nutrition teaching in each of the professional schools in universities, e.g., medicine, dentistry and dental hygiene, nursing, public health, food science and technology, and allied health sciences. In some professional schools, it will be desirable to teach nutrition in a designated course dealing with the basic scientific principles of nutrition and their application to human health. In many schools, nutrition teaching should be incorporated in courses in the basic sciences (such as biology, biochemistry, and physiology); in schools of medicine, nutrition teaching will be incorporated in clinical specialities (such as pediatrics, obstetrics, internal medicine, and surgery). Regardless of the plan of instruction, nutrition should be included in the required or core curriculum.

Currently, in most medical schools, the student learns something about nutrition in courses in several departments, but there is little or no correlation of nutrition teaching. A fragmentary selection of various aspects of nutrition that have relevance to particular clinical subjects is offered, but there are appreciable gaps in nutrition education. A few schools offer elective courses in nutrition, experience in a nutrition clinic or opportunity for nutritional investigation. Many medical students learn only about florid malnutrition, i.e., the deficiency diseases. Little objective assessment of the nutritional knowledge acquired by medical students has been made.

In a medical school with a good nutrition

program, there is usually a strong section or department interested in nutrition or one or more professors with a special interest in clinical nutrition or research.

Recruitment of physicians for a career in nutrition has been difficult due, in part, to lack of subspeciality status for clinical nutrition. Also, there has been a dearth of superior nutrition training programs and of recognition by medical schools and teaching hospitals of the need for such programs.

In professional schools where trained nutrition personnel are not available because of the financial restrictions, the federal government should establish grants to support nutrition teaching. In medical centers where more than one professional school exists, nutrition resources should be pooled through a nutrition unit or coordinating committee. In professional schools where trained personnel are available, nutrition units should be established where advanced training of nutritional specialists can be conducted.

It seems highly desirable to establish a number of new training programs in medical schools throughout the United States to produce the physicians who can be leaders in the development of effective nutrition programs in this country. The Council on Foods and Nutrition of the American Medical Association has made a number of recommendations for nutrition teaching in medical schools.[4] In a conference on this subject in 1962, the importance of nutritional diagnosis as an integral part of medical diagnosis was pointed out, and the profound influence of nutrition in many disease states was discussed. Specific suggestions were made for incorporation of nutrition in the medical curriculum.

Students should work with patients in their homes and in community environments over prolonged periods so that they can develop an understanding of, and concern for, nutrition problems and for the role played by social factors in illness. It is desirable to conduct clinical teaching of nutrition in small groups in hospitals, clinics, and community centers. An interdisciplinary team approach is most valuable. The team might include physicians, dentists, nurses, nutritionists, social workers, and other health personnel. Units in clinical nutrition should be established in teaching hospitals and community centers to demonstrate their value in providing better patient care, in developing preventive medical programs in nutrition, and in attracting young physicians and other health workers to the field of human nutrition.

Special elective courses in both basic and applied nutrition should be developed in all professional schools. More elective time has been made available recently in most curricula. Electives in nutrition can involve participation in programs designed to deliver total health care in poverty areas. Electives in a division of nutritional and metabolic research can serve as an introduction to a career in academic clincial nutrition. A most valuable elective opportunity may be provided by overseas programs in countries where serious malnutrition is common.

Courses of study leading to advanced degrees in nutrition should be available for students of medicine, dentistry, nursing, food science and technology; such courses should also be available for workers in allied health fields. Currently, combined-degree programs are being offered in a few schools; for example, the Master of Science degree in nutrition or the Master of Public Health degree with a major in nutrition can be obtained in conjunction with the M.D. degree. In another program it is possible to obtain both the M.D. and the Ph.D. in nutrition during the prescribed course of study. Other new programs offer the possibility of obtaining both the M.D. and Doctor of Public Health degrees with major emphasis in nutrition. Comparable combined-degree programs should be developed for dental students, nurses, and other allied health workers.

Advanced Academic Training of Other Personnel in Nutrition

Training of Teachers of Home Economics and of Agricultural Extension Workers University units of home economics have traditionally been a site of primary importance for the training of nutrition scientists and practitioners. They have been responsible for basic training of dietitians and public-health nutritionists and have provided most of the nutrition training for agricultural extension workers and teachers of home economics in secondary schools. This latter group of teachers provides nutrition education for the youth of the country. Extension workers bring nutrition directly to the attention of the public and can exert great influence in programs designed to combat malnutrition and improve nutritional health. Today, there is a trend toward changing the orientation of home-economics programs, as well as the name of these academic units. It is essential that nutrition training be given continued recognition and support within new programs as they evolve.

Training of Teachers of Health Education, Physical Education, and Recreation Nutrition and physical fitness are closely associated. Professional personnel in the fields of health and physical education and recreation are in unique positions to contribute to nutrition education, as well as to physical

fitness, as they have regular contact with many of the country's children and youth. Increasing attention is being given to physical education and recreation programs for the poor, for the handicapped, for parents as well as children, and for the aging. Basic nutrition information and its application to health should be included in the curriculum for all personnel in these areas of education and provision should be made for continuing education of this group.

A Summary Statement of Philosophy and Policy

Nutrition is a multifaceted science related to many professional disciplines. The scope of the science of nutrition is difficult to define. One definition of nutrition, as suggested at a conference on nutrition education in medical schools[4] is

> Nutrition is the science of food, the nutrients and other substances therein, their action, interaction and balance in relation to health and disease and the processes by which the organism ingests, digests, absorbs, transports, utilizes and excretes food substances. In addition, nutrition must be concerned with certain social, economic, cultural and psychological implications of food and eating.

Many persons would add to this definition that nutrition includes some aspects of food production, processing, marketing, and distribution. These broad concepts of nutrition indicate that training and research in the science of nutrition, and its application to human health, must be included in many professional disciplines if current problems are to be solved and adequate nutrition is to be provided for all citizens of this country.

REFERENCES

1. White House Conference on Food, Nutrition and Health, 1970. Panel IV-2, *Advanced Academic Teaching of Nutrition*. U.S. Government Printing Office, Washington, D.C.

2. *Minimum Academic Requirements for A.D.A. Membership*, 1969. American Dietetic Association, July 1.

3. *Nutrition Personnel in Public Health*. A report of a Committee of the Faculties for Graduate Training in Public Health Nutrition and the Association of State and Territorial Public Health Nutrition Directors. November, 1969. Ruth L. Huenemann, Chairman. To be published.

4. A.M.A. Council on Foods and Nutrition, 1963. Nutrition Teaching in Medical Schools. *Journal of the American Medical Association* 183:955–957, March 16.

PART 4

Improving Large-Scale
Programs and Agencies

Chapter 20

USDA: Built-in Conflicts

Jean Mayer

Conflicts of interest always have been and still are inherent in the aims and structure of the United States Department of Agriculture. The department is supposed to promote production of agricultural commodities, insure stable (and sufficiently rewarding) prices, and protect farmers. It also administers price-support programs and agricultural subsidies and can retire land into the soil bank. Thus, we end up with a department that simultaneously subsidizes farmers to increase production (through agricultural research and various direct aids to production), pays them not to produce, and fixes prices or subsidies to save them from the consequences of the overproduction (of wheat, corn, cotton, etc.), which would not have occurred had the government-subsidized program not existed. In some extreme cases, money is spent to increase production of crops that are useless (like pitch pine, which became obsolete when the United States Navy decided to replace sailing ships by ironclads over 100 years ago) or harmful (the Department of Agriculture is helping increase tobacco production at the same time that the Department of Health, Education, and Welfare is spending money to decrease tobacco consumption).

Agribusiness versus Small Farmers

Methods developed and subsidized by government programs have increased the sophistication and efficiency of agricultural production. Since the implementation of these methods depends on large amounts of existing or borrowed capital, small farmers are being pushed out of agriculture. The five-billion-dollar subsidy program benefits owners of medium and large farming enterprises and pays nonfarmers to keep land out of production. The disappearance of the small family farm, deplored by sentimentalists, is probably in part inevitable; carried too far, it will mean that we may end up with the minimum number of farmers needed for efficient production, most of it centered in the "farm states" of the Midwest. This is not a desirable trend; biologists recognize that many natural disasters can destroy the productivity of a region or the growth of a crop: weather, floods, plant blights, animal diseases—not to mention man-made emergencies. To have no reserve of farmers, and no knowledge of farming left in "marginal" areas, may be as dangerous as to try to operate a national health system with the very least possible number of physicians and other trained personnel.

It is possible to keep small farmers going. If we put our efforts—and our agricultural subsidies—into the development of additional production of fruits and vegetables (which nutritionally we need far more than we need increased production of wheat, corn, or animal products), we could keep farming in important consumer areas: Pennsylvania, New York, New England, and California. Fruit and vegetable crops do lend themselves to the perpetuation of small enterprises; they employ much more manpower than production of basic cereals or the mass production of beef, pork, poultry, and eggs; but they would need subsidization so that the wages of migrant and other agricultural laborers required could rise to industrial levels without causing a rise of consumer prices, which would defeat the social and nutritional aims. The type of subsidization that should be considered, however, is very different from that presently in effect in our agricultural programs. Like that envisaged by the old "Brannan Plan" (or that in use in the United Kingdom), the program would be designed to keep prices sufficiently rewarding to producers and sufficiently low to the consumers, with the subsidy covering the difference. Present subsidy programs do nothing for the consumers; in fact, existing legislation is often designed—milk is a glaring example—to prevent consumer prices from going down.

It is all too often forgotten that the Department of Agriculture has been given by law extremely important functions that do not fall into the usually-perceived role of the secretary as the helper to and the voice of the farmers and agribusiness but rather into his political role as the chief electoral agent of the President in the farm states. These functions, of course, are his responsibilities in antihunger and proconsumer programs.

Agribusiness versus Welfare Programs

The Secretary of Agriculture administers the food stamp and the donated commodity programs, which together at present keep 15 million Americans from starving. He is also responsible for the National School Lunch Program, which reaches daily about 40 million children. Seven-and-a-half million children receive a free school lunch, and some of them a free breakfast, which may be their best meals of the day. The others pay an average of 30 cents for meals that cost approximately one dollar. There are built-in conflicts of interest in this area as well. Because the donated commodity program (on which 3.5 million poor Americans, the elderly poor in particular, are totally dependent, and which is used as one of the mainstays of communal feeding in schools, vacation camps, and elderly meals programs) is used to help resorb the farm surplus, it often largely consists of inappropriate foods. In some cases the foods are unfamiliar or difficult to cope with—what is a Harlem mother with inadequate kitchen facilities going to do with bags of corn flour? What is an elderly person living alone, often without a refrigerator, to do with canned meat which comes in 30 ounce cans? Other foods are medically inadvisable—lard, high in saturated fat, or high-salt canned goods for the elderly; lack of choice for school programs that have to use whole milk or high-calorie desserts even in urban areas where 20 percent of the children and adolescents may be obese, when skim milk and fruit would clearly be more appropriate. USDA sponsored programs of nutrition education (our main government program in that field) are even more hampered. The mere mention of the words "saturated fat" or "cholesterol" is prevented by powerful dairy and meat pressure groups to which the department always defers. Mention of the risks to health of our 100-pounds-a-year-per-person intake of sugar is another taboo. The answers to these dilemmas continue to be those recommended by the first White House Conference on Food, Nutrition and Health: elimination of the donated food program and its replacement by food stamps, and transfer of the food-stamp program and of the national school lunch program and other community feeding programs to the Department of Health, Education, and Welfare.

Agribusiness versus Consumer Programs

There are even worse conflicts of interest inherent in the department's responsibility as a producer's agent for consumer programs. The Secretary of Agriculture is responsible for meat inspection—a role made more difficult by the fact that the meat producers are the single most affluent and powerful agricultural lobby. For 70 years, reformers—from Upton Sinclair to Father Robert McEwen, S.J.—have fought for effective inspection of the quality and sanitation of our meat supply, all to little avail. Instead of firm leadership in the public interest (which would run contrary to the interests of agribusiness), USDA meat inspection is characterized by (a) unmonitored, unmotivated and often corrupt personnel (over 40 of the 70 USDA meat inspectors in Massachusetts in 1971 were under indictment for allegedly having accepted bribes from slaughterhouses and meat firms); and (b) lax application of medical rules (the department has recently admitted that a proportion of animals are still slaughtered without the required week-long delay after the last injection of diethylstilbesterol being properly observed). In short, the regulatory activities of the USDA are not a credit to our government.

Although the Food and Drug Administration is often criticized, it does a much better job of consumer protection—but then it is in the HEW, which does not have similar built-in conflicts of interest. The solution is either to transfer the food-regulatory activities of USDA to FDA—which is already responsible for monitoring the safety of most of our food supply—including 80 thousand food plants—or else (instead of further enlarging the already over-swollen Department of Health, Education, and Welfare) to transfer both regulatory agencies to a new Department of Consumer Affairs.

No one concerned with the continued health and prosperity of the nation wants the two million farmers on whom the bulk of our food production depends to be neglected or to be deprived of a voice in government. But neither is there a reason why 15 million poor, 40 million school children, or 206 million consumers should always be subordinated to a special interest group, important though it may be.

Chapter 21

Food and Drug Administration

James D. Grant

The Food and Drug Administration has already been mentioned in one or another context in previous chapters. Before discussing FDA's activities in relation to our food supply, it might be helpful to outline the scope of the agency's total functions and responsibilities, which dictate its regulatory and operational philosophy. The Food and Drug Administration is a regulatory body set up to assist, and ensure, citizen compliance with certain federal statutes. A balanced institution, based on scientific probity and impartial administration of regulatory law, FDA administers parts of the Public Health Service Act, the Federal Food, Drug, and Cosmetic Act and, in addition, the Fair Packaging and Labeling Act, the Federal Hazardous Substances Act, the Import Milk Act, the Filled Milk Act, the Federal Caustic Poison Act, and the Flammable Fabrics Act.

To accomplish this mission FDA (1) clears new drugs for safety and effectiveness before they are marketed; (2) establishes safety tolerances for food additives, pesticide residues, and color additives; (3) establishes standards of identity, quality, and container fill for food products; (4) inspects factories, warehouses, and distributors; (5) samples and examines interstate and imported shipments; (6) conducts research; (7) assists in the interchange of scientific information; (8) works with state and local agencies on consumer protection matters; (9) conducts a program of consumer information and education; (10) prevents the use of unfair or deceptive methods of packaging or labeling; (11) works with industry to promote voluntary compliance; (12) tests insulin, colors, and antibiotics before they are sold; (13) evaluates the labeling and safety of household products containing hazardous substances, and prevents the sale of items too hazardous for home use; (14) evaluates state shellfish sanitation programs; and (15) reviews design of sanitary systems for new interstate conveyances and support facilities. In response to the immediate public health needs that fall within its mandate, it also performs the educational function of appropriate dissemination of scientific information to members of the public health profession, educational institutions, and others arms of government.

In sum, FDA is charged with the responsibility of ensuring that foods are safe and wholesome, drugs are safe and effective, household products are safe or carry adequate warning labels, and all of the above are honestly and informatively labeled and packaged for the consumer. Obviously, then, many activities of the Food and Drug Administration have a substantial impact on the national food supply. It is absolutely necessary that all steps taken, both in new directions and in meeting continuing responsibilities, be designed to benefit the American public in two ways: first, by increasing consumer protection, and second, by enabling the free-market economy to continue to provide safe and nutritious food.

FDA and Food

The regulatory or operational philosophy that guides FDA in its food-related activities is this: our first responsibility is consumer protection. This goal can best be achieved when the government acts in cooperation with the food industry, each sector doing those things it can do best, to achieve the common end. It is the responsibility of the government *to ensure* a safe and nutritious food supply and *to see that the consumer is informed* about the quality and contents of the foods that are marketed. It is the responsibility of the food industry *to provide* a safe and nutritious food supply, and *to give the consumer accurate information* on which to base intelligent choices. In the free market, the consumer can then make a choice among many products.

Safety, as the above discussion makes clear, has been, and will continue to be, the primary concern of FDA in all its activities. In its dealings with the food industry and the food consumer, however, the agency finds that insuring good nutrition in our food supply is becoming an increasingly important function. The future food-related activities of the FDA, to be fully effective, must be concentrated on (1) safety, (2) nutritional quality, and (3) truth to the consumer in the marketing of foods. This will necessitate provision of adequate resources in dollars and manpower to the Food and Drug Administration to enable it to carry out these responsibilities.

Safety   One of the most crucial safety problems is food additives: flavoring substances, emulsifiers, preservatives, coloring agents, and a host of other materials having a variety of purposes. There is a great deal of public confusion about additive safety. Many consumers are under the impression that a product is either on the "generally recognized as safe" (GRAS) list, and hence safe, or it is banned. In reality, there are a number of gradations in between. For example, there are certain kinds of tolerances associated with many products on the GRAS list. More importantly, there are many food additives that are permitted pursuant to food-additive petitions. The advantage of this latter approach is that a tolerance can be established which assures reasonable safety based on the best available scientific knowledge and at the same time permits positive control within expected consumption patterns. In the future more products currently on the GRAS list will probably be controlled either through tolerance limitations while leaving them on the list or through food-additive petitions.

With respect to the GRAS list itself, the FDA is undertaking a number of investigations. Under a contract with the Food Protection Committee of the National Academy of Sciences-National Research Council, all available scientific and production data are being collected on the GRAS-list items. This will lead to a full evaluation of all additives on the list.

In addition, FDA is pursuing activities to improve its own understanding of materials on the GRAS list, as well as other food additives. It is conducting an extensive study and evaluation of the scientific information already existing. FDA is increasing the portion of its manpower and dollar resources allocated to food safety and is engaging in new scientific tests and studies.

Further, FDA is reviewing the criteria against which it judges the safety of ingredients. The intent is to publish in the *Federal Register* more scientific guidelines and protocols for the evaluation of food additives. This will enable FDA to define better what it expects of the food industry when they submit scientific data for the review and approval of food additives. In short, FDA is conducting about as deep and intensive a review of food safety as is possible.

This review considers both the question of scientific criteria and the current use of products in food. FDA, however, is not conducting such an intensive effort because it believes foods are now unsafe. If it did, it would be acting against the unsafe additives. This review of food safety is being conducted

to be certain that we are effectively using the best that science has to offer in the seventies as compared with earlier periods when each particular safety determination was made.

The difficulty facing FDA from a scientific standpoint, however, is that safety must always be somewhat relative. Safety can be established scientifically with a high probability, but the probability can probably never be 100 percent—it can never be absolute, or at least not with the present state of our scientific knowledge and understanding. Most of the safety activities just enumerated are essentially concerned with the preclearance of foods, or at least the conditions under which foods will be manufactured before they are admitted to the food supply.

Obviously, the safety question runs far beyond this consideration to include the whole area of surveillance and compliance in the manufacture and distribution of food. Exercising effective consumer protection during the production of food, especially from the standpoint of health and safety, is a growing and complex problem. Manufacturing processes are increasingly based on sophisticated technological systems. Complex quality control systems are becoming the order of the day. A growing proportion of the national diet is composed of manufactured foods, or foods processed to such an extent that their quality control resembles a manufacturing, rather than a straight agricultural process.

In the future, with respect to manufacturing control, FDA will have to rely on surveillance of technical quality control systems as a major adjunct of its traditional plant inspection activities. Another food-safety problem should be alluded to: the percentage of imported foods appears to be increasing. With the advent of the cargo version of jumbo jets, the problem of safety of imported foods will become more complex as many more airports become ports of entry. Working both with its own resources and through international organizations and agreements, FDA must expand its control over imported foods.

Nutritional Quality   Another consideration is nutritional quality. Although the analogy should not be taken too far, we are at a period in development of the food industry that is quite comparable to the period of the mid-sixties in the drug industry. Up until that time in drugs the primary concern was safety. In the early sixties a fundamental change was made. The notion of efficacy was added. This, oversimplified, means the drug must do medically what the manufacturer claims it will do. We are entering a similar period with regard to our food supply. Consumers are saying that, at least for some foods or classes of foods, there must be a positive gain or benefit, and, in the case of a food additive, that there must be a positive reason for its use. Some guidelines on nutritional quality, established by competent scientific and medical groups, are probably the best way to express the usefulness or effectiveness of foods. FDA, obviously, is not about to encourage a nutritional counterpart of the automobile-horsepower race of previous years.

FDA will establish, probably through the Food and Nutrition Board of the National Academy of Sciences-National Research Council, nutritional guidelines for selected classes of foods. FDA is seeking competent medical advice as well. Tentatively, the classes FDA has in mind are: formulated main dishes; new foods, such as analogs for meat products; dairy products and fruit juices; staples that are important in the diet of ethnic groups in whom malnutrition has been found through the surveys; and snack foods.

In selecting these classes, FDA has been guided by the fact that increasing formulation of finished dishes in the factory rather than the kitchen causes the consumer to lose what control there was over the nutritional properties of the end product. The proportions of ingredients are unknown, and in many instances the ingredients themselves are unfamiliar, so that nutrition knowledge, be it formal or folk in nature, is no longer of much help. At the same time, the manufacturer has no guidance in setting up nutritional specifications for the product. In view of the traditional belief of many marketing people that nutrition sells no product and commands no premium, there are many products on the market in which nutritional quality is outside the control of the purchaser and outside the interest of the processor. When foods contribute significantly to the calorie intake, FDA feels that they should also contribute significantly to overall nutrition.

FDA does not propose to set formal standards of nutritional quality. If the guidelines are issued, this should be accomplished within a few years, partly because it will be done on a class basis rather than an individual-food basis. FDA would then expect that commercial pressures and consumer desires would cause processors to make use of the guidelines in formulating and designing their products. If they do so extensively, there will be no reason to consider a mandatory mechanism. The nutritive properties could be achieved, as indicated above, either by controlling formulas and processes so that nutrients normally present in the ingredients, as harvested, would be within the guideline values, or by adding synthetic nutrients in sufficient amounts so that the same purpose would be accomplished.

Informing the Consumer   Obviously, if FDA is going to concern itself with nutritional quality it must be certain that such quality improvements are stated in a meaningful and consistent manner on the label. This leads to the final main concern: nutritional labeling. Here there is increasing consumer interest, but there does not yet seem to be a clear understanding of what would constitute good nutritional labeling or a clear understanding of exactly what the consumer wants. In any event, any effort toward nutritional labeling must be accompanied by an effective program in the media to explain the label to the consumer. There are some nutritional labeling efforts underway now, and they seem to be growing. It is the function of the government to promulgate guidelines and/or regulations for nutritional labeling, taking into account the best outside scientific and professional advice obtainable in developing the guidelines for nutritional quality, as well as within-government sources of scientific and medical advice, like the National Institutes of Health.

FDA expects to develop an overall nutritional labeling policy and to publish some specific actions pursuant to its interest in nutritional labeling.

Need for Support

It is important that we have a strong and stable Food and Drug Administration. Then the consumer and the food industry can know FDA will effectively and efficiently carry out its regulatory responsibilities in an equitable, even-handed manner. If the FDA is weak because of a lack of financial and manpower resources, even-handedness in enforcement becomes very difficult. Further, a strong FDA will result in much greater consumer protection, which, in turn, will mean that the industry clearly understands in advance the FDA position. If we have a strong scientific agency that is trusted both by the scientific community and by the general public, then the food industry will be able to rely on the FDA's scientific and medical determinations. The agency proceeds on the assumption that the consumer and the food industry desire a strong Food and Drug Administration.

But what does it take to provide a strong consumer protection agency? It takes not only effective and efficient management with an outstanding scientific capability, but also the support of Congress and the American people, who, through their control over the laws under which FDA operates and the resources available to FDA, ultimately determine the strength and viability of the agency.

In summary, the new directions and policies at FDA will enable the agency to improve its scientific understanding of and capacity to evaluate food safety; to introduce notions of nutritional quality in a specific manner in the food supply; to take concrete steps to assure truth in marketing food to the consumer; and to increase the resources with which FDA can assure effective and efficient consumer protection.

Chapter 22

Public-Health Nutritionists in State and Local Programs

Ruth Huenemann

Society today needs public-health nutritionists. As indicated in previous chapters, there is need to apply the science of nutrition in the lives of people. This is the work of the public-health nutritionist. He is uniquely trained in the science of nutrition and its application in the life of individuals and communities. This means that he must know how to assess nutrition problems in a community and how to mobilize resources to deal with these problems. He functions alternatively and often simultaneously as an investigator, program planner, promoter, educator, and resource person in the science of nutrition.

A public-health nutritionist does a wide variety of things, of which the following are examples. (1) He identifies nutrition needs of a community in the following ways: by observation; by examination of available health statistics, demographic data, clinic and hospital records, and other health indicators; by talking with people to learn how they perceive their own nutrition needs; by conducting formal nutrition surveys of his community or portions of it through the collection of dietary, biochemical, and clinical data on a sample population. (2) He finds food and educational resources to help meet any needs uncovered by his surveys. He may help people obtain food from private or public sources, such as school feeding programs, food stamps, etc. For the aged and home-bound, he may initiate a home delivered food service. Where feasible, he may encourage home food production. (3) Public-health nutritionists who possess the necessary dietetic skills may help improve the nutrition of institutionalized populations through consultation to nursing and boarding homes, homes for dependent children, prisons, etc. (4) A public-health nutritionist may help bring about necessary food and nutrition legislation. (5) He may advise in regard to food enrichment and fortification.

Throughout his work, education is one of the prime tools of the public-health nutritionist in food supply and eating practices. He may need to educate food purveyors or manufacturers, legislators, health professionals or a multitude of other "gatekeepers" to nutritional health of the population. There are many key people who control eating patterns—for example, the housewife who prepares the family meals, the teen-ager who chooses his own lunch or snacks, the food-service director of a nursing home or small hospital who plans the patients' daily meals. Whom the public-health nutritionist tries to educate will depend largely upon the level of his position and the agency for which he is working.

A number of official and nonofficial agencies employ public-health nutritionists. Chief among these are state, city, and county departments of health. The Agricultural Extension Service employs nutrition specialists at the state and sometimes at the county level. Several departments of the federal government also employ public-health nutritionists, as do certain international agencies. A number of government-funded special health projects are utilizing their services, as are numerous private or semiprivate agencies, such as visiting nurse associations, heart associations, and others. As yet, there is no dearth of positions.

Competencies Required

What kinds of competencies are required by the work of the public health nutritionist? Obviously, they are many and varied, since the field represents a merger of several biological and behavioral sciences. They include, first of all, competence in the science of nutrition itself in order to assure soundness in problem assessment and in program direction. Secondly, since food is the prime tool for implementation of nutrition programs, knowledge of food composition, some understanding of food processing (both home and commercial) and food economics, and an appreciation of the meaning of food in the lives of people is essential. The public-health nutritionist must be able to work with people and to influence their behavior. This means he must have some understanding and a strong appreciation of the social and behavioral sciences. Basic to all else is a genuine concern for the welfare of people. To achieve a leadership position, a public-health nutritionist must be imaginative and resourceful. The field is not for those who want routines, for no two positions are quite the same, and even in the same position, conditions are ever-changing.

Because no one can master all areas in which a public-health nutritionist must be competent, subspecialties have arisen within the field. These include the areas of maternal and child nutrition, chronic disease and aging, mental retardation, institution consultation, handicapping conditions and rehabilitation, nutrition education in schools, and others.

Both specialists and generalists must recognize the contributions other disciplines can and do make to the field of public-health nutrition. A nutritionist must, therefore, be adept at working with other professionals in and outside of the health field.

Training and Education

At the present time, most positions in the field of public-health nutrition require master's level training based on appropriate undergraduate work. A few undergraduate programs are developing, however, to train people for apprenticeships and beginning staff positions. For some positions, a dietetic internship in addition to the master's degree is essential, and a few top positions require the M.D. degree as well as public-health training.

The usual undergraduate requirements include a background in the natural sciences (biology; human physiology; bacteriology; inorganic, organic and physiological chemistry) and the social sciences (sociology, psychology, economics, education and possibly political science) as a foundation for courses in nutrition, foods, dietetics, and public-health nutrition. The requirement of both natural and social sciences tends to attract students with broad interests.

Approved graduate programs in public-health nutrition are offered in schools of public health and other selected graduate schools. Course work includes general public-health courses (epidemiology, biostatistics, environmental health, administration); public-health nutrition, generally accompanied by field projects; advanced nutrition; behavioral sciences and electives. Instruction in public-health nutrition includes study of the nutritional requirements of man at various ages and under varying environmental conditions; study and practice in assessing nutritional status of population groups and nutrition problems in a community; psychological and social aspects of food practices and their implications for change; the planning of nutrition programs in line with biological and social needs at the international, national, and local levels; study of the role of nutrition in programs involving prevention and treatment of disease; evaluation of nutrition programs; research needs and methods. Most programs require at least two months of full-time field work with a community agency. Programs range in length from one to two academic years. Several programs concentrate on training physicians for the field of public-health nutrition, while several others combine a dietetic internship with public-health nutrition training.

Availability of traineeships and scholarships has enhanced the appeal of this type of graduate study.

What kind of student does best in a public-health nutrition curriculum? Fortunately, one who is also most likely to succeed as a public-health practitioner after he finishes his education, namely, one who is concerned for human welfare, likes people and relates well to them, likes and does well in both the natural and social sciences, and who is flexible and innovative. To him, the ever-changing field of public-health nutrition constitutes a challenge and a satisfaction.

Chapter 23

School Lunch Programs

John Perryman

The year 1971 marked the twenty-fifth anniversary of the passage of the National School Lunch Act. For some it was an occasion for self-congratulation. For others it was an occasion for self-evaluation. A quarter century of effort to feed America's school children has certainly witnessed some success—25 million children being served a full meal every school day. That success, however, is tempered by the fact that the 25 million figure represents less than half of the children in American schools.

Two issues loom as vital in looking back a quarter of a century and, more importantly, looking ahead to the demands of the next decade. The first of these issues relates to the unique development of American school food service. The second is concerned with basic alternatives to that development pattern.

Deficiencies in the School-Lunch Program

At the time of its inception in 1946, and for 20 years thereafter, the National School Lunch Program was agriculture-oriented. Its primary purpose was to provide price support for farmers, and the administration of the act clearly reflected the power of farm blocks in Congress. This approach might be called the "spare rib" psychology. A child was given to stick to his ribs what the farmer could spare. Going to Washington year in and year out to testify on behalf of child feeding programs, representatives of school food services would be given perhaps ten or 11 or 12 minutes to appear before the House or the Senate Agriculture Committees. The philosophy of inadequacy was so pervasive that compromise and halfway measures, the concept of hunger by degree, were accepted.

Testimony was given about the amount of money needed just to maintain the program in the face of increased student enrollment from year to year; about the amount of money needed to lower the price for lunch by a few pennies and thus to bring a few more children than last year within the magic circle of American boys and girls who had food in their empty bellies. We continued to look backward, to use as our measuring stick that which had been done in the past, and to applaud ourselves for minimal improvement. Along with the nation as a whole, we accepted hunger by degree. Perhaps because we ourselves had enough to eat.

If those concerned with school food service in the United States accepted the "spare rib" philosophy of Congress, they were inclined as well to accept the "country store" concept in the educational establishment. School food service has acquiesced to the role of an auxiliary service, unrelated to the principal purpose of the American public school—learning. Words about the importance of nutrition education have been many, but actions few.

The Lack of Nutrition Education   Nutrition education—a knowledge of food, a knowledge of what to eat and how to eat and in what combination to eat it, the relationship of food to health, the relationship of food to figure, the relationship of food to physical attractiveness and mental alertness—this can all be a part of school food service. This is not to suggest that a child will absorb such lessons by osmosis simply because he walks through the cafeteria line in school, instead of approaching the drive-in window down the street. Nutrition education has to be a deliberate teaching effort, with its own text materials, carefully and consciously incorporated into the school's curricula. Nutrition education can and should be closely tied to the school food-service operation, which then becomes a living laboratory for lessons being taught, hopefully with the assistance and guidance of the school food service staff.

We are pathetically, tragically unimaginative in our approach to nutrition education—it is little wonder that the subject has not been a favorite one with faculty and students alike. If we can help teen-age boys to translate nutrition education into muscles and teen-age girls to translate it into the swelling curves of womanhood, the pace of the action in the classroom is going to quicken appreciably. If we can help the teen-age girl to realize that the entire nervous system of her baby may well be laid out before she even knows she is pregnant, these vital lessons of the body begin to take on whole new meanings, and both the act and the knowledge of feeding children becomes ever more perceptibly a part of education's job.

Even more debilitating to the rationale for school food service has been the maintenance of an economic-means test. In no other area of public education has there remained such a blatant attempt to discriminate against those unable to pay.

Economic Means Tests   As regards economic-means tests presently incorporated in school-food-service legislation, we are passing through an intermediate, ridiculous, and trying stage of food service in our schools that is both unsound and undesirable from an administrative standpoint. We are saying that some children are pauperized to the point that they may have a free or reduced-price meal, while other children are not. We are saying that we can distinguish between the haves and have-nots and can do so with subtleties and nuances unnoticed by anyone. While we are racking our brains for administrative procedures so secretive as to satisfy the CIA, have we all forgotten the characteristics of children themselves? Have we forgotten the curiosity, the braggadocio and—indeed sometimes the venom of children themselves? There is no administrative method by which an economic-means test can be applied without harming the individual child.

In relation to the hodge-podge and patchwork quilt of federal regulations the economic-means test approaches the extremities of administrative absurdity. We have some food items that we can make available to some hungry children but not to others; we have some monies that we can make available to some hungry children and not to others. We have section-this-of-that-act and section-that-of-this-act, which are applied one way in one state and another way in another, which in turn are applied one way in one school district and another way in another. Above and beyond the straining administrative labyrinth remains the overriding consideration that the stigma of pauperism will no more be removed from a free lunch than it was from free education until both food for thought and food for the stomach are made available equally to one and all. This lesson is not new. These are experiences learned in our own country almost a century and one-half ago as we were struggling with the beginning of free, public universal education in our nation. As an example, after some experiences with public schools in Philadelphia, a labor-union committee found them to be "extremely defective and inefficient." In the National Gazette of 1830, the committee observed:

Their (the public schools) leading feature is pauperism! They are confined exclusively to the children of the poor, while there are, perhaps thousands of children whose parents are unable to afford for them a good private education, yet whose standing professions or connections in society effectually exclude them from taking the benefit of a poor law. There are great numbers, even of the poorest parents, who hold a dependence on the public bounty to be incompatible with the rights and liberties of an American citizen, and whose deep and cherished consciousness of independence determines them rather to starve the intellect of their offspring than submit to become the objects of public charity.

We have only to strike the two words, "the intellect" to apply this same sensitivity of feeling to the free lunch of today. Unfortunately, many an American citizen abhors charity to the point that he would prefer to starve his offspring rather than submit to becoming the object of public charity. Food service for the student during the educational day is a part of education's job.

Food Service as a Part of Education

Recent events in the nation's capital and throughout the nation have sufficient import to alter this tawdry reflection on the past.

The attitude of the Congress of the United States toward child feeding programs has changed so dramatically and so rapidly that it would seem most school administrators and even many school food service leaders have not caught up. We have now the finest opportunity to rid our land of hunger since Chief Massasoit provided a good, hot lunch for the Plymouth settlers. We must not let such an opportunity slip through our hands.

In the entire history of the school-lunch program—from 1946 to 1969—the total federal contribution was approximately 3.6 billion dollars. In 1970 alone the federal involvement in child feeding programs was just over one billion dollars for this one year.

The breakfast program has come of age. It is serving 126 million (1970–1971) meals and is being recognized as perhaps the finest nutritional contribution ever made to the learning process. For the first time in history we have had the courage to say that matching funds for the federal dollar shall not come alone from the nickels and dimes of the children, but also from state-matching funds. For the first time in history we have had the courage to say—as an official commitment by the national government of this nation—that there shall be a school-food-service program physically and financially available—whether he wishes to use it or not—to every child in this nation and in every school in our far-flung network of education for all.

Enormous progress has been made and is being made, but by no stretch of the imagination may we consider the job done. We are still thinking in terms of hunger by degree; we are still limiting our vision of school food service to a world already a generation past.

Recommendations

Two years have passed since the White House Conference on Food, Nutrition and Health was heralded as a breakthrough in child nutrition. Deliberations were lengthy. Discussions were heated. Recommendations were portentous. Section V of the conference dealt with food delivery and distribution as a system. Panel V-4 focused on large-scale meal-delivery systems. The recommendations of that panel, in the light of subsequent events, deserve repetition.

For Immediate, Urgent Action:

a. The President, in recognition of the existence of a national hunger and nutrition emergency, as well as to make real what he has called the "National commitment to put an end to hunger and malnutrition in America," should declare a national hunger emergency to exist in the United States. He should further take all actions possible within existing authority to expand current food programs and establish new programs, in both cases utilizing all available resources and organizations of the American pluralistic economy to feed all hungry Americans this winter and throughout the emergency period.

b. The National School Lunch Program should be immediately funded as a public responsibility, recognized as an integral part of public and nonpublic education and expanded so as to provide school lunches to all economically needy children at no direct cost to any recipient. To the greatest extent practicable, free school lunches should be immediately augmented by free school breakfasts, so as to provide, through secondary school, at least one-third to one-half of the minimal requirements of the Recommended Dietary Allowance. Also, to the greatest extent practicable, school lunch programs should be immediately broadened to include preschool children and the needy in the community, including the elderly, as well as the particularly vulnerable group of migrant children. In all cases, steps should be taken to protect the psyche of the student by not singling out those entitled to free meals as coming from poor families.

c. Both the Legislative and Executive Branches of Government should take all necessary steps to make possible the President's action to combat the national hunger and malnutrition emergency, including all required legislative, financial and administrative changes. Particular attention should be given to facilitate the utilization of all available resources, including the private food-service sector and its extensive capabilities.

For Urgent Action, Based on Immediate Actions:

a. The National School Lunch Program should be expanded so as to provide free lunch (and breakfast where required) to all students, through secondary school, at no direct cost to recipients. This expansion should be such as to provide for meeting all schoolday nutritional needs of all students at no cost to the individual at the earliest feasible date and in no case later than calendar year 1975.

b. Funding for the expansion of school lunch program should be "new money" and identified in categorical budgeting so as to make it invulnerable, and preserve the financial integrity of necessary programs of education in schools.

c. School-lunch programs should be broadened to include positive programs for community center activity and to provide meals at no cost to all those who hunger or are malnourished as a result of poverty, age or condition.

d. The large-scale mass feeding systems expertise of the Armed Forces, the Veterans' Administration, of other governmental agencies and of the private foodservice sector should be utilized in the national commitment to combat hunger and malnutrition. The path should be cleared so as to permit local authorities, including school districts, to utilize all available expertise in developing their antihunger and malnutrition programs with the greatest possible dispatch and in operating their programs with the greatest possible effectiveness and efficiency.

e. At the earliest practicable date, the National Feeding Program should be separated from programs of surplus commodity distribution. Federal Executive responsibility for this "people" program should be assigned by the President to the "people" authority in his cabinet, the Secretary of Health, Education and Welfare. Responsibility for commodity distribution should remain in the Department of Agriculture and with its production-oriented expertise.

f. A national program of impartial and continuing evaluation of progress in the war against hunger and malnutrition should be established to monitor results and insure timely program modification. A National Council for Food and Nutrition should be established in the Executive Office of the President to formulate national policy and to serve the President as a watchdog on the progress of the War on Hunger as well as to insure coordination of national policy with program development. To achieve these ends, we have developed a series of ideas where our current expertise or resources would permit these objectives to be accomplished by reducing waste wherever it is possible and utilizing these savings to assist in paying the total cost of our desired package.

Progress

The sweeping changes urged by this Panel have not been totally realized. But a significant beginning has been made. It was made on March 1, 1971, when H.R. 5291, Universal School Food Service and Nutrition, was introduced in Congress by Representative Carl Perkins of Kentucky. Section 2 of the preamble to that bill "to establish a universal food service and nutrition education program for children" mirrors a new dimension of commitment:

> **a.** The Congress hereby finds that (1) the proper nutrition of the Nation's children is a matter of highest priority, (2) there is a demonstrated relationship between the intake of food and good nutrition and the capacity of children to develop and learn, (3) the teaching of the principles of good nutrition in schools has been seriously inadequate as evidenced by the existence of poor or less than adequate diets at all levels of family income, (4) any procedure or "means test" to determine the eligibility of a child for a free or reduced-price meal is degrading and injurious both to the child and his parents, and (5) the national school lunch and related child nutrition pro-

grams, while making significant contributions in the field of applied nutrition research, are not, as presently constituted, capable of achieving the goal of good nutrition for all children.

b. It is hereby declared to be the policy of Congress to assure adequate nutrition offerings for the Nation's children, to encourage the teaching of the principles of good nutrition as an integral part of the total educational process, and to strengthen State and local administration of food service programs for children. It is further declared to be the policy of Congress that food service programs conducted under this Act be available to all children on the same basis without singling out or identifying certain children as different from their classmates.

Opponents view universal school food service as yet another step toward socialism. They shudder at its cost. But are their arguments any better than those that were initially used against such now well-established programs as child-labor legislation or Social Security?

A hundred years ago, children entered cages that carried them into the bowels of the earth where they dug coal for 12 hours a day in fetid air and unrelieved stench. For a few pennies a day, children toiled all day in lofts in New York and other cities—rolling cigars or assembling rudimentary hand appliances. And the system was defended by those who said that the children would learn to "pay their own way" and that "work builds character," and, ironically, that the exploited children were "learning about the American way of life." This blatant social evil was ended when child-labor laws were enacted, and children came up from the mines and down from the lofts and went to school. But of the children who went to school, some went hungry.

In more recent history, families faced the specter of the Depression. Homes were lost. Jobless days stretched into months and sometimes years. There were haggard faces, empty bellies—and fear. In that time of fear men spoke of a new deal for the elderly. They called it "social security." Through the Social Security program they wished to eliminate the social evil of poverty for the aged, the infirm, and for widows.

Laissez-faire economics, according to which every man looking after his own best interests automatically serves the best interests of society, has already been cast aside by child-labor laws, Social Security, and many other programs designed for the public good. Transportation, national defense, and education are all examples of vital endeavors so vast that they can be accomplished only by common efforts.

Today, the United States finds the cost of a sound diet and of nutrition education for all its children to be too expensive. Yet a truly adequate program of nutrition and nutrition education for our children would require approximately the same expenditure that we make each year to feed our dogs and cats. It would require a billion dollars a year less than we spend each year on horse racing; only one-half of what we spend each year on tobacco; less than one-third of what we spend each year on alcoholic beverages. If we seriously consider our priorities, surely we will decide that a nation that can afford to spend 30 million dollars on candy for its children on one Halloween night can afford to feed the same children a balanced diet throughout the year. We talk too much about the cost of good nutrition and too little about the cost of bad nutrition. The cost of illness in the United States has increased 400 percent in the past ten years and continues to skyrocket. A strong program of nutrition and nutrition education for our youth would cut billions from the medical costs of our nation.

In the spring of 1937, Justice Cardoza, speaking for the Supreme Court, upheld the constitutionality of social-security legislation:

"Needs that were narrow or parochial a century ago may be interwoven in our day with the well-being of the nation. What is critical or urgent changes with the times . . . ."

Conclusion

We are living in extraordinary, exciting, and hopeful times. We are living in an age determined to end war, pollution, and hunger.

The problem of hungry children the world over can be solved. There is enough food in the world today to feed the people of the world. Probably for the first time in the 50-thousand-year history of mankind on earth, hunger and starvation are no longer unavoidable. The fact that hunger still exists is a function not of physical limitations but rather of ignorance. Hunger is a social evil which no longer need plague mankind.

As have other powerful nations before us in history, we grapple with questions of our appropriate role in world leadership. We might use for guidance the words on the marque of a drive-in savings and loan office in a small southern community: "Our youth needs models, not critics." Our world too needs models. If we were to use one-half of 1 percent of our gross national product to build a sound program of nutrition and nutrition education for the children of our nation, we would not only be making a sound financial investment in our own future, we would be giving mankind a model of a valid and effective public response to this major social problem.

Chapter 24

Special Programs for the Very Poor

Robert Choate

Elimination of hunger requires far more than the production of food; it requires regular, dependable delivery of food to the mountain hollow, to the cripple's sixth-floor walkup, to the Indian reservation, and to the home of solitary aged (and perhaps infirm) citizen.

In the United States today, a strange amalgam of institutional meals, delivered dinners, boxed commodities and counterfeit money—food stamps—constitutes an erratic, half-hearted effort to provide food to the nation's poor.

The private food industry has been a reluctant partner in this effort, despite its having one of private enterprise's best success stories. To most citizens, the local supermarket is a highly varied, moderately expensive service station for the body's fuels. Food markets serve best where social stability and economic resources abound. Profits are regular in such areas, and the private-enterprise food system performs more-or-less adequately, providing calories and varied nutrients to over 80 percent of the population.

Beyond the profit perimeter, however, quality goes down, prices go up, labor costs multiply. Major stores are often far apart. Freshness disappears and inefficiency reigns. The calories may still be available, but the nutrient choices are harder to make on a limited budget. Beyond the profit perimeter—whether considered in terms of the individual or of the geographic area, social efforts attempt to ensure that food is available to the poor, the lame, and the bewildered. These nonprofit efforts may have private or governmental backing. The former wear the names "old age homes," "damaged goods stores," "soup kitchens"; the latter wear the labels of "welfare," "surplus commodities," "food stamps" or "school lunches."

No accurate list has been made of the number of private charitable or near-charitable meals served to the poor. Most of these efforts are urban; many are sporadic or demeaning, but a few sparkle with innovation. One might guess that private food services provided by private funds serve one million persons per day.

Child Nutrition Programs

Among the public programs funded by political entities at the local, state, and federal level are school lunches and school breakfasts, now lumped together with their summer-camp counterparts under the title Child Nutrition Programs.

"School lunch" was born in 1946—the product of a desire by Congress to use up war-inflated food production, which supplied world needs during World War II.

To win liberals to the farmer's side, the preamble to the school-lunch legislation cited concern for the needy. But the needy, as was soon discovered, are hard to reach and may have irregular food habits. Thus by 1967 the school-lunch program, funded with a variety of agriculture-benefiting acts, served 16 million children, less than two million of whom were poor children receiving free or cut-rate meals. Noontime meals were *not* served to over 30 million students, five to eight million of whom were poor enough to be considered in food jeopardy.

Stories of poor kids watching the rich eat,

of slum schools without kitchens, and of suburbs with sparkling cafeterias came to light. *Their Daily Bread*—a book produced by five major women's organizations—laid bare the ugly mis-focus of the 1967 school-lunch operation.[1]

Republicans and Democrats in the House of Representatives held hearings in 1967 and 1968 on institutional feeding. The Vanik Bill pressed for day-camp and day-care meals. By 1969, newly elected President Nixon could promise that all needy children would be fed as of Thinksgiving, 1970. Under the dogged eyes of Senators McGovern and Javits, Congress saw to it that the Nixon administration was given the funds and the statutes to deliver on this promise.

But by the spring of 1971, six months after the Thanksgiving deadline, at least 600,000 of the original 6.6 million needy children were not getting free or reduced-price lunches—even though Congress had mandated it. Of the nation's 100,000 public schools, 23,000 still provided no school lunches. In addition, the Department of Agriculture admitted that the 6.6-million estimate might be over a million low. One release by USDA cited 7.9 million as being probably eligible. All figures relating to performance put out by the Department were "preliminary." By spring 1972, 8.2 million children were reached. But it is now obvious that at least one million and perhaps as many as two million very poor children are still not provided for.

The department's commitment to every needy child was erratic; a telegram in the fall of 1970 had notified state school-lunch directors that they "did not have to force feed children." To those disinclined to make the total commitment, this unfortunate phrase seemed to justify inaction. In some ten states, according to the Community Nutrition Institute, food service to the needy exceeded original estimates; in other states, less than 50 percent of the needy were being provided the free or reduced-price meal.

Sometimes it was due to a lack of funds, sometimes to incompetence at the federal or state level. All too often school principals, inconsiderate school boards, and PTA inertia still impede the provision of school lunches, although free band instruments and football uniforms are obtainable by almost any student with the will to play.

School Breakfasts   School breakfasts, considered by some to be more effective and needed than school lunches, never have gotten past the demonstration stage. Middle-class hang-ups with eggs and toast or cereals with milk have sometimes delayed implementation of school breakfasts, particularly in schools with no cafeterias. Despite the recent fortification of rolls, muffins, and cup-cakes to a point where a quarter of the Recommended Dietary Allowance (RDA) of many vitamins and minerals can be obtained when a fortified roll is consumed with a glass of milk, school authorities often find the idea of serving sweet rolls or muffins just too abhorrent to consider.

The Nixon administration's plans for school lunches were laid bare with the publishing of the Fiscal Year 1972 Budget. Now a tried and proven program, school breakfasts were to be given 15 million dollars—an amount identical with the 1971 estimate. In other words, no expansion was provided.

School breakfasts are particularly advantageous for the needy and for those who have long bus rides in to school. School breakfasts reduce truancy and stimulate classroom attentiveness. Yet many schools ignore their promise and convenience.

New York City, according to a January 11, 1971 *New York Times* article, could be tapping 2.1 million dollars to feed breakfast to its 364,000 indigent children. The New York City Board of Education, four months after the funds became available, still had not applied. Claiming breakfast costs at 60 cents per meal, the board either saw the frustrations of serving all the needy only 90 break-fasts in a school year or they overlooked the cheaper but fully nutritious meals now being designed specifically for school breakfasts.

Schools in smaller cities and towns frequently cited janitorial problems, parental responsibilities, or dislike of socialistic programs as reasons for withholding breakfast programs from the needy. Even were they to be interested, 15 million dollars divided by a per-student yearly typical cost of 50 dollars would permit only 300,000 children to be served, of the 50 million who attend our schools.

The Special Milk Program   This program, admitted by the Milk Producers' Federation to be more for the benefit of milk producers than children, again faces efforts to merge it into child nutrition programs. Such efforts have failed in the past, and, as a result, over 104 million dollars' worth of half-pints of milk are given to schools with no regard for whether they benefit the needy or the lunch or breakfast programs.

Camps and Day Care   The day-care and camp-meal program, entitled Nonschool Food in the annual budget, has finally gone up from the 20.8-million-dollar level to only 50 million in 1972.

After three years of attention and improvement, the Child Nutrition Programs thus level off. Despite promises of continued improvements in these programs, the White House apparently has done little to increase the effort.

The Family Feeding Program

The second major supplement to private enterprise's food efforts is considered under the Family Feeding Programs—the direct distribution of commodities and the food stamp program.

Commodities The former originated in 1935 with a compromise piece of legislation originating in a House-Senate Conference made up of such redoubtable characters as Everett Dirksen, Richard Russell, Uncle Joe Cannon, and John McCormack. In return for tariff protection for machinery manufacturers, a special fund—Section 32—was established to:

1. Encourage the exportation of agricultural commodities and products thereof . . .
2. Encourage the domestic consumption of such commodities or products by diverting them . . . from the normal channels of trade and commerce or by increasing their utilization . . . among persons in low income groups as determined by the Secretary of Agriculture; and
3. Re-establish farmers' purchasing power by making payments in connection with the normal production of any agricultural commodity for domestic consumption.

On second-mentioned authority, the Department of Agriculture has seen fit to offer commodities to the poor. In the beginning the food was primarily "surplus." Since the early sixties the commodity direct distribution program has offered ten to 25 of the following items each month:

Apple juice	Orange juice
Beans, dry or canned	Peaches, canned
Butter	Peanut Butter
Cheese	Peas, canned
Corn, canned	Pork, canned
Corn meal	Potatoes, white,
Egg mix	dehydrated
Flour	Raisins
Grapefruit juice	Rice
Grits, corn	Shortening,
Lard/Shortening	vegetable
Meat, canned	Syrup, corn
Milk, evaporated,	Tomato juice
instant or dry	Turkey, canned
Oats, rolled	

Today the program operates in approximately 1,000 counties of the nation's 3,100. There is no tight administration from the federal level. The 1,000 counties seem to produce many variations on the same theme. Many counties offer only a portion of the 25 items now declared by USDA to be available. Some have one warehouse in an area of 1,000 square miles. Others deliver door to door and invite choice-making by recipients. Caloric content is insufficient for a recipient family, particularly if children are present. Nutrient balance is a myth. Improvements have taken place during the past two years, particularly in regard to the variety of foods offered, but impending or threatened dismemberment of the program in favor of food stamps has put off major reforms. The recent House of Representatives debate on food stamps included an effort to improve the quality and services of the commodity program, but that effort too failed.

Of more than passing interest is the fact that the Senate Select Committee on Nutrition and Human Needs, despite a three-year interest in hunger, has never really investigated USDA's operation of the direct distribution program.

The primary recipient complaints are difficulties of acquiring and transporting food, lack of variety and quality, and certification barriers. In counties like New York's Nassau County, the program was operated with computer-aided efficiency. (The poor in that area did not appreciate being ordered by the state legislature to shift over to food stamps.) San Diego offers commodities with an interesting nonprofit distribution mechanism. Fourteen agencies certify recipients; another 14 warehouse the food at convenient locations.

Today, as in 1968, some 3.8 million individuals gain a good part of their food supply from warehouses established to store and distribute the country's excess food items.

Bought primarily to correct a soft market-price condition, with little attention to nutritional balance, these foods seem frequently to offer government-mandated malnutrition.

Food Stamps   Since 1964 the federal government has been printing food stamps to be used in lieu of money to purchase domestic edibles. The philosophy of the food-stamp program is unique; originated for the dollar-short poor, it requires that the poor *purchase* their federal benefits. According to a set formula based on family income and family size, a household can purchase food stamps, for less than face value, for use at retail food markets (see Table 1). In December 1969, the Nixon administration announced major reforms in the "formula" by which the poor could buy this federal largesse. Until then, Congress and the Department of Agriculture actually boasted of helping the poor with $6.74 worth of food per month—to those who would obey the program's edicts. With the new formula inviting joiners to overcome the red tape, participation jumped from 3.2 million in May of 1969 to 9.8 million in March of 1971.

In mid-1969, the U.S. Senate drastically overhauled the food-stamp-program legislation and defined vastly improved levels and terms of assistance. The bill passed the Senate only to lie dormant in the House of Representatives for 14 months. Under the ultra-conservative eye of Congressmen Robert Poage (Tex-D) and Page Belcher (Okla-R), the reform was held up until Christmas week, 1970. Congressmen Thomas Foley (Wash-D) and Albert Quie (Minn-R), concerned over the harshly restrictive terms of the offered committee bill, drafted a substitute which became progressively more conservative as the sides jockeyed for legislative opportunity. On December 20, the Quie/Foley substitute failed, more because of competing Christmas parties than on its own merits. With festive Congressmen within a mile of the House floor, the conservative House Agriculture Committee Bill was enacted with a vote of 119 to 116 on the critical issue.

TABLE 1 The 1972 Schedule of Food-Stamp Benefits per Month (Abbreviated).

	Purchase Requirement	
Monthly Net Income (After Deductions)	*Four Persons in Household (Coupon Allotment: $112.00)*	*Eight Persons in Household (Coupon Allotment: $192.00)*
$ 0 to 19.99	$ 0.00	$ 0.00
20 to 29.99	0.00	0.00
30 to 39.99	4.00	5.00
40 to 49.99	7.00	9.00
50 to 59.99	10.00	12.00
60 to 69.99	13.00	16.00
—	—	—
150 to 169.99	45.00	45.00
170 to 179.00	47.00	51.00
—	—	—
360 to 389.99	88.00	108.00
390 to 419.99	can't buy	117.00
—	—	—
630 to 659.99	can't buy	152.00
over 659.99	can't buy	can't buy

The newly enacted Food Stamp Amendments do offer some valued reforms. For the first time, national standards of eligibility are created; no more than 30 percent of one's income can be paid out for participating (it previously had been as high as 50 percent); if family income is under $30 a month, stamps for a family of four are free; self-certification of families on welfare is permitted; a 60-day carry-on clause extends benefits for mobile families moving to new certification jurisdictions; deductions are permitted to pay for stamps from welfare checks; and stamps can be used for meals by the elderly, if the meals are delivered to their homes. One billion, 75 million dollars are authorized for fiscal 1971 with open-ended authorization thereafter. Over two billion dollars were obtained for the Fiscal Year 1972 budget. This amount did assure almost 12 million of the nation's 25 million poor food-stamp relief. In fiscal 1973, the plans are to reach at the most 13 or 14 million poor with food stamps.

Accompanying these cautious improvements, are amendments that Congressman Foley, Agriculture Committee member, termed "vicious." The wording of the amendments may seem bland, but the discussion that accompanied their development revealed the mentality of the authors. Apparently the drafters felt the puritan ethic—that one should profit only by the sweat of one's brow —should supersede any belief that one should be his brother's keeper.

Groups of individuals living together now are highly restricted in their access to food stamps. (Hippies, communes, and student groups: Stay Out.) A willingness to work was also sought among food-stamp recipients— those who apply for stamps not only must register for work but must accept any employment offered at the state or federal minimum wage or $1.30 per hour, whichever is greater.

Administered in an equitable manner, such amendments could prove constructive. However, in many places they are administered by a reactionary and hostile overseer. In the absence of cautionary clauses better defining the maximum distance of the job from the applicant's residence, the hours to be worked, the suitability of the employment for the employee or the matching of prevailing wages, such an amendment becomes a tool for local warping of the food-stamp theory to make inhuman demands on persons needing food. It is evident that in many parts of the United States, perhaps in 500 of our 3,100 counties, the participation of the poor in food programs is less than 20 percent. Such statistics reflect local disinterest or even outright hostility toward the poor. In such areas fearsome rumors will build around the work-provision amendment and accomplish what administrative hostility cannot—the poor will avoid the program in droves even as their children's diets suffer.

The outcome of the legislative struggle over the work provision represented more than a legislative setback for reform—it was a major defeat. Reformers had heavily influenced the food programs between 1967 and the beginning of 1971. With the enactment of the work provision, the preponderately conservative Agriculture Committee, often openly racist and antipoor, regained a major measure of influence over the administration of these programs.

In 1970 the Office of Economic Opportunity expended almost 50 million dollars in an effort to extend the bureaucracy-laden efforts of USDA into counties where red tape needed to be cut. As budgetary pressures tightened during the drafting of the Fiscal Year 1972 Federal Budget, the wizards of the Office of Budget and Management claimed that none of their bookkeepers could understand the EFMS role. Thus came the extermination of the Emergency Food and Medical Services (EFMS) effort, with zero dollars sought for operations beyond the existing appropriations. EFMS had reached over 750 counties of the United States and was responsible for some of the most imaginative food programs in the country. These efforts were dying by the fall of 1971. They have not been revived since.

Conclusion

Thus we come to a period of uncertainty. President Nixon's first draft budgets for the 1973 fiscal year seem to indicate an Executive Branch slowdown on food reform.

OEO's Emergency Food and Medical Services program is on its way to oblivion. Day-care feeding and school breakfasts are developing at best extremely slowly. Summer programs are underfunded. Representing Mr. Nixon's most successful domestic improvements—in a field strewn with failures—the drive for better food programs for the poor apparently may have been abandoned on the 40-yard line, for in 1972 only 60 percent of the poor can be considered out of food jeopardy.

REFERENCE

1. Committee on School Lunch Participation, 1968. *Their Daily Bread.* Sponsored by Church Women United, National Board of the Y.W.C.A., National Council of Catholic Women, National Council of Jewish Women, and National Council of Negro Women. McNelley-Rudd Printing Service, Inc., Atlanta, Georgia.

Chapter 25

Income Maintenance

Alvin L. Schorr

Confused and, indeed, infuriating conversations about "income maintenance" arise from unexpressed differences about the meaning of that awkward term. In the older and technical sense, income maintenance means all cash, goods, and services provided by the government that are generally intended to be used for subsistence. For example, free public education or government subsidy intended to encourage shipbuilding are not included, and social security, public assistance, food stamps, and Medicare are included. More recently, income maintenance has, in some discussions, come to mean cash payments to people below a specified income level. It is a substitute term for "relief" or "public assistance" that emphasizes the search for a more decent and inclusive system.

Using one definition or the other subtly but powerfully influences one's conclusions. The very organization of such a book as this inclines readers to the newer definition of income maintenance. The book deals with malnutrition among specific groups; one is led to think about a cash program for the poor. This approach to the problem contains its own conclusion—a large, sanitized public-assistance program, with only its levels and inclusiveness remaining to be settled. The older and broader definition is more difficult, complicated, flexible, and powerful. It deals with programs distributing over 100 billion dollars a year to American citizens, and does not necessarily lead one to favor a large new program. The broader definition and the conclusions it encourages appear to be preferable.

Designing a Program

There are seven issues to be settled in designing an income-maintenance program. Although this may seem excessively didactic, it may be refreshing for once to set out all the relevant assumptions and biases. These are the major issues: efficiency, income-testing, inadvertent side effects, adequacy, dynamism, incentive, and cash versus goods or services. It will rapidly appear that the issues are intertwined. Therefore, they will be outlined in somewhat overlapping fashion, capitalizing a word when a new issue is introduced.

About two-thirds of the social-security funds paid out to the aged go to people who are or otherwise would be poor. If reaching poor people is considered the sole objective, then Social Security is 66 percent EFFICIENT. Food stamps are not given to people unless they demonstrate that they are poor; that represents 100 percent efficiency. When money is limited (a way of viewing the matter that we shall attempt somewhat to undermine), obviously efficiency is desirable.

Unfortunately, efficiency is hard to come by, as public assistance will illustrate. Some years ago, families were given exactly the amount of money that agencies said they needed to meet minimum requirements. If a divorced husband began to send support payments or a mother began working, welfare payments were reduced by the same amount. The program was 100 percent efficient, but left recipients no financial incentive to work or develop other income. Over

the years, therefore, INCENTIVE arrangements were introduced into the programs. For example, now a welfare mother who works has her grant reduced only by two-thirds the amount of her earnings; one-third of her earnings is her net gain. This means that money may be retained in excess of the amount the agency has determined she needs; the program is no longer entirely efficient.

In programs like public assistance, it is possible to achieve high efficiency and incentive at very low levels of ADEQUACY. (Adequacy is the extent to which the level of payment seems likely to support decent living). For example, the President's original Family Assistance Program provided $1,600 for a family of four (low adequacy) and permitted retention of 50 percent of earnings (moderately satisfactory incentive). No four-person family with income over $3,920 would have received F.A.P. As that is approximately the poverty level, the proposal achieves nearly 100 percent efficiency. As soon as one moves to a level that is more nearly adequate, either incentive or efficiency must suffer. For example, the President's Commission on Income Maintenance Programs proposed a program that would pay $3,600 to a family of four with no other income. The incentive arrangement would permit retention of 50 percent of earnings, so people with total income over $7,000 would receive some payment. Such a program would be only 36 percent efficient.

In short, a program that gives money only to people who are poor can achieve high efficiency, but *only if* adequacy or the incentive arrangement is poor. One can also attempt to achieve efficiency through quite another approach from making payments only to people who are poor. For example, some OEO benefits were provided freely in so-called poverty areas. Quite reasonably, it was assumed that virtually everyone in the neighborhood would be poor. Therefore, it was cheaper administratively and seemed better to give benefits freely than to weed out those who were not poor. Social security achieves moderate efficiency for somewhat similar reasons. As such a large proportion of the aged or widowed are likely to be poor, retirement and survivors insurance achieve at least moderate efficiency. (The British, who have preferred this approach to achieving efficiency, call it "selectivity.")

One of the problems in using efficiency to evaluate programs is that it tends to deal with matters at a single moment in time. The underlying assumption is that money is limited and, viewed at any given moment, of course it is. But some programs are likely to stagnate and wither, while others have a DYNAMISM that leads them to expand and improve. From the point of view of poor people, it may be better to accept a smaller share in such a dynamic program than to have a fixed sum all to themselves. That is often precisely the choice that must be made, and those who opt for efficiency in their behalf do them no favor.

For example, payments to old people under social security and under public assistance were virtually equal in 1940—$20.25 and $22.10 per person. But the average social-security payment had increased $73 by 1968, and the average assistance payment only $49—a difference of 50 percent in the rate of increase.*

In 1935, when Congress was deciding how to allocate money, obviously efficiency would by itself have represented a misleading criterion. Public assistance would have given poor people more money in the earlier years but, because of its dynamism, poor people did better with social security in later years even though they were sharing with people who were not poor.

Why does one program stagnate and another grow? One answer is that social security is a popular program and Old Age Assistance or public assistance is less popular. That is a somewhat circular answer, to be sure, as social security is popular in part because its administration has been kept decent and its payment levels advanced. A possibly related answer is that Old Age Assistance draws on the political power of old, *poor* people, while social security draws on the political power of *all* old people. The former rely on the charity of legislators, the latter on their wish to be reelected. This suggests that efficiency may in some sense be counter to the long-term interests of poor people. The more efficient, the more a program depends on their political power alone. Poor people may do well with efficiency at a time of widespread guilt or reformist zeal, but over the long run they do better to join their interests with those of more powerful groups.

In the discussion of issues so far, we have, without acknowledging it, been weaving in and out of a discussion of INCOME-TESTING. The unique quality of income-tested programs is a demonstration that a person or family has less than a specified sum of money. Upon that demonstration, income-tested programs fill the deficit or, if they contain an incentive arrangement, some-

*Another comparison that takes account of broadening coverage as well as rising payment levels is in terms of the total amounts paid out. In 1940, Old Age Assistance paid out 473 million dollars and retirement insurance 17 million dollars. But by 1968, OAA was paying out 1.7 billion dollars and retirement insurance 16 billion dollars. One might argue that the increases were more rapid in social security because it is a social insurance program, while funds for public assistance come from general revenue. During this period, however, social-security beneficiaries were receiving far larger benefits than insurance considerations would require. They were not being paid out of general revenue but neither were they being paid out of their own contributions. (Beneficiaries were being paid out of the contributions of *current* wage earners, not out of their own *past* contributions. That is quite a different matter.) The choices were being made by Congress and, for both social security and public assistance, were plainly responsive to political considerations.

what overfill it. Income-maintenance programs that are not income-tested provide money for a variety of other reasons—because a man reaches a stipulated age and has worked for some period of time (retirement insurance under social security), because he has been dismissed from work (unemployment insurance), because he has performed specially valued services (veterans' benefits), because he is disabled (disability insurance), and so forth. None of these criteria for eligibility is linked as a matter of law or regulation to a showing of inadequate income.

Income-testing was the first possibility noted as a way to achieve efficiency: programs might be limited to those who are poor or, in other words, a demonstration of need might be required. It is a plausible approach. Unfortunately, income-tested programs have historically been administered in such a manner as to deter poor people from applying and to make many of those who received assistance miserable. Public housing, medical care in public clinics, Aid to Dependent Children—all were originally designed by reformers to serve poor people. Obviously, none has succeeded in serving them well. The issue ran through the struggle in the sixties to enact Medicare. Under the pressure to offer some proposal, opponents of Medicare argued that need should be made the basic criterion in a new national program. At some risk of getting no program at all, old people opposed a program that would apply an income test. Wilbur J. Cohen explained, in a quote from the Michigan News Service, May 12, 1960, "We need a system which creates no invidious distinctions based on income—one where an individual is entitled to receive benefits on the basis of his general contributions to society . . ."

The recurrent failure of income-tested programs for poor people to operate reasonably, whatever their designers intended, must lead us to ask whether the problem lies deeper than original intentions. More likely, the inevitable political impotence of the poor, already noted, and a deep-seated distrust of poor people in American ideology produce the equation, "Poor people's programs are poor programs." That equation has long-range and immediate consequences. Benefit levels do not improve and entitlement is not liberalized. And more personally, applicants are put off for weeks and months, wait their turns for hours on hard benches, and are addressed by their first names. They suffer themselves to be counselled and taught when experience with decent living standards would be more to the point. Unless we see signs about us of some new birth of wisdom and humanity, we may do well not to multiply or greatly expand income-tested programs. Rather, we would select other approaches such as social security and design them to accomplish our purposes.

The issue of INADVERTENT SIDE EFFECTS arises most sharply in connection with income-tested programs. In their nature, income-tested programs pay off for lack of money. One therefore wonders whether parents separate or adults fail to work in order to secure the payoff. The tendency of couples to separate in order to secure a benefit has been much exaggerated. We are a more sentimental people than public discussion recognizes; money does not nakedly determine our relationships. Nor is money liberally extended when a mother has shed a husband. His whereabouts and the reason for the separation are extensively examined; she must swear out a warrant for his arrest. There has been much talk and few studies of the matter, and no evidence that such desertion is more than an occasional anecdote.

In any event inadvertent side effects have to be recognized and dealt with. Incentive arrangements are one kind of attempt to avoid the side effect of discouraging work. Most income-tested programs address the matter more directly, defining who should work or enter training and querying people about why they do not. Those whose answers are unsatisfactory may lose all or part of their benefits. Similarly, the effort to discourage marital separation leads to considerable attention to sexual and marital relationships. Clearly this is one of the reasons that income-tested programs become onerous: as such programs appear to invite exploitation, regulations are devised and multiplied to avoid exploitation. These regulations compound bureaucracy, and, at worst, discourage people from pursuing their applications for assistance.

Other kinds of programs may also have side effects, however. For example, by providing income to old people, social security has accelerated the tendency of the aged to live separately from their children. Few regret the development, even though it is unplanned, and so nothing has been done about it. Another example arose from the fact that widows' benefits under social security are higher than those of the wives of retired men. Consequently, it appeared that aged widows were living with aged men without getting married in order to retain the higher benefits. An amendment permitting them to retain the higher benefit level despite remarriage has presumably wiped out this side effect.

We are left, finally, with the issue of CASH PAYMENT. Historically, goods and services have been provided directly for a variety of reasons. They have been thought so important, as in the case of food, that people should be allowed no option to buy other things instead. They have been so expensive, as in the case of medical care, that poor people could not really be expected to meet the cost out of periodic cash payments. They have been unavailable for purchase, as in the case of housing or public education, unless the government itself organized their provision. On the other hand, if too many things are provided *as things*, people find

themselves without real choices to make at all. It has been argued that they cannot learn self-reliance, but that argument may be subsidiary. They are in fact not free in the way we intend Americans to be free.

The issue has specifically been argued in terms of nutrition policy. On one hand, poor people given cash may not spend as much for food as nutritionists think they should. (Obviously, this means that, at some nutritional level, *they* think rent or electricity or clothing more important—the point that touches one's philosophy about the rights of individuals.) On the other hand, available devices for providing food have intrinsic difficulties. Distributing commodities is ineffective and wastefully inefficient. Food stamps with a purchase requirement bring upon themselves a buyer's strike. While some are seduced by the arrangement into using more food, others avoid food stamps entirely and so get no benefit at all.

The Importance of the Definition of Income Maintenance

To sum up so far, it appears that choosing the direction to go in income maintenance can be a complex and difficult task. If one defines income maintenance as more or less equivalent to public assistance, choices are limited, but that is partly because some decisions are implicit in the definition: (1) Adequacy, efficiency, and incentive must be traded off against one another in a game that cannot be won. (2) The interests of the poor must be divided from the more general and more powerful interests of other income-maintenance beneficiaries. (3) We must doggedly gamble that a large income-tested program can be successful in the United States. Accepting those implicit limitations, choices can then be made about how many people to include, at what precise level of benefits, how tightly to tie them to the labor market, and so forth. Certainly the choices that remain to be made are important to the people whom they will affect, but surely the intrinsic limitations that have been indicated portend failure.

The Better Definition   The alternative is to define income maintenance as all the range of programs that transfer money to people for subsistence. A complicated range of programs has to be understood and combined into a pattern that, among other things, erases inadequate income as a reason for malnutrition. Such an approach has the advantage of dealing with 100 billion dollars a year in transfer payments rather than the five or ten billion dollars available for public assistance. It has the advantage that it can provide income as a matter of right to prevent poverty rather than as charity to alleviate poverty. And complexity lends this approach flexibility. That is, we are not trapped in a single design that must meet all needs. The appropriate ideology is that of social security, and its elements would be as follows.

An Income Maintenance Program

At given times in the past, we have identified what appeared to be major risks to income—old age, disability, widowhood, being orphaned, unemployment—and have devised programs that would guard against each risk. Public assistance has a place in this framework of programs as a way of helping people with special, temporary needs. Existing features of this system should be strengthened and the new programs that our times require and our wealth permits should be identified. Such a revised system should be planned and monitored to do the maximum that is possible for people who would otherwise be poor.

Strengthening the System   To strengthen the existing system, we would take two steps.

(1) The minimum social-security benefit for an aged person should be doubled. It is now $77. (Bills to raise the minimum level to $110 have already been introduced in Congress.) Benefits for those with higher than minimum earnings should also be raised, but not as quickly at first. (2) In addition, perhaps one million aged people, who are not now covered by social security or similar public systems, should be provided status under social security, following the precedent of an amendment in 1965 that "blanketed" people over 72 into social security. These two steps would not, between them, be very expensive. In large measure, they would simply mean that millions of aged people would no longer deal with two programs (Social Security and Old Age Assistance) but would rely on one (Social Security) alone. But at the same time these two reforms would very nearly wipe out poverty among the aged.

Provision for other social-security beneficiaries would also be strengthened. Because of a family maximum written into the law, a widow with three or four children may receive as little as $116 a month under social security. Obviously, the family maximum in such cases requires improvement. The social-security definition of who is gravely disabled needs to be liberalized. Benefits under unemployment compensation need to be brought in line with present levels of income, and uncovered groups brought into the program. And, of course, we are already engaged in the legislative struggle that will lead to insured medical care for those who are younger than 65. The Commissioner of Social Security has estimated that, by steps such as these, one-third to one-half of the poverty now existing in the United States could be avoided.

Expanding the System   When we have visualized what might be achieved by such improvements, two major omissions would probably strike us. One is the group of people between middle age and retirement—

say, people between 45 to 65. When wage earners lose their jobs at these ages, they have inordinate difficulty in finding new work. They may be unemployed for months; continued unemployment in turn becomes an obstacle to finding work. The problem of this middle-aged group brought pressure to provide social security benefits at younger ages than 65. But that solution in turn produces a problem. Reduced benefits are provided at 62; retirement at younger ages would provide even smaller benefits; so those retiring early augment the ranks of the aged poor. Instead, we need a federal program that specifically insures against long-term unemployment. In its nature, it would combine income support and retraining arrangements. People still unemployed when benefits under existing state programs are exhausted—generally after six months—would be eligible for the new program. Such a program would insure against a large and growing risk to income security. At the same time, it would free retirement insurance to operate adequately for the retired, without distortion in an attempt to meet the risk of unemployment.

The other major omission in our income-maintenance system is a program to assure income for children, a point that has been underscored in the national debate about assisting the "working poor." Two out of five poor families are headed by a person working full time. This statistic simply reflects the fact that a man working full time at the minimum wage is, if he has as many as two children, nevertheless poor. Fitting wages to family size is not a problem only for poor people, to be sure. Most young families have a problem because the man is starting out, and with young children at home the woman cannot work. Their need is highest when their income is least. All families except the moderately well-to-do suffer, if they have more than two or three children, from straitened budgets for long periods of time. Substantial British evidence

indicates that even at moderate incomes, children in such families show measurable deficiencies—in height, in weight, and in school performance.[1,2,3,4]

The foremost nominee as a method of providing income to children would be a program of children's allowances. Such a program would eliminate the income-tax exemption for children—a government subsidy that pays more to those who have more—and replace it with a cash payment for every child regardless of income. At a payment of $50 a month, three-fourths of all family poverty would be wiped out. At the same time, substantial aid would be given to families with marginal and moderate incomes. Well-to-do families would not benefit, as the cash payment would simply replace their present gain from income-tax exemptions. So far as one can tell from all available evidence, such a program would not increase the birth rate.[5,6] Nor would it get entangled in the problems that bedevil income-tested programs—incentive, inadvertent side effects, and isolation of poor people as a beneficiary group.

In the end, we would need a small income-tested program for those people whose risk had not been met in any other way. At the poverty level, such a program would deal with three or four million people—no more. (By contrast, the income-tested program proposed by the President in 1969 would have dealt with 23 million people. And it did not include all needy people, let alone bring everyone to the poverty level.) This comparatively small income-tested program would be far easier to operate than now, when so many different kinds of people require assistance. It would include some single individuals not sufficiently handicapped to be covered by other programs, some small families without fathers, and a scattering of others. It would not include the working poor, for their income problem would be prevented by the children's allowance. Therefore, we would not have to struggle so hard to retain incentive; a modest incentive arrangement would do. We would not have to trade off incentive against adequacy, which is to say that adequate payments could more readily be provided. Food programs would be retained until the essential components of the program had been assembled at a reasonable level of adequacy. They could then be phased out on the assumption that everyone has at least the essential cash that is needed.

Summary

The combination of programs that is outlined could be assembled in five to eight years. Despite the absence of details, certain advantages may be evident. (1) Most people would receive money, without feeling or having the public feel that they were being indulged. (2) Just as in present retirement insurance, poverty would be prevented instead of being alleviated. (3) In the long run, poor people would receive more money than under income-tested programs. (4) There would be no programmatic schism between the majority and a large have-not minority. (5) Everyone would have cash with which to buy food and other necessities. Whatever its complexity, from the point of view of wiping out hunger and uniting the country this course is the prescription of choice.

REFERENCES

1. **Butler, N. R., and Bonham, D. G.,**   1963. *Perinatal Mortality.* E & S Livingstone, Ltd., Edinburgh.

2. **Lambert, R.,**   1964. *Nutrition in Britain 1950–1960.* G. Bell & Sons Ltd., London.

3. London City Council, 1961. *Report on Heights and Weights (and other Measurements) of School Pupils in the County of London in 1959.*

4. **Douglas, J. W. B.,**   1964. *Home and School.* MacGibbon & Kee, Ltd., London.

5. **Whitney, V. H.,**   1968. Fertility Trends and Children's Allowance Programs. In Burns, E. M., ed., *Children's Allowances and the Economic Welfare of Children.* Citizens Committee for Children, New York.

6. **Whitney, V. H.,**   1966. *Income and the Birth Rate.* In Schorr, A. L., ed., *Poor Kids: A Report on Children in Poverty.* Basic Books, Inc., New York.

Conclusion

Jean Mayer

The authors of these chapters have spoken for themselves, and if the reader has arrived at this point he or she will have formed his or her own conclusion about the future shape of our nutrition policy. An editorial summary is unnecessary; generalizations are of necessity subjective. Nevertheless, for what they are worth, the following comments seem justified.

First, the complex industrial food supply of a country of over 200 million can no longer be allowed to evolve solely in response to "the forces of the market." Because food is intimately linked to the health of the nation—particularly to that of the vulnerable groups—and because the nutritional value of the processed and new foods can no longer be assessed by traditional criteria evolved in thousands of years of trials and errors, we need constant surveillance of the nutritional status of our population. We need, in particular, to monitor the nutritional health of growing children and adolescents, of pregnant and nursing mothers, and of the elderly—all groups that traditionally have been "vulnerable" either because their needs are particularly great or because they are not in a position to fend for themselves, or for both reasons simultaneously. We need to develop special policies for their protection. Groups that have been the object of centuries-long discrimination or have been reduced to a state of tutelage from which they are but slowly emerging, and who are still clearly administered by (and sometimes at the mercy of) the United States Government need special help—at least until they achieve real social and economic equality.

Secondly, as more and more of our citizens, freed from the threat of the nutritional diseases of poverty, fall prey to the nutritional diseases of abundance, we need to develop new nutritional policies. If we don't use science and a greater degree of foresight to save ourselves from the damages already inflicted by the unguided technology of the past, we shall spend a greater and greater proportion of our resources just to stay at the same place (in regard to health) that we occupy now. The nation's health no longer lends itself to much improvement simply by the piecemeal "problem solving" approach. We must evolve nutritional policies which will clearly be part and parcel of an overall program in preventive medicine.

Third, to realize these aims we must have a measure of national agreement on the evolution of our food supply, shared by consumers, manufacturers, and distributors. Our food supply must not only be abundant and safe, it must be nutritious. Because, for better or for worse, the physical activity of our people has decreased in the past century as a result of the mass availability of individual transportation and labor-saving devices, our average food intake has decreased. That it has not decreased fast enough to prevent a rise in the prevalence of obesity should not obscure the cardinal point that, in order to maintain an adequate nutrient intake in the presence of decreased caloric requirements, we must have foods that are more nutritious than ever before. Yet the post-World War II period has seen an invasion of our food intake by "fun foods," soft drinks, and other sources of "empty calories" that we can afford less than when our aver-

age intake was higher. The chapters on foods show clearly that, once again, we have all the technology we need to correct this new threat. Indeed, since the White House Conference on Food, Nutrition and Health, there have been encouraging signs that many large manufacturing firms have taken up very seriously the challenge of using technology for improving nutrition. Extension of enrichment techniques to a large proportion of snack foods, development of a number of imaginative high protein, high-nutrient new foods and beverages, improvements of old foods (like macaronis) give hope that a corner has been turned. Because we want to preserve freedom of consumer choice, because we don't know everything and are thus not ready to rely entirely on enrichment of processed foods, we need policies that will encourage the intelligent consumption of basic, "primary" agricultural products and also permit comparison between various types of processed foods. Grading policies, nutritional labeling, and other means of consumer information are the necessary informational counterparts of the agricultural and industrial amelioration of our food supply. The chapters on foods and the consumer give a general blueprint for such a food policy for the nation—a mixture of more extensive regulations and more extensive information that represents a reasonable balance between the exercise of intelligent authority and that of intelligent choice.

That "consumer" information should be part of a more general program of national education comes out of the chapters on nutrition education policy. These deal with three categories—professionals, without whose leadership no program will long endure; the general public, the main target of this effort; and as everywhere in this book, the very poor emerge as the first socioeconomic priority—not necessarily because they know less but because, being poor, they suffer more from any nutritional mistake;

indeed, in some perverse fashion, they are forced to know more than the rich in order to feed their families adequately on a restricted income.

Any thoughtful and compassionate American who has considered the problems of the least fortunate of our fellow citizens has come to the conclusion that we need to insure some form of income maintenance. Opinions on the mode of administration, the support level, work incentives and guarantees vary, but without money, food money such as food stamps and food programs, there can be no nutrition policy for at least 20 million of our fellow citizens. The marked improvement realized since the conference has mitigated, but by no means eliminated, the urgent need for a federal policy in this crucial matter. Two chapters specifically deal with this problem, but it has come back over and over again as a *leitmotif* throughout the book.

Food and nutrition policies, income policies, education policies, are in turn dependant on government departments and services at all levels. These must also be responsible for the constant reassessment of these policies through the monitoring and evaluation of their results. Four crucial levels and approaches have been singled out: local government, state government, the Department of Agriculture, the Food and Drug Administration. There may well be, in the near future, a reapportionment of responsibilities. Indeed, there have been discussions in Washington about the possibility of major changes in the structure of the cabinet and of regulatory agencies. Even should these changes take place in the near future, which seems not altogether likely, the types of responsibilities that would have to be as-

sumed by the reorganized departments or agencies and the thrust of the necessary policies would remain.

At the closing session of the White House Conference, I expressed what I believe was the common feeling of all present, that until then all of us in the past had spoken too exclusively with the same sorts of persons we were—in terms of age, color, profession, and economic position. The conference was a gigantic national conversation in which voices were sometimes loud and agreement was not always reached, but at last we were speaking frankly about our daily bread. We discovered that young, old, men, women, liberals, conservatives, businessmen, consumers, health professionals, blacks, whites, Indians, Spanish-speaking Americans, citizens of American dependencies, teachers, students, activists, farmers, ministers, government officials—all of us had many aspirations in common. We wanted all Americans to be able to enjoy the fruit of our bountiful crops and the ingenuity of our industry so that hunger should be eliminated from our land. We wanted our food supply to be as wholesome and nutritious as our science and technology should permit so that malnutrition, like hunger, should disappear from America.

It is our hope that this book will contribute to the continuing national discussion of policies that will implement this consensus. Our food supply is the most visible symbol of our national interdependence; it is, in a very deep sense, the national communion table. Insuring good nutrition for all Americans is a necessary first step if we want all of them to feel that they are truly entitled to life, liberty, and the pursuit of happiness.

Biographical Notes

Editor

Jean Mayer, Ph.D., D.Sc., is Professor of Nutrition and Lecturer on the History of Public Health at Harvard University, Boston, Massachusetts. His experimental work has dealt with various aspects of nutrition, but preeminently with the mechanism of regulation of food intake and the etiology of obesity. He was the first Chairman of the National Council on Hunger and Malnutrition in the United States (1968–1970) and has been a Special Consultant to the President (1969–1970). He was Chairman of the first White House Conference on Food, Nutrition and Health and presided over the one-year-after follow-up meeting of the conference in 1971. He was Chairman of the Nutrition Section of the Second White House Conference on Aging (1971). He is a member of the President's Consumer Adivsory Council and Chairman of its Health Section. He is at present editing a volume that will deal with U.S. nutrition policies abroad.

Contributors

Jean Mayer's co-authors include twelve persons who were chairmen or vice-chairmen of panels at the White House Conference on Food, Nutrition and Health, two who were leading staff members, and several who were key participants.

John C. Ayres, Ph.D., is Chairman of the Food Science Division of the College of Agriculture at the University of Georgia, at Athens. His major research interests are the microbiological deterioration of foods, the presence of toxicants and pathogens in foods, and food technology. He is author or editor of over 200 publications dealing with these subjects. He served as a member of the Panel on Food Safety at the First White House Conference on Food, Nutrition and Health.

Gordon Falk Bloom, Ph.D., LL.B., is Senior Lecturer at the Sloan School of Management, Massachusetts Institute of Technology, Cambridge, Massachusetts. He is a board member and member of the Executive Committee of the National Association of Food Chains and a member of the Food Retailing Advisory Commission of the Office of Emergency Preparedness. He is author of *Productivity in the Food Industry* (MIT Press, Cambridge). He was a member of the Panel on Problems of Budgeting, Marketing, and Pricing at the White House Conference.

George M. Briggs, Ph.D., is Professor of Nutrition at the University of California, Berkeley, California, and Executive Editor of the *Journal of Nutrition Education*. He has served as President of the Society for Nutrition Education (1968–1969), and, at the White House Conference, as Chairman of the Panel on Nutrition Education in Elementary and Secondary Schools.

Robert B. Choate is Chairman of the Council on Children, Media, and Merchandising, Washington, D.C. He is now concentrating on advertising to and through children in all fields, particularly including the advertising of edible products. He acted as a Consultant for Community Affairs on the staff of the White House Conference on Food, Nutrition and Health.

Julius M. Coon, Ph.D., M.D., is Professor of Pharmacology and Chairman of the Department at Thomas Jefferson University, Philadelphia, Pa. He is a member of the Food Protection Committee of the National Academy of Sciences-National Research Council, and Chairman of the Subcommittees on Toxicology and Non-nutritive Sweeteners. He is also a member of the Committee on Radiation Preservation of Foods and of the Subcommittee on Naturally Occuring Toxicants in Foods. He serves on the World Health Organization's Expert Advisory Panel on Food Additives. Dr. Coon was Chairman of the Panel on Food Safety at the White House Conference.

Effie O. Ellis, M.D., is Special Assistant to the Executive Vice President, American Medical Association, Chicago, Illinois. At the time of the White House Conference on Food, Nutrition and Health, Dr. Ellis was Director of Maternal and Child Health for the Ohio State Department of Health. A pediatrician, she has extensive experience in the specialized health care needs of the poor. She served as Chairman of the Panel on the Family as a Delivery System: The Role of Nutrition in Reinforcing the Family Structure, Special Problems of Poor People.

Mary C. Egan, B.S., M.S., is Chief of the Nutrition Section of the Maternal and Child Health Service, Health Services and Mental Health Administration, U.S. Department of Health, Education, and Welfare, Rockville, Maryland. She served at the White House Conference on Food, Nutrition and Health as a Consultant for the Panels on Pregnant and Nursing Women and Young Infants, and on the Family as a Delivery System.

Samuel J. Fomon, M.D., is Professor of Pediatrics at the College of Medicine, University of Iowa, Iowa City, Iowa, and Consultant in Medical Nutrition, Maternal and Child Health Service, U.S. Department of Health, Education, and Welfare. He directs a research program in infant growth and nutrition that is currently particularly concerned with factors influencing food intake by normal infants. He also directs a training program in pediatric nutrition sponsored by the Maternal and Child Health Service. A second edition of his textbook, *Infant Nutrition*, is in preparation. Dr. Fomon acted as Chairman of the Panel on Children and Adolescents at the White House Conference on Food, Nutrition and Health.

Grace A. Goldsmith, M.D., M.S. in Medicine, is Dean of the School of Public Health and Tropical Medicine at Tulane University and Consultant Physician, Charity Hospital and Touro Infirmary, New Orleans, Louisiana. She is Chairman of the Council on Foods and Nutrition of the American Medical Association, member of the Governing Council of the American Public Health Association, and President of the American Society for Clinical Nutrition. She served as Chairman of the Panel on Advanced Academic Teaching of Nutrition at the White House Conference.

Richard S. Gordon, Ph.D., is President of the Institute for Urban Development and Visiting Professor of Management at Washington University in St. Louis, Missouri, as well as Senior Consultant to the Office of the Commissioner of the Food and Drug Administration. As a result of his experience at the White House Conference on Food, Nutrition and Health, he organized the Institute for Urban Development to help citizens, professionals, and various agencies and businesses to come together to develop public policy and to plan and execute specific projects in housing, education, public health and nutrition, environmental quality, and economic development. He served at the Conference as Chairman of the Panel on New Foods.

James D. Grant, B.S., M.B.A., served as Deputy Commissioner of the U.S. Food and Drug Administration from January 1970 through May 1972. He is the author of articles on nonprofit research and development organization, on systems and government, and on national food, drug, and product safety policies, programs, and issues as they affect the American public. He was Vice President of the National Institute of Public Affairs, a nonprofit educational organization, when he left to act as Deputy to Jean Mayer at the First White House Conference on Food, Nutrition and Health.

D. Mark Hegsted, Ph.D., is Professor of Nutrition at Harvard University, Boston, Mass. He served as Head of the Food and Nutrition Board, National Academy of Sciences-National Research Council, from 1968 to 1972, and is President of the American Institute of Nutrition. His major research interests, the availability and utilization of protein, iron, and calcium, have led to his present concern with development of a dependable and sensitive survey method for large populations at risk of malnutrition. He was Chairman of the Panel on Standards of Dietary and Nutritional Evaluation at the White House Conference.

Ruth L. Huenemann, D.Sc., is Professor of Public Health Nutrition at the University of California, Berkeley, California. She is engaged in the education and training of nutritionists for the public health field, directing a Master of Public Health Program that combines academic work with field experience. Graduates are working in local, state, and national health programs in the United States and other countries. She has also had extensive experience with nutrition programs in many countries around the world. At the White House Conference she acted as a member of the Panel on Advanced Academic Teaching of Nutrition.

Howard N. Jacobson, M.D., is Director of the Joint Boston College School of Nursing-Harvard Medical School Program (The Macy Program) and is Associate Professor of Obstetrics and Gynecology at the Boston Hospital for Women, Harvard Medical School, Boston, Massachusetts. He is Chairman of the National Research Council Committee on Maternal Nutrition. Results of the Committee's Workshop on Nutrition Supplementation During Pregnancy will be published in the fall of 1972. Dr. Jacobson served as Vice-Chairman of the Panel on Pregnant and Nursing Women and Young Infants at the White House Conference.

Michael C. Latham, M.B., M.P.H., is Professor of International Nutrition at the Graduate School of Nutrition, Cornell University, Ithaca, New York. He has worked extensively with the populations of developing countries, and is at present conducting a joint study with Harvard and Bogotá, Colombia, on malnutrition and mental development. He is author of *The Planning and Evaluation of Applied Nutrition Programmes* (WHO/FAO, Rome, 1972). He served at the Conference as Vice-Chairman of the Panel on Groups for Whom the Federal Government has Special Responsibilities.

Varnum D. Ludington, M.S., is a retired Vice President of General Foods Corporation. He acts as a Consultant for Development and Future Planning, making his headquarters in Greenwich, Connecticut.

As Director of General Foods' Center for Applied Nutrition, he was instrumental in developing a low-cost, high-protein pasta that has been successfully marketed in many countries. He is a member of the AID Research Advisory Committee and is especially concerned with food-fortification projects in Thailand, the Middle East, Guatemala, North Africa, and Chile. He also participates in the food development projects of UNIDO. He acted as a Consultant for the Panel on Food Manufacturing and Processing.

Robert J. McEwen, S.J., Ph.D., is Professor of Economics at Boston College, Chestnut Hill, Massachusetts, and President of the Association of Massachusetts Consumers, Inc. He is consultant to the Food and Drug Administration in Washington, and has been leading Massachusetts consumers in evaluating and monitoring the Price Commission actions, with special reference to food prices. He has conducted two surveys on the observance of price-posting regulations and testified at the Boston hearing conducted by the Price Commission on April 21, 1972. He acted as Chairman of the Consumer Task Force at the White House Conference on Food, Nutrition and Health.

Robert B. McGandy, M.D., is Associate Professor of Physiology at the Harvard School of Public Health, Boston, Massachusetts. His major interests, experimental and clinical, are in the primary prevention of heart disease. He has recently taken part in studies at boys' schools in Massachusetts, which were done to determine whether substitution of low-cholesterol foods in the daily menu can influence the rise in serum cholesterol often seen in adolescent males. He was a Member of the Panel on Traditional Foods.

Emil M. Mrak, Ph.D., is Chancellor Emeritus of the University of California at Davis. He is Chairman of the Hazardous Materials Advisory Committee of the Environmental Protection Agency, Trustee of The Nutrition Foundation, member of the Advisory Council of the Nestle Foundation to improve nutrition in underdeveloped nations, and Chairman of the Assembly Science and Technology Advisory Council of the California Legislature. At the White House Conference he served as Chairman of the Panel on Food Quality.

Vera G. Mrak, Ph.D., acts as Nutrition and Consumer Consultant for the Food and Drug Administration. Her interests lie in the field of food chemistry, freezing storage, and organoleptic difference testing.

Susan H. Mills, B.A., is Administrative Assistant to the Macy Program, of which Dr. Jacobson is Director. She is co-author of the chapter on Pregnancy and Lactation.

John N. Perryman, Ph.D., is Executive Director of the 50,000 member American Food Service Association, Denver, Colorado. (The Association is the professional organization for school food service personnel in the United States and is a major force in support of U.S. programs and legislation concerned with child health and education. It is also engaged in foreign consultant work, with members contributing their services throughout the world.) He has worked with the Brazilian government in their child feeding programs since 1966, and has participated in several White House Conferences on youth and nutrition, and in the Second World Food Congress, 1970. He was a member of the Panel on Large-Scale Meal Delivery Systems at the White House Conference on Food, Nutrition and Health.

Alvin L. Schorr, B.S.S., M.S.W., is Dean of the Graduate School of Social Work, New York University, New York. He has been Director of Research at the Office of Economic Opportunity and Deputy Assistant Secretary of the U.S. Department of Health, Education, and Welfare. In 1967 and 1970, he directed a project providing consultation to national organizations and model cities about their income-maintenance programs. He is the author of *Poor Kids* (Basic Books, Inc., N.Y.), which sets forth alternative approaches to providing income for children.

Albert J. Stunkard, M.D., is Professor and Chairman of the Department of Psychiatry at the University of Pennsylvania, Philadelphia. As part of his clinical and experimental studies on human obesity, now in their twentieth year, Dr. Stunkard is conducting a large-scale study with TOPS, the national self-help group for obesity, to try to determine whether behavior modification or traditional treatment methods are more effective, and also whether professional or lay group leaders are more effective in applying the techniques. He is also studying social factors in obesity, particularly their influence in childhood, and exploring new medications for treating obesity. He was a member of the Panel on Adults in an Affluent Society: The Degenerative Diseases of Middle Age.

Helen D. Ullrich, M.A., R.D., is Editor of the Journal of Nutrition Education and Education Director of the Society for Nutrition Education, Berkeley, California. In the latter capacity, she directs the National Nutrition Education Clearinghouse for the Society. Mrs. Ullrich was formerly a nutrition specialist for the Agricultural Extension Service of the University of California.

Donald M. Watkin, M.D., M.P.H., is Acting Chief of the Spinal Cord Injury Center of the Veterans Administration Hospital, West Roxbury, Massachusetts, and Research Associate in Nutrition at the Pathology Foundation, Boston. In 1971 he acted as Chairman of the Technical Committee on Nutrition and a member of the Planning Board for the White House Conference on Aging, for which he organized a workshop on solutions to the nutrition problems of the aged. He is preparing a position paper for the American Public Health Association on nutritional assessment, and is co-author of a book to be published on training allied health personnel in academic settings and on-the-job projects. At the White House Conference on Food, Nutrition and Health, he served as Vice-Chairman of the Panel on the Aging.

Bibliography

Adair, John, and Deuschle, Kurt W., 1970. *The People's Health: Medicine and Anthropology in a Navajo Community.* Appleton-Century-Crofts, New York.

Allsworth, Edward, ed., 1971. *The Aged, the Family and the Community.* Columbia University Press, New York.

American Chemical Society, 1966. *Organic Pesticides in the Environment.* American Chemical Society, Washington, D.C.

Ayres, John C., et al., eds., 1969. *Chemical and Biological Hazards in Foods.* Hafner Publishing Company, Inc. New York.

Batchelder, Alan B., 1971. *The Economics of Poverty,* Second Edition. John Wiley & Sons, Inc., New York.

Berry, W. T. C., 1971. *Portfolio for Health.* Oxford University Press, London.

Bicknell, Franklin, 1970. *The Chemicals in Your Food.* Emerson Books, Inc., New York.

Bigwood, E. J., and Gerard, A., 1970. *Fundamental Principles and Objectives of a Comparative Food Law,* Vol. 3, Elements of Structure and Institutional Elements. Albert J. Phiebig, White Plains, New York.

Blakeslee, Alton L., and Stamler, Jeremiah, 1963. *Your Heart Has Nine Lives: Nine Steps to Heart Health.* Prentice-Hall, Inc. Englewood Cliffs, New Jersey.

Bloomberg, Warner, Jr., and Schmandt, Henry J., eds., 1968. *Power, Poverty, and Urban Policy.* Urban Affairs Annual Reviews. Sage Publications, Inc., Beverly Hills, California.

Bloomberg, Warner, Jr., and Schmandt, Henry J., eds., 1970. *Urban Poverty: Its Social and Political Dimensions.* Sage Publications, Inc., Beverly Hills, California.

Brody, Eugene B., 1968. *Minority Group Adolescents in the United States.* Williams & Wilkins Company, Baltimore.

Brophy, William A., and Aberle, Sophie D., eds., 1969. *The Indian: America's Unfinished Business.* Report of the Commission on the Rights, Liberties, and Responsibilities of the American Indian. University of Oklahoma Press, Norman, Oklahoma.

Burgess, Anne, and Dean, R. F., 1963. *Malnutrition and Food Habits.* Free Press, New York.

Buzzell, R. D., and Nourse, R. E., 1967. *Product Innovation in Food Processing 1954–1964.* Harvard Business School, Division of Research, Boston.

Charm, Stanley E., 1971. *Fundamentals of Food Engineering,* Second Edition. Avi Publishing Company, Westport, Conn.

Ciba Foundation Study Group No. 31, 1968. *Nutrition and Infection.* Williams & Wilkins, Baltimore.

Citizens Board of Inquiry, 1968. *Hunger USA.* Beacon Press, Boston.

Clark, Margaret, 1970. *Health in the Mexican-American Culture: A Community Study.* University of California Press, Berkeley.

Coles, Robert, 1967. *Children of Crisis: Study of Courage and Fear.* Little, Brown & Company, Boston.

Coles, Robert, 1971. *Migrants, Sharecroppers and Mountaineers.* Vol. 2 of *Children of Crisis.* Little, Brown & Company, Boston.

Coles, Robert, 1971. *Children of Crisis: the South Moves North.* Little, Brown & Company, Boston.

Coles, Robert, and Clayton, A. 1969. *Still Hungry in America*. W. W. Norton & Company, Inc, New York.

Coles, Robert, and Erikson, Jon, 1971. *The Middle Americans: Proud and Uncertain*. Little, Brown & Company, Boston.

Coles, Robert, and Piers, Maria, 1969. *Wages of Neglect: New Solutions for the Children of the Poor*. Quadrangle Books, Inc., Cleveland, Ohio.

Cross, Jennifer, 1970. *The Supermarket Trap: The Consumer and Food Industry*. Indiana University Press, Bloomington, Indiana.

Cummings, Richard O., 1970 (reprint of the 1940 edition). *The American and His Food: A History of Food Habits in the United States*. Arno Press, New York.

Davidson, L.S.P., Passmore, R., and Brock, J., 1972. *Human Nutrition and Dietetics*, Fifth Edition. Livingstone, Edinburgh. Williams & Wilkins, Baltimore.

Day, Mark, 1971. *Forty Acres—Cesar Chavez and the Farm Workers*. Praeger Publishers, New York.

De Beauvoir, Simone, 1972. *The Coming of Age: The Study of the Aging Process*. G. P. Putnam's Sons, New York.

Desrosier, Norman W., 1970. *The Technology of Food Preservation*, Third Edition. Avi Publishing Company, Westport, Conn.

Desrosier, Norman W., and Desrosier, John, 1971. *Economics of New Product Development*. Avi Publishing Company, Westport, Conn.

Deutsch, Ronald M., 1971. *The Family Guide to Better Food and Better Health*. Meredith Publishers, Des Moines, Iowa.

Division of Biology and Agriculture, National Academy of Sciences, 1969. *Use of Drugs in Animal Feeds*. National Academy of Sciences, Washington, D.C.

Durfee, David A. [N.D.]. *Poverty in an Affluent Society: Personal Problem or National Disgrace*. Prentice-Hall, Inc., Englewood Cliffs, New Jersey.

Earle, R. L., 1966. *Unit Operations in Food Processing*. Pergamon Press. Inc. Elmsford, New York.

Final Report, White House Conference on Food, Nutrition and Health, 1970. U.S. Government Printing Office, Washington, D.C.

Follow-up Report, White House Conference on Food, Nutrition and Health, 1971. U.S. Government Printing Office, Washington, D.C.

Food and Agriculture Organization of the United Nations, 1970. *Pesticide Residues in Food*. Available from UNIPUB, INC. New York.

Food and Nutrition Board, National Academy of Sciences, 1966. *Dietary Fat and Human Health*. National Academy of Sciences, Washington, D.C.

Food and Nutrition Board, National Academy of Sciences, 1970. *Maternal Nutrition and the Course of Pregnancy*. National Academy of Sciences, Washington, D.C.

Food Protection Committee, National Academy of Sciences, 1965. *Chemicals Used in Food Processing*. National Academy of Sciences, Washington, D.C.

Food Protection Committee, National Academy of Sciences, 1964. *Evaluation of Public Health Hazards from Microbiological Contamination of Foods*. National Academy of Sciences, Washington, D.C.

Food Protection Committee, National Academy of Sciences, 1966. *Toxicants Occurring Naturally in Foods*. National Academy of Sciences, Washington, D.C.

Frazier, William C., 1967. *Food Microbiology*, Second Edition. McGraw-Hill Book Company, New York.

Galbraith, John Kenneth, 1969. *The Affluent Society*, Second Edition. Houghton-Mifflin, Inc., Boston.

Gale, E., and Goodman, M. [N.D.]. *What Americans Really Eat*. Fleet Press Corporation, New York.

Glazer, Nathan, and Moynihan, Daniel P., 1970. *Beyond the Melting Pot: the Negroes, Puerto Ricans, Jews, Italians and Irish of New York City*, Second Edition. MIT Press, Cambridge.

Goldston, Iago, ed., 1969 (reprint). *The Family: A Focal Point in Health Education*. International Universities Press, Inc., New York.

Graham, Frank, Jr., 1970. *Since Silent Spring*. Houghton-Mifflin, Inc., Boston.

Graham, Frank, and Graham, Ada, 1969. *The Great American Shopping Cart*. Simon and Schuster, New York.

Graham, H. D., ed., 1968. *Safety of Foods-A Symposium*. Avi Publishing company, Westport, Conn.

Grieg, W. Smith, ed., 1971. *Economics of Food Processing*. Avi Publishing Company, Westport, Conn.

Gunther, Francis A., ed., 1962–1971. *Residue Reviews: Residues of Pesticides and Other Chemicals in Foods and Feeds*. In 35 volumes. Springer-Verlag, Inc., New York.

Harrington, Michael, 1970. *The Other America: Poverty in the United States*. Macmillan Company, New York.

Harris, Robert, and von Loesecke, Harry, 1971 (reprint of 1960 edition). *Nutritional Evaluation of Food Processing*. Avi Publishing Company, Westport, Conn.

Jacobs, Jane, 1969. *The Economy of Cities*. Random House. Inc. New York.

Joint Commission on Mental Health of Children, 1969–1970. *Crisis in Child Mental Health: Challenge for the 1970's*. Harper & Row Publishers, Inc., New York.

Jokl, Ernst, 1964. *Nutrition, Exercise, and Body Composition*. Charles C Thomas, Publishers, Springfield, Illinois.

Josselyn, Irene M., and Joint Commission on Mental Health of Children, 1971. *Adolescence*. Harper & Row Publishers, Inc. New York.

Kosa, John, et al., 1969. *Poverty and Health: A Sociological Analysis*. Harvard University Press, Cambridge.

Kotz, Nathan, 1970. *Let Them Eat Promises: The Politics of Hunger in America*. Prentice-Hall, Inc., Englewood Cliffs, New Jersey.

Liener, I. E., 1969. *Toxic Constitutents in Plant Foodstuffs*. Academic Press, New York.

Longree, Karla, 1967. *Quantity Food Sanitation*. John Wiley & Sons, Inc., New York.

Margolius, Sidney, 1971. *The Great American Food Hoax*. Walker & Company, New York.

Martin, Ethel A., 1971. *Nutrition Education in Action: A Guide for Teachers*, Third Edition. Holt, Rinehart & Winston, Inc. New York.

Matthiessen, Peter, 1970. *Sal si Puedes: Escape if You Can. Cesar Chavez and the New American Revolution*. Random House, Inc., New York.

Mayer, Jean, 1972. *Human Nutrition: Its Physiological, Medical and Social Aspects*. Charles C Thomas, Publishers, Springfield, Illinois.

Mayer, Jean, 1968. *Overweight: Causes, Cost and Control*. Prentice-Hall, Inc., Englewood Cliffs, New Jersey.

McWilliams, Margaret, 1967. *Nutrition for the Growing Years*. John Wiley & Sons, Inc., New York.

Meyer, William, 1971. *Native Americans: the New Indian Resistance*. International Publishers Company, Inc., New York.

Miller, Herman P., 1971., *Rich Man—Poor Man*. Thomas Y. Crowell Company, New York.

Moynihan, Daniel P., ed., 1968, 1969. *On Understanding Poverty*. Basic Books, Inc., New York.

Orr, Larry L., and Hollister, Robinson G., eds., 1971. *Income Maintenance: Interdisciplinary Approaches to Research*. Institute for Research on Poverty Monograph Series. Markham Publishing Company, Chicago.

Pen, Jan, 1971. *Income Distribution: Facts, Theories, and Policies*. Praeger Publishers, New York.

Pyke, Magnus, 1970. *Food and Society*. Transatlantic Arts, Inc. Levittown, New York.

Pyke, Magnus [N.D.]. *Man and Food*. World University Library Series. McGraw-Hill Book Company, New York.

Pyke, Magnus, 1971. *Synthetic Food*. St. Martin's Press, Inc. New York.

Reed, Gerald, 1966. *Enzymes in Food Processing*. Academic Press, New York.

Reiss, I. L., 1971. *The Family System in America*. Holt, Rinehart & Winston, Inc., New York.

Roe, Francis J., 1971. *Metabolic Aspects of Food Safety*. Academic Press, New York.

Rogers, Edward, 1965. *Poverty on a Small Planet: A Christian Looks at Living Standards*. Macmillan Company, New York.

Sapeika, Norman, 1969. *Food Pharmacology*. Charles C Thomas, Publishers, Springfield, Illinois.

Schorr, Alvin L., 1966. *Poor Kids: A Report on Children in Poverty*. Basic Books, Inc., New York.

Segal, Judith A., 1970. *Food for the Hungry: The Reluctant Society*. Johns Hopkins University Press, Baltimore.

Sorkin, Alan L., 1971. *American Indians and Federal Aid*. Brookings Institution, Washington, D.C.

Stone, Robert. [N.D.] *Family Life Styles Below the Poverty Line*. D. C. Heath & Company, Indianapolis, Indiana.

Subcommittee on Economy in Government, 1970 (reprint of 1969 edition). *America's Indians, Facts and Future. Toward Development for the Native American Communities*. Arno Press, New York.

Taylor, Clara M., and Riddle, Katherine P., 1971. *Annotated International Bibliography of Nutrition Education: Material, Resource, Personnel, and Agencies*. Teachers College Press, Columbia University, New York.

Theobald, Robert, ed., 1966. *Guaranteed Income: Next Step in Economic Evolution*. Doubleday & Company, Inc. Garden City, New York.

Townsend, Claire, 1971. *Old Age: The Last Segregation*. Ralph Nader's Study Group Report on Nursing Homes. Grossman Publishers, Inc., New York.

Tompkins, Dorothy C., 1970. *Poverty in the United States during the Sixties, a Bibliography*. University of California, Institute for Governmental Studies, Berkeley.

Turner, James S., 1970. *The Chemical Feast: A Report on the Food and Drug Administration*. Grossman Publishers, Inc., New York.

van Arsdel, W. B., et. al., eds., 1969. *Quality and Stability of Frozen Foods: Time-Temperature Tolerance and Its Significance*. John Wiley & Sons, Inc., New York.

Waxman, Chiam I., ed., 1968. *Poverty, Power, and Politics*. Grosset and Dunlap, Inc., New York.

Weisbrod, Burton A., ed., 1965. *Economics of Poverty: An Economic Paradox*. Prentice-Hall, Inc., Englewood Cliffs, New Jersey.

Winter, Ruth, 1969. *The Poisons in Your Food*. Crown Publishers, Inc., New York.

Wohl, Michael G., and Goodhart, Robert S., eds., 1973. *Modern Nutrition in Health and Disease*, Fifth Edition, Lea & Febiger, Philadelphia.

Yudkin, John, 1972. *Sweet and Dangerous*. Peter Wyden Company, New York.

Index